The Commercial Determinants of Health

THE COMMERCIAL DETERMINANTS OF HEALTH

Edited by
Nason Maani
Mark Petticrew
and
Sandro Galea

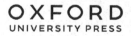
OXFORD
UNIVERSITY PRESS

OXFORD
UNIVERSITY PRESS

Oxford University Press is a department of the University of Oxford. It furthers
the University's objective of excellence in research, scholarship, and education
by publishing worldwide. Oxford is a registered trade mark of Oxford University
Press in the UK and certain other countries.

Published in the United States of America by Oxford University Press
198 Madison Avenue, New York, NY 10016, United States of America.

Library of Congress Cataloging-in-Publication Data
Names: Maani, Nason, editor. | Petticrew, Mark, editor. | Galea, Sandro, editor.
Title: The commercial determinants of health / edited by Nason Maani,
Mark Petticrew, and Sandro Galea.
Description: New York, NY : Oxford University Press, [2023] | Includes
bibliographical references and index.
Identifiers: LCCN 2022020930 (print) | LCCN 2022020931 (ebook) |
ISBN 9780197578759 (paperback) | ISBN 9780197578742 (hardback) |
ISBN 9780197578773 (epub) | ISBN 9780197578780
Subjects: MESH: Social Determinants of Health | Commerce | Health
Inequities | One Health | Social Control Policies
Classification: LCC RA418 (print) | LCC RA418 (ebook) | NLM WA 30 |
DDC 362.1—dc23/eng/20220810
LC record available at https://lccn.loc.gov/2022020930
LC ebook record available at https://lccn.loc.gov/2022020931

DOI: 10.1093/oso/9780197578742.001.0001

9 8 7 6 5 4 3 2 1

Paperback printed by Lakeside Book Company, United States of America
Hardback printed by Bridgeport National Bindery, Inc., United States of America

CONTENTS

SECTION 3. Case Studies by Industry

SECTION 4. Cross-Industry Mechanisms

SECTION 5. Advancing Science and Scholarship

ACKNOWLEDGMENTS

We would like to thank all our colleagues who contributed so willingly to each of the chapters, this book has been a pleasure to work on in large part due to their dedication, sincerity, and incisiveness. We are indebted to the editorial guidance of Sarah Humphreville and Emma Hodgdon at Oxford who have supported our work with speed, warmth, and good humour. Above all we thank our families for their support as we took on this book amidst many other ongoing projects and commitments.

CONTRIBUTORS

Salma M. Abdalla, MBBS, MPH
Research Fellow
Department of Epidemiology
Boston University School of
Public Health
Boston, MA, USA

Peter J. Adams, PhD
Professor
School of Population Health
University of Auckland
Auckland, NZ

**Luke N. Allen, MBChB, MPH,
PGCert Clin Edu, PGDip Health
Res, MRCGP, FHEA**
Research Fellow
Department of Clinical Research
London School of Hygiene &
Tropical Medicine
London, UK

Julia Anaf, PhD
Research Fellow
Stretton Health Equity, Stretton
Institute
School of Social Sciences, Faculty of
Arts, University of Adelaide
Adelaide, AU

George J. Annas, JD, MPH
Warren Distinguished Professor and
Director, Center for Health Law,
Ethics & Human Rights
Department of Health Law, Policy,
and Management
Boston University School of
Public Health
Boston, MA, USA

Pepita Barlow, DPhil
Assistant Professor
Department of Health Policy
London School of Economics and
Political Science
London, UK

Fran Baum, PhD
Professor
Stretton Institute
University of Adelaide
Adelaide, AU

Lisa Bero, PhD
Professor
Center for Bioethics and
Humanities, Schools of Medicine
and Public Health
University of Colorado Anschutz
Medical Campus
Aurora, CO, USA

Rebecca Cassidy, BA, MPhil, PhD
Professor
Department of Anthropology
Goldsmiths
London, UK

Sally Casswell, PhD
Professor and Co-director
SHORE & Whariki Research Centre,
College of Health
Massey University
Auckland, NZ

Jeff Collin, PhD
Professor of Global Health
Global Health Policy Unit, School of
Social & Political Science
University of Edinburgh
Edinburgh, UK

Eric Crosbie, PhD, MA
Assistant Professor
School of Public Health
University of Nevada, Reno
Reno, NV, USA

**Katherine Cullerton, B App Sci,
Grad Dip Nut&Diet, MPH, PhD**
Senior Lecturer
School of Public Health, Faculty of
Medicine
The University of Queensland
Herston, AU

Sarah Dance, MSc
Research Assistant
Tobacco Control Research Group,
Department for Health
University of Bath
Bath, UK

Alice Fabbri, MD, PhD
Research Fellow
Department for Health
University of Bath
Bath, UK

Matt Fisher, PhD
Senior Research Fellow
Stretton Health Equity, Stretton
Institute, School of Social Sciences
The University of Adelaide
Adelaide, AU

Gary Fooks, PhD, MA, LLB
Reader in Sociology and Policy
Sociology and Policy
Aston University
Birmingham, UK

Nicholas Freudenberg, DrPH
Distinguished Professor of
Public Health
Department of Community Health
and Social Sciences
City University of New York
Graduate School of Public Health
and Health Policy
New York, NY, USA

Sandro Galea, MD, DrPH
Dean, Robert A Knox Professor
School of Public Health
Boston University
Boston, MA, USA

**Anna B. Gilmore, MBBS (hons),
DTM&H, MSc (dist), PhD**
Professor of Public Health
Department for Health
University of Bath
Bath, UK

Muluken Gizaw, PhD
Assistant Professor
Department of Preventive Medicine
School of Public Health, Addis Ababa
University
Addis Ababa, ET

Eduardo J. Gómez, PhD
Department of Population and
Community Health
College of Health
Lehigh University
Bethlehem, PA, USA

Benjamin Hawkins, PhD
Senior Research Associate
MRC Epidemiology Unit
University of Cambridge
Cambridge, UK

Sarah Hill, PhD, MPH, MBChB
Senior Lecturer
Sydney School of Public Health
University of Sydney
Sydney, AU

Shona Hilton, PhD, MSc, BSc
Professor of Public Health Policy
CSO/MRC Social and Public Health
Sciences Unit
University of Glasgow
Glasgow, UK

Erin Hobin, PhD
Senior Scientist
Department of Health Promotion,
Chronic Disease, and Injury
Prevention
Public Health Ontario
Toronto, ON, CA

Adnan A. Hyder, MD, MPH, PhD
Senior Associate Dean for Research,
Professor of Global Health &
Director of Center on Commercial
Determinants of Health
Milken Institute School of
Public Health
George Washington University
Washington, DC, USA

Vinu Ilakkuvan, DrPH, MSPH
Founder and Principal Consultant
PoP Health
Fairfax, VA, USA

**Alexandra Jones, PhD, LL.M
(Global Health Law), BA/LLB**
Senior Research Fellow (Food Policy
and Law)
Food Policy
The George Institute for Global
Health, UNSW
Sydney, AU

Nora Kenworthy, PhD
Associate Professor
School of Nursing and Health Studies
University of Washington Bothell
Bothell, WA, USA

Cécile Knai
Professor of Public Health Policy
London School of Hygiene &
Tropical Medicine
Faculty of Public Health and Policy
Tavistock Place, London, UK

Jim Krieger, MD, MPH
Clinical Professor
Health Systems and
Population Health
University of Washington
Seattle, WA, USA

Jennifer Lacy-Nichols, PhD
Research Fellow
Centre for Health Policy, Melbourne
School of Population and
Global Health
University of Melbourne
Melbourne, AU

Cassandra de Lacy-Vawdon,
BHSc (Hons)
Lecturer, PhD Candidate
School of Psychology and Public
Health, School of Public Health and
Preventive Medicine
La Trobe University, Monash
University
Melbourne, AU

Joana Madureira Lima, MD,
MSc, PhD
Health Policy Adviser
World Health Organization
Regional Office for Europe
Lisbon, KG

Nason Maani, BSc (Hons),
MSc, PhD
Lecturer in Inequalities and Global
Health Policy
Global Health Policy Unit, Social
Policy (or GHPU/Soc Pol)
School of Social and Political
Sciences
University of Edinburgh
Edinburgh, UK
Adjunct Assistant Professor
Department of Epidemiology
Boston University School of
Public Health
Boston, MA, USA

Martin McKee, CBE, MD, DSc
Professor of European Public Health
Department of Health Services
Research and Policy
London School of Hygiene &
Tropical Medicine
London, UK

Mélissa Mialon, PhD, MSc, BSc
Assistant Professor (Research)
Trinity Business School
Trinity College Dublin
Dublin, IE

Rob Moodie, MBBS,
MPH, FAFPHM, FRACGP,
DTMH, DRACOG
Professor of Public Health
Melbourne School of Population and
Global Health
University of Melbourne
Melbourne, VI, AU

Marion Nestle, PhD, MPH
Professor, Emerita
Nutrition and Food Studies
New York University
New York, NY, USA

Leona Ofei, MPH
Graduate Student
Department of Community
Health Sciences, Fielding School of
Public Health
University of California,
Los Angeles (UCLA)
Los Angeles, CA, USA

Nino Paichadze, MD, MPH
Assistant Research Professor
Department of Global Health
Milken Institute School of Public
Health, the George Washington
University
Washington, DC, USA

Mark Petticrew, PhD
Professor
Department of Public Health,
Environments and Society
London School of Hygiene &
Tropical Medicine
London, UK

Simone Pettigrew, PhD,
MComm, BEc
Professor
Food Policy
The George Institute for Global Health
Sydney, AU

Rob Ralston, PhD
Research Fellow
Global Health Policy Unit
University of Edinburgh
Edinburgh, UK

Natalie Savona, BA (Hons), MA,
MPhil, PhD
Assistant Professor
Faculty of Public Health and Policy
London School of Hygiene and
Tropical Medicine
London, UK

May CI van Schalkwyk,
MBBS, MPH
NIHR Doctoral Fellow and Public
Health Specialty Registrar
London School of Hygiene &
Tropical Medicine
London, UK

Laura Schmidt, PhD, MSW, MPH
Professor
Philip R. Lee Institute for Health
Policy Studies and Department of
Humanities and Social Sciences
School of Medicine
University of California
San Francisco, CA, USA

Tim Stockwell, PhD, MA
(Oxon), MSc
Scientist and Professor
Canadian Institute for Substance
Use Research
University of Victoria
Victoria, BC, CA

Katerini Tagmatarchi Storeng, PhD
Associate Professor
Centre for Development and the
Environment
University of Oslo
Oslo, NO

Nancy Tomes, PhD
Distinguished Professor
Department of History
Stony Brook University
Stony Brook, NY, USA

Martin White, MD, MSc, MB
ChB, FFPH
Professor of Population Health
Research
MRC Epidemiology Unit
University of Cambridge
Cambridge, UK

William H. Wiist, DHSc, MPH, MS
Courtesy Faculty
Global Health Program, School of
Biological and Population Health
Sciences, College of Public Health
and Human Sciences
Oregon State University
Corvallis, OR, USA

Marco Zenone, MSc
PhD Candidate
Faculty of Public Health and Policy
London School of Hygiene and
Tropical Medicine
London, UK

SECTION 1

Why Commercial Determinants?

CHAPTER 1

Commercial Determinants of Health

An Introduction

NASON MAANI, MARK PETTICREW, AND SANDRO GALEA

Our health is to a large degree shaped by the world around us—that is, by the conditions in which we are born, grow, work, and live. As described in pivotal reports in recent years, most notably by the World Health Organization in its report on the social determinants of health in 2008,[1] it is these conditions that are largely responsible for health and for the health inequalities observed within and between countries.[2] Subsequent approaches informed by this understanding, such as Health in All Policies[3] or One Health,[4] have sought to close health gaps through coordinated action on policy beyond health.

The world around us is shaped by forces beyond government policy. In particular, in the modern era, the economic and political power of the private sector influences our physical and social environments, the evidence surrounding problems and their solutions, and even the nature of public discourse and understanding.[5,6] In the era of social media, the private sector often provides the structures and the fora in which public debates take place. The private sector could also be said to influence health at every level of society, directly and indirectly. Whereas international organizations or national governments might do so with a view to promoting "Health in All Policies," the private sector is by definition driven by "Profit in All Policies." Considering the relative influence of private sector actors, it is more important than ever to understand their role in shaping health and policy, particularly where there may be a conflict between profits and health.

Nason Maani, Mark Petticrew, and Sandro Galea, *Commercial Determinants of Health* In: *The Commercial Determinants of Health*. Edited by: Nason Maani, Mark Petticrew, and Sandro Galea, Oxford University Press.
© Oxford University Press 2023. DOI: 10.1093/oso/9780197578742.003.0001

Commercial actors, particularly large, multinational commercial actors, have the social, economic, and political gravity to shape the world in ways health departments and even entire national governments cannot. Certainly, commercial actors can shape our health as individuals and as populations, but beyond that, they can shape how we define ourselves, live our lives, interact with others, and how we perceive problems and solutions. Despite the ubiquity of commercial forces, however, until recently, the commercial determinants remained largely absent from our conceptual frameworks of the social determinants of health.[7]

There are also challenging gaps in the empiric evidence. To date, much research on the commercial determinants of health has focused on the tobacco industry and, to a lesser extent, on aspects of the food and alcohol industries. Thus, there are important questions about the extent to which a focus on a narrow range of products can be extrapolated to informing our understanding of other sectors and industries, where the harms and benefits are less well-defined and their business activities less well-described and understood.

Particularly at a time when public–private partnerships are viewed as a cost-effective way to tackle urgent problems, it is imperative we have the theoretical frameworks and the evidence base to understand and predict the activities of private sector actors in ways that avoid harms, maximize any potential benefits where possible, and guide us around the proximal and distal pitfalls of partnerships between those concerned with promoting the health of populations and those engaged in commercial activity.

Research on this subject is growing but faces a number of challenges.[5,8] First, agreement is needed on a common, inclusive definition of the commercial determinants of health. Most existing research is generated in industry-specific silos, with a focus on a specific product category, such as tobacco or alcohol. This risks missing the cumulative effects of such actors in areas such as regulatory approaches or the framing of policy options, with potential downstream consequences for population health and health equity. Second, we need more empirical work of an interdisciplinary nature, but also new fora that might allow cross-disciplinary communication and collaboration on these issues. Third, we need to address emergent gaps in our understanding, particularly how they pertain to low- and middle-income countries. It is our hope that this book contributes toward such goals by seeking to synthesize current definitions, frameworks, and empirical research into a coherent research and translational entity, and by providing an accessible entry point for a wider number of scholars who can help the field make the leap to its next level for the benefit of science and society.

This book provides an introduction to this field. It is intended to provide a conceptual understanding and a review of the empirical evidence on these issues, in a way that is accessible to academics and policymakers. It includes case studies that highlight the common and disparate aspects of a variety of industry actors, and it aims to help inform research and action at a critical time in our history to help lay the foundations for studying a core contributor to our health that influences individuals, communities, and societies at all levels. It aims to distill some of the main themes emerging in the field and, in doing so, aid in its definition, structure, and growth.

The book begins with chapters that provide a grounding for the reader, discussing why it is that such determinants constitute a foundational component of the social determinants of health and introducing the concept of commercial determinants as both directly and indirectly affecting health and health equity. The following chapters then adopt an interdisciplinary approach to describe the various ways in which commercial actors shape the upstream drivers of health, such as through shaping policy, evidence, and public discourse. Having developed this broader interdisciplinary lens for the reader, the chapters in the following section offer examples of how this lens has been applied to a variety of industries that serve as case studies.

In some cases, these are areas in which the evidence base is relatively well developed. In others, such as fossil fuels or gambling, the case studies serve as examples to the reader of how useful the triangulation of evidence and theory from other arenas might be in the study of these less well-research industries, as well as what the unique features might be that require further empirical research.

Having given examples of the similarities and differences of a range of different commercial sectors, the next portion of the book widens the reader's perspective to consider the cumulative, distal effects of such commercial activities, beyond individual sectors, on health and equity. This includes cumulative effects on policy, the evidence base, and public discourse. By cumulative effects, we refer to the shifting of aspects of the policy and public conversation environment, through the combined effects of many corporate actors, by, for example, moving away from regulatory approaches, limiting transparency, accountability or oversight, reducing tax burdens and legal liability, or otherwise affecting barriers to political influence.

Taken together, the sections of the book up to this point aim to give the reader a firm grasp of the conceptual and empiric state of the field and some of the possibilities for cross-fertilization and shared learning. Having offered an overview of key concepts, mechanisms of influence, examples and cumulative effects in previous sections, the last two sections of the book seek to outline the future for scholarship and action on the commercial determinants of health.

Overall, this book aims to present cross-cutting ideas and evidence bases in a way that brings a field of study together, describes the state of that field of study, and considers its future direction and potential impact. The field of commercial determinants research remains one in development, with early evidence of research funders taking interest in the broader consequences of commercial activity on health and policy, and developing initial frameworks and courses, but with few dedicated conferences, journals, or books to support junior scholars as they move into this rapidly growing field. It is hoped that this book is the next stop on this journey, bringing together past and recent evidence across a range of disciplines in a way that demonstrates the utility of a commercial determinants lens, offers an accessible reference point for scholars, helps give this field shape and direction, and helps establish a foundation for future research and translation efforts.

REFERENCES

1. Commission on Social Determinants of Health. *Closing the Gap in a Generation: Health Equity Through Action on the Social Determinants of Health.* World Health Organization; 2008.
2. Dahlgren G, Whitehead M. The Dahlgren–Whitehead model of health determinants: 30 years on and still chasing rainbows. *Public Health.* 2021; 199: 20–24.
3. Puska P. Health in all policies—From what to how. *Eur J Public Health.* 2014; 24(1): 1.
4. Mackenzie JS, Jeggo M. The One Health approach—Why is it so important? *Trop Med Infect Dis.* 2019; 4(2): 88.
5. Maani N, McKee M, Petticrew M, Galea S. Corporate practices and the health of populations: A research and translational agenda. *Lancet Public Health.* 2020; 5(2): e80–e81.
6. Madureira Lima J, Galea S. Corporate practices and health: A framework and mechanisms. *Global Health.* 2018; 14(1): 21.
7. Maani N, Collin J, Friel S, et al. Bringing the commercial determinants of health out of the shadows: A review of how the commercial determinants are represented in conceptual frameworks. *Eur J Public Health.* 2020; 30(4): 660–664.
8. Freudenberg N, Lee K, Buse K, et al. Defining priorities for action and research on the commercial determinants of health: A conceptual review. *Am J Public Health.* 2021; 111(12): 2202–2211.

A Systems Perspective on the Pathways of Influence of Commercial Determinants of Health

CÉCILE KNAI AND NATALIE SAVONA

2.1 INTRODUCTION

The understanding that corporate actors affect people's health, often negatively, is not new. In Henrik Ibsen's 1882 play "An Enemy of the People," the local doctor recommends closing the Norwegian town's lucrative spa because the surrounding waters are contaminated from nearby tanneries, causing ill health in patrons. He is met with angry opposition by those with interests in the spa, who argue that "the matter in this instance is by no means a purely scientific one; it is a combination of technical and economic factors," dubbing the doctor a "public enemy."[1] Likewise in his 1906 novel *The Jungle*, Upton Sinclair exposed the exploitation of factory workers in Chicago's meatpacking plants through the story of Lithuanian immigrants, following their difficult journey after arriving in America. The book caused public outcry in response to his account of contaminated meat and unhygienic processing methods, leading to the nation's first meat inspection and the introduction of food safety regulations.[2]

Then and now, action to allay public health harms due to unhealthy commodities may cause the industries that produce them to incur financial losses[3] and thus to invest in strategies to promote and protect their interests. Their products and such strategies are what is meant by the commercial determinants of health (CDOH), an issue that sits within multiple, complex spheres of influence and interest. The main proposition of this chapter, therefore, is that

Cécile Knai and Natalie Savona, *A Systems Perspective on the Pathways of Influence of Commercial Determinants of Health* In: *The Commercial Determinants of Health*. Edited by: Nason Maani, Mark Petticrew, and Sandro Galea, Oxford University Press. © Oxford University Press 2023. DOI: 10.1093/oso/9780197578742.003.0002 a study of CDOH requires a complex systems perspective to clarify the pathways of influence of corporate actors on health, providing an opportunity to properly understand competing interests, design and resilience of unhealthy systems, and consequences of policy interventions, intended or not.

The study of CDOH includes analyses of unhealthy commodity industries (UCIs), their products, and their marketing and corporate political strategies. It is an increasingly established field of research, the focus of which includes the production of unhealthy commodities,[4,5] the adverse health impacts attributable to commercial activities,[4] and the strategies employed by commercial actors to promote products that can damage health.[4-8] The study of CDOH has been described in literature focused on addiction, global health, health governance, health promotion, systems thinking, and other domains.[6,9]

Although few influences are purely negative in an absolute sense, the well-documented, overwhelmingly negative impact of UCI products and practices[4-8] should be the focus of health research, with a degree of urgency, given the burden of death and disease to which they contribute. It is now well-documented that global ill health due to unhealthy commodity use or consumption has become a chronic, complex, pervasive problem.[5,10,11]

2.2 A COMPLEX SYSTEM OF INFLUENCE

What do we know about how corporate actors shape health? Unhealthy commodities and the influence of UCI on health policymaking are major upstream determinants of health i.e., macro drivers, such as economic and structural factors. The causal pathways linking commercial products and practices with health are complex. The complexity of the problem is not limited to understanding just the drivers of unhealthy commodity consumption; it extends to the way in which corporate actors shape wider systems to support their business interests.[5] Various explanatory models set out how commercial actors negatively affect population health[4,12-14] via a range of market and non-market strategies. The non-market practices employed by individual UCIs to influence health and health policies are well-documented—for example, corporate political activities (CPAs) are used to shape government policy in ways favorable to them.[4,15-19] There is also clear evidence of strong business links across UCIs,[4] relationships between UCIs and the public sector, such as with "revolving doors,"[4] and commonalities in CPAs employed across UCIs. All these are used to support market goals by leveraging political and social influence to affect policy in their favor.[20-23] These strategies include complex and subtle tactics such as the spread of misinformation.[24] A recent study demonstrates how alcohol industry organizations mislead the public about the associations between alcohol and cancer by misrepresenting the evidence through denial or omissions that alcohol consumption increases cancer risks, by distortion of risks, and by distraction, diverting consumer attention from the evidence of a negative relationship.[25]

The growing evidence of the existence and pathways of influence of CDOH is often met with resistance by the commercial sector and with a slow response by those responsible for protecting population health.[9] One reason for this is the public health community's relatively narrow approach to public health problems, despite understanding and acknowledging the importance of prioritizing the broad upstream determinants of ill health.[5] The conception of risk, the design of public health interventions, and policy responses overall continue to consider the impact of UCIs on population health in a linear way, focusing on individual-level choices. Public health research and practice are likely to have more impact by taking a systems perspective —that is, viewing ill health as a result of the aggregation of, and interactions between, diverse actors, factors, and their environments.[26]

Much complexity also lies within the functioning of corporate power and influence. It can take the form of exertion of direct influence on decision-makers via, for example, lobbying, longer term processes to shape norms, political ideas and public opinion over time, and more subtle expressions of power such as appeasement.[27] For example, UCIs use the rhetoric of cooperation to normalize their role in research and policy settings,[28] to the point where it has become the accepted norm for corporations directly contributing to ill health to be included in global scientific and health policy fora for resolving it. This has led to further normalization and wide acceptance of phenomena such as public–private partnerships to improve health and voluntary mechanisms whereby commercial actors design and monitor their own standards of conduct. These approaches have consistently been found ineffective at addressing public health problems created by UCIs,[22,29] and they are reflective of perhaps the most complex aspect of these pathways of influence—that is, the positioning of corporate actors as legitimate partners in population health,[28] as credibly "part of the solution."[30]

Thus, given the intricacies and multiple spheres of influence, conventional linear thinking is inadequate for looking to solve chronic, complex social problems such as the adverse effects of CDOH.[31] A complex systems approach, however, has long been acknowledged as the most appropriate way to analyze how corporate actors work to influence health and health policy and what can be done to mitigate their power.[4,32]

2.3 A COMPLEX SYSTEMS APPROACH TO EXAMINE COMMERCIAL DETERMINANTS OF HEALTH

The notion of a system is a heuristic, a conceptual tool used to examine a complex issue. A systems approach theorizes that the behavior of an element in the system depends on other conditions in the system, rather than the mechanisms or characteristics of that specific element alone.[33] Thus, UCI actions and interactions between them are greater than the sum of their parts and have an effect across the system. A systems approach posits that the behavior of a system is shaped by the interactions between its parts so that any attempt to improve its performance must take account of the many parts of the system, *as* a system, not separately.[34]

The environmental scientist and systems thinker Donella Meadows proposes that a system can be conceptualized as a set of elements (e.g., individuals or physical structures) interconnected (characterized by feedback loops) in such a way that they produce their own pattern of behavior over time, with some expected, desirable consequences and others that are unintended or unwanted. A complex systems approach helps visualize our work in public health as part of a wider system,[35] and it gets us to acknowledge the interconnections, or relationships that hold the elements together, and the function or purpose of the system by observing how it behaves.[36]

Meadows explains system thinking by citing a Sufi parable[36]: "You think that because you understand 'one' that you must therefore understand 'two' because one and one make two. But you forget that you must also understand 'and.'" In public health research and practice, we tend to focus on the "ones," or the elements of a system, because they are the most tangible, concrete, visible parts, such as individuals (as consumers), individual behaviors (e.g., online gambling), skills (e.g., reading a food label), and physical structures (e.g., a supermarket). Interventions targeting such individual elements make up the bulk of our actions. We tend to intervene with a new activity or approach without fully considering how it may impact on the wider system, its actors, and their interests and influence.[35] However, Meadows cautions that most responses to complex problems occur at the level of system elements because they are the most visible, tangible, and concrete, and thus the easiest points of intervention—the notorious "low-hanging fruits"—yet they are the least effective at bringing about change. In contrast, intervening to change the system's function or paradigm—its most deeply held beliefs, or the trunk of the tree, to continue the fruit analogy—is enormously challenging but commensurately effective because it manages to "hit a leverage point that totally transforms the system," with lasting impacts such as the establishment of new cultural or dietary norms.[36]

Additional to complex systems' heterogeneous, nonlinear characteristics is the principle that the behavior of one component of the system is affected by the behavior of others. So, for example, the promotion of a new type of burger (through ads across multiple media, formulated in specific ways for specific people, with financial and other incentives) incites people to buy and consume more of that burger. Another principle is that the capacity of any part of the system must be able to withstand the complexity of its task[37]: One "task" expected of individuals within the system dominated by the UCIs is to engage in behaviors that optimize their health—to eat healthily, to not smoke, to drink alcohol or gamble only in moderation—yet their autonomy is affected by other components of the system, particularly the corporations that make, market, and sell these products. Indeed, the continuing prevalence of unhealthy commodity-related diseases highlights the difficulty for individuals in making truly "responsible" decisions given their capacity, or power, within the UCI system as it stands. While the system remains high functioning in favor of UCIs, it is unrealistic to expect individuals to resist their products on the basis of future, uncertain health outcomes.

Another important principle to consider is that a system is dynamic and adaptive so that it responds to or resists external changes. As illustrated in Figure 2.1, the global system functions in favor of UCIs and their interests; the previous description of the complex pathways of influence goes some way to explain how they are able to resist or adapt to external pressures such as threat of regulation and to diversify to survive and thrive. The system is not functioning well from a public health perspective because most interventions designed to address ill-health created by UCI consumption or use fail to do so. Part of the challenge in finding effective actions is that solutions using traditional theories of change rather than a systems approach are easier to conceptualize and operationalize.[38] But most theories of change suffer from pitfalls including linear thinking, simple chains of cause and effect, and relying on a fixed plan that ironically forfeits change when other things adapt around the intervention.[39] Failing to account for the wider system—including corporate practices—means we do not account for its potential resilience and capacity to absorb "shocks" such as public health interventions, which then themselves fail. An example of this is the "shock" of a food safety scandal when lead was found in instant noodles packets in India; though a temporary decrease in sales was observed,[40] trust and brand loyalty were largely unaffected. This was in large part due to the combined strategies of manufacturer, which made instant noodles transformative in changing dietary and cooking norms across India.[41] Thus, when the crisis happened, the "system" was resilient from the perspective of the manufacturer: It protected noodle sales through its capacity to adapt and absorb the dangers.[5]

Ideally, a systemic theory of change, or other systems analysis, discerns the drivers of CDOH and prompts a strategy that effectively integrates the identified leverage points.[31]

(a)

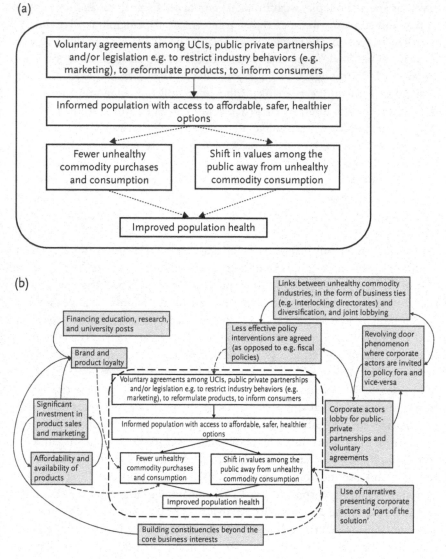

(b)

Figure 2.1 Demonstrating differences between linear (a) and systems (b) thinking in approaching commercial determinants of health through the example of voluntary agreements between unhealthy commodity industries (UCIs) and governments.

2.4 HOW DOES A SYSTEMS APPROACH WORK IN PRACTICE?

Systems analyses of complex problems can be conducted in a range of ways, from using a systems' lens to conceptualize a problem to specific systems methods.[42]

A systems approach is a lens, a way of thinking, a way of conceptualizing and scrutinizing a problem. It can lead to a practical illustration of the complexity of pathways of impact, how different factors interact, and leverage points for change that may not appear in linear logic models or traditional theories of change as well as potential unintended consequences of an intervention.[31] An example of taking a systems approach is the creation of a system map through a range of methods, such as group model building (GMB). GMB is a participatory, structured format that brings together stakeholders in a given problem and that leads them in the creation of causal loop diagrams to illustrate the complexity of the problem's drivers. System maps then help inform responses to the issue, helping explain visually how factors are interrelated and where leverage points for change or intervention might be found. A recent study of adolescent obesity employed GMB with young people to capture their experience of the drivers of obesity, generating system maps that very clearly highlighted the importance of (among other pathways) social media and influencers in young people's life and how they relate to depression and anxiety, which in turn were described to reduce motivation to eat healthily and exercise.[43]

Systems methods draw on systems and complexity science, using processes such as computer modeling to investigate complex problems—for example, simulating how an intervention might interact with the wider system.[42] They also include what has been referred to as "systems framing" or using systems thinking to frame an analysis[42]; examples include clarification of systems concepts through worked examples related to CDOH,[4,5] systems evaluations of public–private partnerships,[35] and the formulation of concrete methodological implications of a complexity perspective when conducting systematic reviews and guideline development.[44]

As described above, typical linear approaches to public health challenges, using conventional theories of change, emphasize inputs and outputs rather than elements and how they interconnect to create the existing problematic situation. Figure 2.1 illustrates the contrast between linear thinking to address CDOH to improve population health (Figure 2.1a) and the dismantling of linear thinking when starting to think in systems (Figure 2.1b).

Figure 2.1b is by no means comprehensive but is evidence-based, drawing on recently published reviews and analyses[4,5,35]; it demonstrates a range of reasons why a portfolio of potentially effective policy interventions rarely achieves population health aims, due to the effective strategies employed by corporate actors. This starts with them negotiating the retraction—or at least weakening—of otherwise effective policies and gradually results in a fading impact on improving population health. Thus, Figure 2.1b indicates that the increasingly normalized choice of using voluntary agreements and public–private partnerships with UCIs to address complex public health problems is not effective at doing so; one way in which power and influence are imposed is through creating opportunities for interlocking directorates (when an individual linked to one organization sits on the board of directors of another)[45]—and "revolving doors" between the public and private sector. This practice, illustrated at length by Knai et al.,[4] works to undermine trust in the public sector because of real or perceived conflicts of interest. Thus, Figure 2.1b illustrates a part of the current system that is designed to benefit commercial interests at the expense of health and is thus highly resilient to public health interventions.

2.5 CONCLUSION

Public health researchers and practitioners do instinctively think in "systems," yet most interventions and the way they are evaluated remain entrenched in conventional linear thinking. For example, warnings on advertisements for gambling or other products to be "responsible" ignore the many other factors that drive gambling addiction; food package labeling of fats, sugars, and salt ignores the other reasons people choose such products beyond their health value. A systems approach to the CDOH goes some way to exposing, conceptualizing, and acting on these multiple spheres of influence. A systems approach is the best way to expose, understand, and analyze fully the practices of the commercial sector and to situate them in the orbit of the public health "system"—to help make sense of the "mess." Use of a piecemeal, linear approach does population health an injustice.

REFERENCES

1. Ibsen H. *An Enemy of the People. The Wild Duck. Rosmersholm.* Oxford University Press; 1882. Translated with an introduction by James McFarlane, 1960 edition.
2. Ebbeling C, Pawlak D, Ludwig D. Childhood obesity: Public-health crisis, common sense cure. *Lancet.* 2002; 360: 473–482.
3. Leviton C, Needleman C, Shapiro M. *Confronting Public Health Risks: A Decision Maker's Guide.* SAGE; 1998.
4. Knai C, Petticrew M, Capewell S, et al. The case for developing a cohesive systems approach to research across unhealthy commodity industries. *BMJ Glob Health.* 2021; 6(2): e003543.
5. Knai C, Petticrew M, Mays N, et al. Systems thinking as a framework for analyzing commercial determinants of health. *Milbank Q.* 2018; 96(3): 472–498.
6. Kickbusch I, Allen L, Franz C. The commercial determinants of health. *Lancet Glob Health.* 2016; 4(12): e895–e896.
7. Maani N, McKee M, Petticrew M, Galea S. Corporate practices and the health of populations: A research and translational agenda. *Lancet Public Health.* 2020; 5(2): e80–e81.
8. de Lacy-Vawdon C, Livingstone C. Defining the commercial determinants of health: A systematic review. *BMC Public Health.* 2020; 20(1): 1022.
9. Buse K, Tanaka S, Hawkes S. Healthy people and healthy profits? Elaborating a conceptual framework for governing the commercial determinants of

non-communicable diseases and identifying options for reducing risk exposure. *Global Health*. 2017; 13(1): 34.

10. World Health Organization. Noncommunicable diseases: Fact sheet. 2021. https://www.who.int/news-room/fact-sheets/detail/noncommunicable-diseases

11. Cassidy R. How corporations shape our understanding of problems with gambling and their solutions. In: Kenworthy N, MacKenzie R, Lee K, eds. *Case Studies on Corporations and Global Health Governance Impacts, Influence and Accountability*. Rowman & Littlefield; 2016: 89–101.

12. Baum FE, Sanders DM, Fisher M, et al. Assessing the health impact of transnational corporations: Its importance and a framework. *Global Health*. 2016; 12(1): 27.

13. Madureira Lima J, Galea S. Corporate practices and health: A framework and mechanisms. *Global Health*. 2018; 14(1): 21.

14. Mialon M. An overview of the commercial determinants of health. *Global Health*. 2020; 16(1): 74.

15. Savell E, Fooks G, Gilmore AB. How does the alcohol industry attempt to influence marketing regulations? A systematic review. *Addiction*. 2016; 111(1): 18–32.

16. Mialon M, Swinburn B, Sacks G. A proposed approach to systematically identify and monitor the corporate political activity of the food industry with respect to public health using publicly available information. *Obes Rev*. 2015; 16(7): 519–530.

17. Ulucanlar S, Fooks GJ, Gilmore AB. The policy dystopia model: An interpretive analysis of tobacco industry political activity. *PLoS Med*. 2016; 13(9): e1002125.

18. Hancock L, Ralph N, Martino FP. Applying Corporate Political Activity (CPA) analysis to Australian gambling industry submissions against regulation of television sports betting advertising. *PLoS One*. 2018; 13(10): e0205654.

19. Scott C, Hawkins B, Knai C. Food and beverage product reformulation as a corporate political strategy. *Soc Sci Med*. 2017; 172: 37–45.

20. Dorfman L, Cheyne A, Friedman LC, Wadud A, Gottlieb M. Soda and tobacco industry corporate social responsibility campaigns: How do they compare? *PLoS Med*. 2012; 9(6): e1001241.

21. Cassidy R, Loussouarn C, Pisac A. Fair game: Producing gambling research. *The Goldsmiths Report*. 2013. http://www.gold.ac.uk/media/documents-by-section/departments/anthropology/Fair-Game-Web-Final.pdf

22. Knai C, James L, Petticrew M, Eastmure E, Durand MA, Mays N. An evaluation of a public–private partnership to reduce artificial trans fatty acids in England, 2011–16. *Eur J Public Health*. 2017; 27(4): 605–608.

23. Hawkins B, Holden C, Eckhardt J, Lee K. Reassessing policy paradigms: A comparison of the global tobacco and alcohol industries. *Glob Public Health*. 2016: 1–19.

24. Suarez-Lledo V, Alvarez-Galvez J. Prevalence of health misinformation on social media: Systematic review. *J Med Internet Res*. 2021; 23(1): e17187.

25. Petticrew M, Maani Hessari N, Knai C, Weiderpass E. How alcohol industry organisations mislead the public about alcohol and cancer. *Drug Alcohol Rev*. 2018; 37(3): 293–303.

26. Petticrew M, Shemilt I, Lorenc T, et al. Alcohol advertising and public health: Systems perspectives versus narrow perspectives. *J Epidemiol Community Health*. 2017; 71(3): 308–312.

27. Lacy-Nichols J, Marten R. Power and the commercial determinants of health: Ideas for a research agenda. *BMJ Glob Health*. 2021; 6(2): e003850.

28. Lie AL. "We are not a partnership"—Constructing and contesting legitimacy of global public–private partnerships: The Scaling Up Nutrition (SUN) movement. *Globalizations.* 2021; 18(2): 237–255.

29. Kunkel DL, Castonguay JS, Filer CR. Evaluating industry self-regulation of food marketing to children. *Am J Prev Med.* 2015; 49(2): 181–187.

30. Nixon L, Mejia P, Cheyne A, Wilking C, Dorfman L, Daynard R. "We're part of the solution": Evolution of the food and beverage industry's framing of obesity concerns between 2000 and 2012. *Am J Public Health.* 2015; 105(11): 2228–2236.

31. Stroh D. *Systems Thinking for Social Change.* Chelsea Green Publishing; 2015.

32. Holder H. *Alcohol and the Community: A Systems Approach to Prevention.* Cambridge University Press; 1998.

33. Diez Roux AV. Complex systems thinking and current impasses in health disparities research. *Am J Public Health.* 2011; 101(9): 1627–1634.

34. Newell B, Proust K. *Introduction to collaborative conceptual modelling.* Working paper. ANU Open Access Research. 2012. https://digitalcollections.anu.edu.au/handle/1885/9386

35. Knai C, Petticrew M, Douglas N, et al. The public health responsibility deal: Using a systems-level analysis to understand the lack of impact on alcohol, food, physical activity, and workplace health sub-systems. *Int J Environ Res Public Health.* 2018; 15(12): 2895.

36. Meadows D. *Thinking in Systems: A Primer.* Earthscan; 2008.

37. Finegood DT, Merth TD, Rutter H. Implications of the foresight obesity system map for solutions to childhood obesity. *Obesity.* 2010; 18(Suppl 1): S13–S16.

38. ActKnowledge. Theory of change. 2011. https://www.theoryofchange.org/wp-content/uploads/toco_library/pdf/2011_-_Montague-Clouse_-_Theory_of_Change_Basics.pdf

39. NPC. Thinking big: How to use theory of change for systems change. 2018. https://www.thinknpc.org/resource-hub/thinking-big-how-to-use-theory-of-change-for-systems-change

40. Cherry L, Rosemary G, Suneetha K, et al. Purchase trends of processed foods and beverages in urban India. *Glob Food Sec.* 2019 Dec; 23: 191–204.

41. Baviskar A. Consumer Citizenship: Instant Noodles in India. *Gastronomica.* 2018; 18(2): 1–10.

42. McGill E, Er V, Penney T, et al. Evaluation of public health interventions from a complex systems perspective: A research methods review. *Soc Sci Med.* 2021; 272: 113697.

43. Savona N, Macauley T, Aguiar A, et al. Identifying the views of adolescents in five European countries on the drivers of obesity using group model building. *Eur J Public Health.* 2021; 31(2): 391–396.

44. Petticrew M, Knai C, Thomas J, et al. Implications of a complexity perspective for systematic reviews and guideline development in health decision making. *BMJ Global Health.* 2019; 4(Suppl 1): e000899.

45. Mizruchi M. What do interlocks do? An analysis, critique, and assessment of research on interlocking directorates. *Annu Rev Sociol.* 1996; 22: 271–298.

CHAPTER 3

Global Health and Equity Burden of Commercial Determinants of Health

JULIA ANAF, FRAN BAUM, AND MATT FISHER

3.1 INTRODUCTION

In this chapter, the review and understanding of commercial determinants of health (CDOH) are based on the definition by Kickbusch et al.[1] of CDOH as "the strategies and approaches used by the private sector to promote products and choices that are detrimental to health." The proximal impacts of CDOH are conceived as the result of the marketing and consumption of unhealthy products that are known to be risk factors for noncommunicable diseases (NCDs). Distal impacts accrue from strategic political and business practices that are designed to place corporate profits ahead of public health.

In conceptualizing and researching CDOH, particular attention must be paid to large national and transnational corporations (TNCs) because of their large and growing influence on the conditions of daily living and the broader sociopolitical conditions that determine health and health equity.[2-4] Thus, in this chapter, the conception of CDOH is also informed by a corporate health impact assessment framework[3] that includes the global economic, political, and regulatory context in which TNCs operate; their structure, products, and operations; and their health-related impacts on daily living conditions. This understanding also draws upon the Commission on Social Determinants of Health conceptual framework of social determinants of health (SDOH) and health inequities.[2] According to these frameworks, current evidence on the CDOH falls into four main categories: health behaviors and choices related to risk factors for chronic disease, other SDOH factors affecting daily living conditions, corporate political and business practices influencing regulatory

Julia Anaf, Fran Baum, and Matt Fisher, *Global Health and Equity Burden of Commercial Determinants of Health* In: *The Commercial Determinants of Health*. Edited by: Nason Maani, Mark Petticrew, and Sandro Galea, Oxford University Press. © Oxford University Press 2023. DOI: 10.1093/oso/9780197578742.003.0003 environments, and the globalized political and economic environment sanctioning corporate activities.

3.2 HEALTH BEHAVIORS AND CHOICES RELATED TO RISK FACTORS FOR CHRONIC DISEASE

Health behaviors and choices related to risk factors for chronic disease are strongly influenced by the lucrative marketing and sale of unhealthy commodities, including food and beverages, alcohol, gambling, and tobacco.[5,6] Individual choices are heavily influenced by the manipulative techniques and images used by those marketing and advertising these products. As markets become saturated in high-income countries, these industries have turned their attention to low- and middle-income countries. For example, the displacement of traditional food systems in Latin America, Asia, and Africa by ultra-processed and low-nutrient products, marketed by TNCs and operating mainly from the United States and Europe, has been rapidly increasing since the 1980s. There are implications for health equity due to the potential for these commodities to undermine public health and public institutions in countries that are unable to afford health care costs associated with NCDs.[7]

3.3 OTHER SOCIAL DETERMINANTS OF HEALTH AFFECTING DAILY LIVING CONDITIONS

In addition to the well-known behavioral risk factors for chronic disease, private sector activities affect a number of other daily living conditions. Equity of access to affordable, appropriate health care is a known SDOH. Ideally, health systems emphasize health promotion and disease prevention. Access to health services is adversely affected by increasing privatization of health care systems and the dominance of biomedical strategies partly based on the power of pharmaceutical corporations to promote the use of their products.[8]

Another relatively recent concern is the impact of corporate social media on public attitudes and behaviors and also on psychological conditions. A study concerning impacts of social media indicates that prolonged use may relate to negative symptoms of anxiety, stress, and depression.[9] Although diverse media platforms offer important information and evidence, they also promulgate and enable misinformation, political interference, and mistrust of science.[10] By enabling cyberbullying, computer hacking, frauds and scams, and reputational damage, digital media TNCs can have a major impact on risks for poor mental health (see also Chapter 20).[11]

Health-related impacts of private sector activities on daily environmental conditions include exposure to hazardous wastes, despoilation of the lands of Indigenous peoples, and industrial disasters caused by extractives industries.[12] The clearing of forests for commercial purposes including intensive farming has been linked to the increasing number of zoonotic viruses including SARS-CoV-2, which causes COVID-19.[13]

Social conditions are affected by the operations of TNCs and their impacts on local goods and services and the quality of local community life. The presence of TNCs may often weaken local industries that reflect the culture and history of a place to a much greater degree than large global companies.

Whereas safe, secure, and adequately paid work benefits health, there has been an increase in insecure forms of work that adversely affect health, resulting from business strategies that fragment traditional employment models.[14,15] TNCs engage in labor hire and "sham contracting" whereby employers disguise employment relationships as contracting arrangements across a range of industry sectors.[16] These employment practices contribute to increasing health inequities.

TNCs also affect daily living conditions due to their power over international, national, or local economies, public revenue, and local production systems. This corporate power, along with binding trade agreements and increasing capital mobility, has diminished the capacity of individual countries to guarantee that economic activity by TNCs and other business entities contributes to, or at least does not erode, health equity.[2]

The effects of TNCs on daily living conditions may increase health and social inequities within and across groups and countries. Examples from the fast-food industry include the epidemics of NCDs that mainly affect the Global South.[7] In higher income countries, TNCs strategically place fast-food outlets in areas of lower socioeconomic status with implications for low-income and other populations living in vulnerable circumstances.[17] Extractives industries apply unfair and inconsistent operating standards globally, exploiting limited, or poorly enforced, regulatory frameworks in different jurisdictions (see Chapter 28).[18]

3.4 CORPORATE POLITICAL AND BUSINESS PRACTICES INFLUENCING REGULATORY ENVIRONMENTS

Research on CDOH has expanded to also examine corporate business, political, and marketing strategies that influence regulatory environments in ways that are relevant to health or health equity. These include political lobbying and donations, and influencing international agreements and regulations.

3.4.1 Political Lobbying and Funding

Key corporate strategies to foster commercial interests include political lobbying and funding, especially through representative industry organizations such as in the food and beverage and extractive industries.[19,20] This may also involve use of "front" groups—organizations that purport to represent one agenda while in reality serving some other parties or interests whose sponsorship is mostly hidden.[21] The power of lobbying and funding by big business can impose a chilling effect on policies or agreements that are seen to adversely affect corporate interests. For example, the food industry has undermined public health regulation by opposing introduction of "sugar taxes" in many jurisdictions and lobbying instead for weaker voluntary measures such as food labeling.[22]

Similarly, powerful fossil fuel industries act to prevent political action on climate change by lobbying to manufacture doubt and using "greenwashing" or corporate social responsibility strategies to present an environmentally responsible public image.[23]

Another way for private sector actors to control the policy agenda is by influencing research on health-related features of products or practices.[24] Such influence is achieved by corporate funding, with commercial imperatives driving the research agenda away from public health priorities.[24] Further influence is achieved through "revolving doors," or the movement of politicians, senior bureaucrats, and senior staffers into industry and vice versa. Elected representatives leaving government often take up roles as lobbyists or consultants or take positions on corporate boards, using contacts and insights gained in prior roles to foster their best interests.[25]

3.4.2 Influencing International Agreements and Regulations

Through their historic involvement in international business, TNCs have the capacity to influence international relations and trade agreements[26] in ways that have implications for public health. These include investor–state dispute settlement (ISDS) conditions that allow TNCs to challenge government regulations in different jurisdictions. The threat of ISDS can be a disincentive to governments that seek to enact laws for protecting environmental and public health.[27] For example, the tobacco TNC Philip Morris used an ISDS clause in a trade agreement with Hong Kong to challenge the Australian High Court judgment supporting plain packaging for tobacco products.[28]

The impact of global patent regulation in the form of the World Trade Organization's Trade-Related Aspects of Intellectual Property Rights agreement has wide-reaching effects on pharmaceutical research and global public healt.[29] Large pharmaceutical TNCs focus on more profitable product lines, with fewer medications developed for largely overlooked but devastating diseases that, in most cases, affect people living in the developing world.[30] This lack of global public investment, despite pharmaceutical TNCs receiving tax breaks and public funding for basic research, adversely affects health equity.

The size and power of TNCs also allow them to shift their assets and corporate ownership between jurisdictions for tax minimization purposes.[31] The lack of effective global regulation on TNCs' financial operations reduces the capacity and revenues of national governments to improve health and social welfare, make other public investments, and work to reduce inequity.

3.5 COMMERCIAL DETERMINANTS OF HEALTH AND THE COVID-19 PANDEMIC

During the COVID-19 pandemic, diverse industry sectors have used the changed global environment to further their financial interests in ways that can affect public health. For example, fast-food industries used even more nuanced, sophisticated marketing techniques to specifically align their products with the efforts and acclamation of front-line health and emergency services workers.[32] Industries sought to shape the regulatory environment by lobbying for their particular commodities, including for alcohol and extractive products to be designated as "essential."[32] Technology corporations profited from the increased demand for people to work remotely and use online conferencing and shopping. These technological trends are likely to continue postpandemic and further consolidate corporate power.[32]

3.6 GLOBALIZED POLITICAL AND ECONOMIC ENVIRONMENT SANCTIONING CORPORATE ACTIVITIES

Global health and equity burdens from CDOH stem from the foundation and changing iterations of capitalism.[33]

3.6.1 Theorizing Corporate Power

Lima and Galea[34] apply a power lens to the operations of TNCs, using a radical theory of power developed by Lukes[35] for understanding the ways in which TNCs impose their power. They highlight the different dimensions of power, the vehicles by which it is exerted, and corporate practices of power. They argue that the distal outcome of exertion of TNC power is an imbalance in the macrosocial determinants of health that ultimately affects the incidence of risk factor for disease (see Chapter 22). The proximal impact is a decline in population health and increase in health equity.[34]

3.6.2 The History of Corporate Power

Large-scale extraction of goods and labor have been occurring for centuries, relying on colonized, subjugated, and enslaved labor driven by the profit motive across workshops and slave plantations.[36] There has been a long history of wealth extraction without fair payment to workers, contributions to social or economic infrastructure, or regard for resulting environmental problems.

Today, TNCs dominate many global supply chains. Through these chains, they play a similar role to the many free-trade merchants who formed alliances with those who deployed slave labor to produce the commodities (e.g., tobacco, cotton, and sugar cane) upon which the trading system of their era relied.

3.6.3 The Rise of Neoliberal Economic Theory and Expansion of Transnational Corporations

Subsequent changes to capitalism were reflected in the rise of neoliberal economic theory, which gained political prominence especially by the responses to the economic recessions of the 1970s and 1980s by U.S. President Ronald Reagan and UK Prime Minister Margaret Thatcher. Neoliberalism has subsequently been imposed globally through structural adjustment programs promoted by the International Monetary Fund (IMF), the World Bank, and the World Trade Organization, which have all promoted the growth of TNCs within a global neoliberal policy environment.[37] The operations of the World Bank and the IMF have been challenged in relation to issues of democratic governance, human rights, and the environment. Their bias toward fiscal consolidation, the private sector, and debt servicing restricts the space for public policy that fosters government finance of health, social, and physical infrastructure.[38] TNCs have expanded the reach of their products, practices, and thus health impacts through a process of globalization. The imposition of austerity measures on the public, while at the same time lowering corporate taxation rates and trade tariffs, has promoted private ahead of public interests and also increased inequities.[38] The expansion of TNCs in this global political and regulatory environment has been facilitated by corporate mergers and acquisitions, the promise of unlimited growth,[39] and a corporate identity with a narrow focus on profit maximization.

3.6.4 The Financialized Global Economy

The latest iteration of capitalism is a financialized global economy.[40] Corporate profits are increasingly accrued through financial channels rather than through more tangible commodity production and trade. Under financialized capitalism, policymakers have reduced taxes and sanctioned tax evasion for corporations and wealthy individuals.[41] At the micro-level, financialized capitalism affects daily experiences, or the "financialization of the everyday," with a shift toward financial markets providing even the most basic human needs.[41]

One of the crucial questions concerning the capitalist system is understanding the role of the world's largest country—China. Chinese governments have embraced features of capitalism, although its style is presented as state capitalism. There is no doubt that the economic development of China has reduced inequities between China and high-income countries. Understanding its mode of commercial determinants will be an essential task for future scholars. Most political economy analyses of China now agree that China is a developing form of state-centric capitalism.[42] Chinese policies of slowly recognizing private enterprise and property rights have involved both entrepreneurialism and the crucial role of the state[42]; this is but one more model of capitalism that will affect the health of populations in the future, but it is not covered in this chapter.

3.7 CHALLENGING CORPORATE POWER

Challenging corporate power to support health and health equity involves multiple strategies. TNCs have both global and local reach, and it is necessary to think globally in response.[43] A range of governance tools may be drawn upon, including national and international regulation of market activities, using effective binding instruments and voluntary codes.

The power of civil society is the "capacity to organize to affect positive change."[44] Civil society organizations have developed a range of actions that act as potentially strong vehicles for mitigating the adverse health impacts of TNCs.[19] Strategies include shareholder activism, threatening reputational damage, product boycotts, public protest or awareness-raising activities, the disruption of company operations, lobbying governments to restrict TNC activities and/or impose appropriate penalties, or taking legal action.[45,46] Such "grassroots" activism has expanded globally, triggered by a range of factors, including new norms regarding social justice and human rights, greater openness to political activity,[47] and growing employee demands for ethical corporate practices. The People's Health Movement (PHM) cited commercial determinants in its People's Health Charter (formulated in 2000)[48] without using the term when it drew clear links between TNCs and the global political economy:

> The world's resources are increasingly concentrated in the hands of a few who strive to maximize their private profit. Neoliberal political and economic policies are made by a small group of powerful governments, and by international institutions such as the World Bank, the International Monetary Fund and the World Trade Organisation. These policies, together with the unregulated activities of transnational corporations, have had severe effects on the lives and livelihoods, health and well-being of people in both North and South.[49]

The movement's foresight in naming the problem has meant that the PHM has been at the forefront of public health interest in advocating for action on the CDOH.

3.8 CONCLUSION

This chapter has highlighted the growing evidence on the health and health equity impacts of CDOH. Future research needs to expand beyond a focus on corporate marketing and sale of unhealthy products to consider a range of direct and more distal effects of private sector activities on public health, considering industry sectors as well as individual TNCs. Commercial enterprise has many social and economic benefits, and health impacts of CDOH are not necessarily negative. However, the current global environment affected by CDOH presents major risks for public health in a range of areas, including climate change, socioeconomic inequities, health behaviors, and risks of NCDs. Other research considerations are the roles of state-controlled corporate entities under rising global powers such as China, with its unique form of capitalism, that need to be considered with respect to health and health equity.

REFERENCES

1. Kickbusch I, Allen L, Franz C. The commercial determinants of health. *Lancet Global Health*. 2016; 4(12): e895–e896.
2. Commission on the Social Determinants of Health. *Closing the Gap in a Generation: Health Equity Through Action on the Social Determinants of Health. Final Report of the Commission on Social Determinants of Health*. World Health Organization; 2008.
3. Baum F, Sanders D, Fisher M, et al. Assessing the health impact of transnational corporations: Its importance and a framework. *Global Health*. 2016; 12: 27.
4. Mialon M. An overview of the commercial determinants of health. *Global Health*. 2020; 16(1): 74.

5. Moodie R, Stuckler D, Monteiro C, et al. Profits and pandemics: Prevention of harmful effects of tobacco, alcohol, and ultra-processed food and drink industries. *Lancet*. 2013; 381(9867): 670–679.

6. Freudenberg N. *Lethal But Legal: Corporations, Consumption, and Protecting Public Health*. Oxford University Press; 2014.

7. Monteiro C, Cannon G. The impact of transnational "big food" companies on the South: A view from Brazil. *PLoS Med*. 2012; 9(7): 1–5.

8. Dew K. As pharmaceutical use continues to rise, side effects are becoming a costly health issue. *The Conversation*. February 21, 2019.

9. Karim F, Oyewande AA, Abdalla LF, Chaudhry Ehsanullah R, Khan S. Social media use and its connection to mental health: A systematic review. *Cureus*. 2020; 12(6): e8627.

10. Center for Countering Digital Hate. The disinformation dozen: Why platforms must act on twelve leading online anti-vaxxers. 2021. https://www.counterhate.com/disinformationdozen

11. Akram W, Kumar R. A study on positive and negative effects of social media on society. *Int J Comput Sci Eng*. 2017; 5(10): 347–354.

12. Adeola FO. *Hazardous Wastes, Industrial Disasters, and Environmental Health Risks*. Palgrave Macmillan; 2011.

13. Climate and COVID-19: Converging crises. *Lancet*. 2021; **397**(10269): 71.

14. Green F. Health effects of job insecurity. *IZA World of Labor*. 2020; 212.

15. Kim TJ, von dem Knesebeck O. Is an insecure job better for health than having no job at all? A systematic review of studies investigating the health-related risks of both job insecurity and unemployment. *BMC Public Health*. 2015; 15(1): 985.

16. Australian Council of Trade Unions. *Australia's Insecure Work Crisis: Fixing It for the Future*. Australian Council of Trade Unions; 2018.

17. Anaf J, Baum F, Fisher M, Harris E, Friel S. Assessing the health impact of transnational corporations: A case study on McDonald's Australia. *Global Health*. 2017; 13(1): 7.

18. International Consortium of Investigative Journalists. Australian mining companies digging a deadly footprint in Africa. 2015. Accessed August 20, 2018. https://www.icij.org/investigations/fatal-extraction/australian-mining-companies-digging-deadly-footprint-africa

19. Wiist W. The corporation: An overview of what it is, its tactics, and what public health can do. In: Wiist W, ed. *The Bottom Line or Public Health: Tactics Corporations Use to Influence Health and Health Policy, and What We Can Do to Counter Them*. Oxford University Press; 2010: 3–71.

20. West M. *Corporate lobbying a billion dollar business*. Michael West Media; 2017.

21. Center for Media and Democracy. Front groups. 2020. Accessed December 14, 2020. https://www.sourcewatch.org/index.php/Front_groups#:~:text=A%20front%20group%20is%20an,of%20the%20third%20party%20technique

22. Baker D, Lawrence M. Sweet power: The politics of sugar, sugary drinks and poor nutrition in Australia *The Conversation*. May 3, 2018.

23. Oreskes N, Conway E. *Merchants of Doubt: How a Handful of Scientists Obscured the Truth on Issues From Tobacco Smoke to Global Warming*. Bloomsbury; 2010.

24. Fabbri A, Lai A, Grundy Q, Bero LA. The influence of industry sponsorship on the research agenda: A scoping review. *Am J Public Health*. 2018; 108(11): e9–e16.

25. Michael West Media. *Revolving doors: Australia's fossil fuel networks*. Michael West Media; 2018.

26. Friel S. *Trade-related pathways to nutrition and health*. PowerPoint presentation. 2014.
27. Townsend R. When trade agreements threaten Australian sovereignty: Australia beware. *The Conversation*. November 15, 2013.
28. Friel S, Hattersley L, Townsend R. Trade policy and public health. *Annu Rev Public Health*. 2015; 36(1): 325–344.
29. Townsend B, Schram A. Trade and investment agreements as structural drivers for NCDs: The new public health frontier. *Austr N Z J Public Health*. 2020; 44(2): 92–94.
30. Citro B, Grover A, Lander F, Mankad M. Pharmaceutical companies and global lack of access to medicines: Strengthening accountability under the right to health. *J Law Med Ethics*. 2012; 40(2): 234–251.
31. Henn M. *Tax Havens and the Taxation of Transnational Corporations*. Friedrich Ebert Stiftung; 2013.
32. Collin J, Ralston R, Hill S, Westerman L. *Signalling Virtue, Promoting Harm: Unhealthy Commodity Industries and COVID-19*. Spectrum and NCD Alliance; 2020.
33. Jones A, Lacy-Nichols J, Baker P, et al. Disrupting the commercial determinants of health. *Med J Austr*. 2021; 274.
34. Lima J, Galea S. Corporate practices and health: A framework and mechanisms. *Global Health*. 2018; 14: 21.
35. Lukes S. *Power: A Radical View*. 2nd ed. Palgrave Macmillan; 2005.
36. Higginbottom A. Enslaved African labour: Violent racial capitalism. In: Ness I, Cope Z, eds. *The Palgrave Encyclopedia of Imperialism and Anti-Imperialism*. Cham, Switzerland: Springer; 2019: 1–16.
37. Labonté R. Globalization and health. *International Encyclopedia of the Social & Behavioral Sciences* 2015: 198–205.
38. Bretton Woods Project. *What are the main criticisms of the World Bank and the IMF?* 2019.
39. Korten D. *When Corporations Rule the World*. Earthscan; 1995.
40. Freudenberg N. *At What Cost? Modern Capitalism and the Future of Health*. Oxford University Press; 2021.
41. Sell SK. 21st-century capitalism: Structural challenges for universal health care. 2019. https://pubmed.ncbi.nlm.nih.gov/31775788
42. McNally CA. Theorizing Sino-capitalism: Implications for the study of comparative capitalisms. *Contemp Politics*. 2019; 25(3): 313–333.
43. Baum F. *The New Public Health*. 4th ed. Oxford University Press; 2015.
44. Turner J. Explaining the nature of power: A three process theory. *Eur J Social Psychol*. 2005; 35(1): 1–22.
45. Reed D. Resource extraction industries in developing countries. *J Business Ethics*. 2002; 39(3): 199–226.
46. Baazil D, Miller H, Hurst L. Shell loses climate case that may set precedent for Big Oil. *Financial Review*. May 27, 2021.
47. Green G. *Citizen activism and Civil Society: How Change Happens*. Oxford University Press; 2016.
48. People's Health Movement. *People's charter for health*. Cape Town, South Africa: People's Health Movement; n.d.
49. Third World Network. People's charter for health. 2021. Accessed October 18, 2021. https://www.twn.my/title/charter.htm

SECTION 2

*How Do Commercial Determinants
Shape Upstream Drivers of Health?*

CHAPTER 4

The Role of Policy in Studying the Commercial Determinants of Health

BENJAMIN HAWKINS

4.1 INTRODUCTION

In his seminal article, Baron[1] differentiated between "market" and "non-market" strategies as key components of an integrated corporate strategy. While the former refers to the aspects of business behavior that we perhaps most intuitively place under the rubric of strategy—including marketing and promotional and product pricing—the latter refers to the various other activities entered into by companies to ensure an amenable commercial environment conducive to profit. This includes what we can term corporate political activity, namely attempts to shape policy and policymaking processes.[1,2] Baron's contribution was to highlight the importance of non-market strategies, placing them on an equal footing with market strategies in his conceptualization of corporate activity and the determinants of success. In so doing, he more accurately reflects the importance of regulatory environments—and the resources dedicated by individual businesses and their collective bodies to influencing them—than much of the literature on the commercial determinants of health (CDOH) would suggest. These insights highlight the importance of public policy, and corporate engagement in policy processes, as a key determinant of health outcomes and an important object of study. This in turn requires engagement with theories and concepts from the field of policy studies in order to fully appreciate the ways in which corporate political actors shape policy regimes and, thereby, health outcomes. This chapter begins

Benjamin Hawkins, *The Role of Policy in Studying the Commercial Determinants of Health* In: *The Commercial Determinants of Health*. Edited by: Nason Maani, Mark Petticrew, and Sandro Galea, Oxford University Press.
© Oxford University Press 2023. DOI: 10.1093/oso/9780197578742.003.0004

by introducing the field of policy studies and examining the main approaches to studying the policy process. This includes placing national policy debates in their international context via theories of multilevel governance. It then examines how these theories and approaches have been applied to the study of CDOH through the example of alcohol and tobacco regulation and the activities of these health-harming industries to shape policy regime at the national and supranational levels.

4.2 STUDYING PUBLIC POLICY

Public policy is the term used to refer to the range of policies put in place by governments to regulate affairs within their territorial space, including health policy and other social policies (e.g., welfare) of relevance to health outcomes. Public policy also includes the range of measures designed to regulate potentially health-harming activities of private sector actors such as the production, sale, and marketing of tobacco, alcohol, and unhealthy processed food and drink, as well as environmental degradation and wider structural determinants of population health. Perhaps the most important and remarkable observation about the policy studies literature, with regard to CDOH, is just how little attention the political interventions of the business sector has received by political scientists in relation to other actors and issues.[3] This omission appears even more anomalous when we consider the degree of focus placed on business activities in related fields such as microeconomics or management science, their enormous economic importance, and the wider veneration of businesses and business leaders within capitalist societies. It is in the area of health policy, and the study of health-harming industries, where the political influence of the business sector has received perhaps the most scholarly attention, albeit often from a public health perspective, as opposed to a policy studies or political science perspective.[4] More recently, this literature has been supplemented by the increasing engagement of political scientists and health policy scholars with the issue of corporate political activity and the deployment of policy theory to add greater analytical depth and nuance to public health accounts of CDOH.[5-8]

Theories of the policy process seek to identify the conditions under which policy change does and does not occur. This involves a focus on the institutional context in which policies are made, the key decision-makers and other actors involved in that process, as well as the policy advocates that seek to influence it. Policymaking has been conceptualized and studied from a range of different perspectives, which reflect the broader range of approaches within the social sciences. These include differences between those who emphasize either structure or agency. Institutionalist scholars understand politics to be explainable mainly in terms of contextual or structural factors, highlighting the formal laws and rules, as well as informal norms that set the "rules of the game" and limit what can and cannot be done within a policy setting. In contrast, rational choice theorists take an actor-centered approach, viewing policy development as the result of policy actors seeking to change the course of events, while others seek to oppose this and defend the status quo. In reality, policymaking is a complex interplay of both structure and agency in which policy actors are both constrained by and at the same time reinforce and/or reshape and reinterpret, the policy setting in which they are embedded.

Other scholars have focused instead on the *process* of policy, identifying a series of "stages" through which policy debates may pass.[9] This begins with an *agenda-setting phase* in which a particular social issue, practice, or outcome becomes defined as a "policy problem," an issue that is the legitimate object of government intervention or for which governmental response is necessary and required. In the agenda-setting phase, policy advocates will seek to define the issue with which they are engaged as a policy problem and seek to gain sufficient political traction among key policy actors for it to enter onto the relevant government's policy program. Following the agenda-setting phase, policy processes involve a *policy development* stage, in which solutions to an identified policy problems are identified; an *enactment and legitimation* stage, in which relevant laws and other regulatory measures to address the policy problem are put in place and endorsed by relevant bodies, such as national parliaments; an *implementation phase*, in which the policy measure is brought into effect; and an *evaluation phase*, in which its effects are measured. Although the stages model has been criticized as offering an overly simplistic account of the highly complex policymaking process,[10] it nevertheless offers a useful heuristic device or ideal type through which to analyze policy debates.

John Kingdon conceptualized the potential for policy change through his multiple streams framework, focusing on what he termed the *problem*, *policy*, and *politics* streams of the policy process.[11] Only where these three streams converge—that is, in terms of problem definition, available solutions, and political will to implement these—is policy change possible (see Chapter 5). Kingdon places a strong emphasis on the role of what he terms "policy entrepreneurs" in opening these "policy windows."

The advocacy coalition framework (ACF) focuses on the role of policy advocates in arguing for a particular policy change or agenda.[10] The ACF seeks to identify relevant groups of policy actors committed to a particular issue or solution to a policy problem within a policy subsystem. These groups coalesce around a set of "deep core," "policy core," and "secondary" beliefs that they share. Other frameworks used to examine policymaking in the field of health include the "3Is" model, in which policy change is explained in terms of the key *ideas* in circulation and *interests* at play within the particular *institutional* context in which policy decisions are taken. In the arena of global health, Walt and Gilson's "policy triangle" places policy actors at the center of their concep-tualization of the policymaking terms of *content*, *context*, and *process*.[12]

Whereas the approaches outlined above seek to identify consistencies and generalizations, the field of interpretative policy analysis (IPA) eschews the idea of there being universal laws of the policy process that pertain over time and space. Drawing on critical and post-structuralist theories, IPA scholars argue that each empirical case must be analyzed in its own terms, and expla-nations for policy change (or the absence of change) must be sought in the specificities of the particular case at hand.[13]

A key focus of many analyses in the field of IPA is the use of language and the generation of meaning in policymaking contexts. In other words, how do key policy actors make sense of the issues with which they are engaged, the aims of policy, and the right or capacity of governments to intervene effec-tively in citizens' lives? Others have identified the ways in which policy actors seek to frame policy debates and the key terms and issues within these in ways amenable with their underlying interests and objectives. The ability to shape policy debates in this way is a powerful means of influencing outcomes, including in the area of health.[14] For example, a systematic review of the cor-porate political strategies of the global alcohol industry identified framing strategies, along with policy influencing and lobbying strategies, as a key com-ponent of the overall influencing activities.[15] Consequently, framing analyses and discourse analyses are a critical part of the methodological toolkit to be employed by policy scholars seeking to understand CDOH.

4.3 MINIMUM ALCOHOL PRICING IN THE UNITED KINGDOM

Developments in UK alcohol policy in the past decade offer a valuable case study for understanding the ways in which different approaches to the policy process can be applied to studying different aspects of an extended policy process. Since the late 1990s, the United Kingdom has had a devolved polit-ical structure in which certain areas of public policy are set independently in England, Scotland, Wales, and Northern Ireland. Within this system, health policy is devolved to individual nations, whereas taxation policy is decided centrally for the entire United Kingdom in London. In 2008, the Scottish government announced its intention to introduce a minimum unit price for alcohol (MUP) sold in Scotland. This created a floor price for each standard measure of alcohol (or "unit") with the aim of reducing population-level con-sumption. The measure was designed to address significant health inequalities both within its borders (e.g., between the East End of Glasgow and its wealthy satellite towns) and between Scotland and other parts of the United Kingdom. The minority Scottish National Party (SNP) administration's attempt to pass legislation for this failed in 2010, but following the 2011 election in which the SNP gained an overall majority in the Scottish Parliament, the legislation eventually passed in 2012. This was immediately challenged by the alcohol industry under the auspices of the Scotch Whisky Association (SWA). Although the case, heard in the Scottish, UK, and European level courts, failed to block MUP coming into force, it managed to delay the implementation of MUP by 6 years.

The alcohol policy process in the United Kingdom and the attempts by industry actors to oppose the introduction of MUP have been studied in detail by political scientists.[16] This included analysis of the ways in which health policy advocates and industry actors sought to frame the policy debate in the agenda-setting and policy development phases, in ways that facilitated and opposed the shift toward "whole population" measures such as MUP.[17] It also identified the importance of an emerging advocacy coalition between different alcohol, health, and other policy actors able to coalesce around a core policy objective of MUP as a mechanism for delivering multiple health and other public policy objectives, within a specific policy subsystem. Analysis of the first attempt to pass MUP into law in 2010 examined the various points of access in the policy process and the policymaking architecture,[18] and it emphasized the importance of a distinct "policy style" and political culture in post-devolution Scotland.[19] Following the passage of MUP into law in Scotland in 2012, Kingdon's policy stream model was used to explain how a policy window opened up for this policy transfer to occur to other parts of the United Kingdom and why it closed up again so quickly. The introduction of MUP in Scotland broke the previous UK-wide alcohol policy consensus and created momentum for the introduction of similar measures in England, as well as offered a clear precedent that alcohol policy advocates in England could cite. Following pressure from back bench MPs in his own Conservative Party, and faced with other short-term political pressures, Prime Minister David Cameron was convinced to adopt MUP as government policy in England via the UK Government's 2012 alcohol strategy. However, plans to implement the measures were abandoned in July 2013 following industry opposition.[6]

The agenda-setting, policy development, and enactment phases are the focus of much scholarship in the field of policy studies because these offer researchers empirical developments and "tangible" events that are amenable to research. However, the example of MUP demonstrates that this emphasis underplays the importance of the implementation and evaluation stages of the process. The importance of implementation, and the opportunities this affords corporate political actors to at least delay unfavored policies, is obvious in the case of MUP and the legal challenge mounted by the SWA.[7] The application of a stages heuristic to the case of UK alcohol policy also highlights the interconnections that exist between the different stages of the policy process.[8] This was evident in policymakers' and advocates' views that the prospect of legal challenge had cast a shadow over the whole policy process. The mere possibility of judicial review, which had been articulated to Scottish ministers by industry actors at the very earliest stage of the policy process, shaped the approach taken by the Scottish government to the legislation and the design of the policy. This led to the inclusion of robust evaluation processes for the policy and a "sunset clause" in the legislation, which means the Scottish Parliament must act to renew the policy 5 years after its implementation. Both these elements offer industry actors new opportunities to influence the perception and continuation of the policy and create a clear additional "veto point" at which it can be challenged and potentially repealed.

4.4 THE INTERNATIONAL DIMENSION

Recent innovations in the study of corporate activity have focused on the international component of public policy debates and the extent to which public policy at the national level is shaped and constrained by regional and global governance arrangements. Political scientists conceptualize the relationship between the subnational, national, and supra-national levels of decision-making via the concept of multilevel governance (MLG). This identifies the ways in which relevant policy decisions are made at differ levels of abstraction but that these have implications for policymaking elsewhere and at other levels. MLG has been a particularly important theoretical innovation in the context of the European Union (EU) given the existence of a highly developed supranational policy-making and enforcement competences within established supranational institutions, including European Commissions, the European Parliament, and the Court of Justice of the European Union.

In the case of MUP, the concepts of MLG and policy "spillover" are crucial to understanding alcohol pricing policy in the United Kingdom. They allow us to examine how MUP came on to the agenda first in Scotland via policy entrepreneurship facilitated by devolution and how it subsequently spread to different areas of the United Kingdom.[6] In addition, the legal challenge to MUP highlights the relevance that laws made at different levels have for those elsewhere. The decision to adopt MUP (as opposed to other pricing measures) reflects the powers available to the Scottish government and those retained by Westminster.[8] Moreover, it demonstrates the need for Scottish law to comply with those at the UK and European levels, and potentially also the global trade regime and the ability to sue decision-making venues (i.e., courts) at other levels to challenge policies in Scotland. Finally, MLG helps us to understand cooperation between policymakers and advocates at the Scottish, UK, and European levels to support the policy while industry actors were able to draw on similar alliances to oppose the policy during the legal hearings at all these levels.[7]

Drawing on theories and concepts from international law and political science, Hawkins and Holden[5] have argued that the international sphere is characterized by an increasing tendency toward constitutionalized forms of governance, in which the interactions between states and between private actors (including corporations) are governed and shaped by quasi-constitutional legal orders and dispute resolution procedures. This is evident in the World Trade Organization's dispute resolution mechanisms as well as investor–state dispute resolution mechanisms (see Chapter 9). In addition, these agreements often contain regulatory cooperation chapters whereby new laws introduced by national governments, which have potential implications for the functions of an agreement or their commitments under this, must be notified to other parties to offer them the chance to raised objections. This creates the potential for large corporations to feed directly into domestic policy processes. As such, each trade agreement entered into by a government creates potential "veto points."[20,21]

This is particularly important with regard to noncommunicable disease policies given the evidence base in support of measures to restrict the sale, marketing, and consumptions of products (e.g., tobacco, alcohol, and processed food/drinks) identified as key drivers of these diseases and to curtail the activities of the associated producer industries.[22] Policies that impose price increases and restrictions on product packaging could potentially infringe investor rights and protections against the expropriation of intellectual property contained in International trade and investment agreements (TAIs) and leave governments open to legal challenges. These issues came to the fore in two such cases initiated by cigarette producer Philip Morris International against the governments of Uruguay and Australia to oppose enhanced warning and packaging requirements for cigarettes in each domain.[23] In Australia, this included the introduction of "standardized packaging" (SP), in which all color branding and logos are removed from the packs, which must be a uniform color across brands.[23,24]

The concept of MLG and its relevance for health policy was evident in the agreement of the EU's 2014 Tobacco Products Directive (TPD) and parallel developments in tobacco control policy with EU member states.[25] Initial proposals for the TPD included a commitment to introduce SP for all cigarette sales throughout the EU. After strong industry opposition, these proposals were dropped in favor of enlarged graphic health warnings on all tobacco products. However, the directive included an explicit recognition that these measures represented a minimum requirement and that member states had the right, within the confines of EU law, to go beyond this to introduce SP at the national level. The governments of Ireland and the United Kingdom (which was an EU member state at the time) proceeded to develop domestic SP laws in parallel with the TPD. These were challenged, unsuccessfully, by tobacco industry actors in court on the basis that they infringed key aspects of single market law. Thus, although the TPD fell short of introducing SP, it created both a political impetus for member states to pursue this and legal protection for those that did within a core piece of single-market legislation.[24]

4.5 CONCLUSION

This chapter has examined the ways in which the discipline of policy studies, and the key concepts and theoretical perspectives in that domain, can be applied to the study of the CDOH. It focused principally on health-harming industries and drew on examples of corporate actors research from the fields of alcohol and tobacco control in the United Kingdom, at the European level, and internationally. Although the empirical focus of the chapter is quite specific, it is relevant to other aspects of the broader corporate determinants agenda. The insights here can be applied to other industries and decision-making context, including those discussed elsewhere in this volume. As previous studies have suggested, the strategies identified in relation to the global tobacco and alcohol industries are similar to those employed by other industries, and thus provides stimulus to conduct similar research in other policy areas.[26] Furthermore, the concepts and theories introduced here have been underutilized by researchers in public health and can usefully be applied to other industries and policy context to move the research agenda beyond description of industry-related harms to more in-depth understandings of the nature of commercial power in these contexts.

REFERENCES

1. Baron DP. Integrated strategy: Market and nonmarket components. *California Manage Rev.* 1995; 37(2): 47–65.
2. Eastmure E, Cummins S, Sparks L. Non-market strategy as a framework for exploring commercial involvement in health policy: A primer. *Social Sci Med.* 2020; 262: 113257. https://doi.org/10.1016/j.socscimed.2020.113257
3. Wilks S. *The Political Power of the Business Corporation.* Elgar; 2013.
4. McKee M, Stuckler D. Revisiting the corporate and commercial determinants of health. *Am J Public Health.* 2018; 108(9): 1167–1170.
5. Hawkins B, Holden C. A corporate veto on health policy? Global constitutionalism and investor-state dispute settlement. *J Health Polit Policy Law.* 2016; 41(5): 969–995.
6. Hawkins B, McCambridge J. Policy windows and multiple streams: An analysis of alcohol pricing policy in England. *Policy Polit.* 2020; 48(2): 315–333. https://doi.org/10.1332/030557319X15724461566370
7. Hawkins B, McCambridge J. UK alcohol policy, multi-level governance and corporate political strategy: The campaign for minimum unit pricing in Edinburgh,

London and Brussels. *Br J Polit Int Relat.* 2021; 23(3): 391–409. https://journals. sagepub.com/doi/pdf/10.1177/1369148120959040

8. Hawkins B, McCambridge J. "Tied up in a legal mess": The alcohol industry's use of litigation to oppose minimum alcohol pricing in Scotland. *Scottish Affairs.* 2020; 29(1): 3–23. https://www.euppublishing.com/doi/full/10.3366/scot.2020.0304

9. Pressman J, Wildavsky A. *Implementation.* University of California Press; 1973.

10. Sabatier PA, Jenkins-Smith HC. *Policy Change and Learning: An Advocacy Coalition Approach.* Westview; 1993.

11. Kingdon JW. *Agendas, Alternatives, and Public Policies.* Little, Brown; 1984.

12. Walt G, Gilson L. Reforming the health sector in developing countries: The central role of policy analysis. *Health Policy Planning.* 1994; 9(4): 353–370.

13. Yanow D. Interpretation in policy analysis: On methods and practice. *Critical Policy Analysis.* 2007; 1(1): 110–122.

14. Koon AD, Hawkins B, Mayhew SH. Framing and the health policy process: A scoping review. *Health Policy Planning.* 2016; 31(6): 801–816.

15. McCambridge J, Mialon M, Hawkins B. Alcohol industry involvement in policy-making: A systematic review. *Addiction.* 2018; 113(9): 1571–1584.

16. McCambridge J, Hawkins B, Holden C. The challenge corporate lobbying poses to reducing society's alcohol problems: Insights from UK evidence on minimum unit pricing. *Addiction.* 2014; 109(2): 199–205.

17. Hawkins B, Holden C. Framing the alcohol policy debate: Industry actors and the regulation of the UK beverage alcohol market. *Crit Policy Stud.* 2013; 7(1): 53–71.

18. Hawkins B, Holden C. "Water dripping on stone?" Industry lobbying and UK alcohol policy. *Policy Polit.* 2014; 41(1): 55–70.

19. Holden C, Hawkins B. "Whisky gloss": The alcohol industry, devolution and policy communities in Scotland. *Public Policy Admin.* 2013; 28(3): 253–273.

20. Immergut E. *Health Politics: Interests and Institutions in Western Europe.* Cambridge University Press; 1992.

21. Tsebelis G. *Veto Players: How Political Institutions Work.* Princeton University Press; 2002.

22. Jahiel RI, Babor TF. Industrial epidemics, public health advocacy and the alcohol industry: Lessons from other fields. *Addiction.* 2007; 102: 1335–1339.

23. Hawkins B, Holden C, MacKinder S. A multi-level, multi-jurisdictional strategy: Transnational tobacco companies' attempts to obstruct tobacco packaging restrictions. *Global Public Health.* 2019; 14(4): 570–583. https://doi.org/10.1080/17441692.2018.1446997

24. Hawkins B, Holden C, MacKinder S. *The Battle for Standardised Cigarette Packaging in Europe.* Palgrave; 2020.

25. Holden C, Hawkins B. Law, market building and public health in the European Union. *Global Social Policy.* 2017; 18(10): 45–61.

26. Kenworthy N, MacKenzie R, Lee K, eds. *Case Studies on Corporations and Global Health Governance: Impacts, Influence and Accountability.* Rowman & Littlefield; 2016.

CHAPTER 5

Understanding the Politics of the Commercial Determinants of Health

EDUARDO J. GÓMEZ

5.1 INTRODUCTION

Understanding the politics of the commercial determinants of health is a new area of scholarly inquiry. More than ever, policymakers and public health researchers realize that industries, including the tobacco, alcohol, soda, and ultra-processed food corporations, have had a considerable amount of political power and health policy influence, facilitated through favorable international and domestic economic contexts.[1-3] In recent years, this realization has contributed to a new area of business and public health research, namely the corporate political activity (CPA) literature. The CPA literature discusses the multitude of corporate industries, from tobacco to pharmaceuticals and even the information technology sector, that have inserted themselves into the politics of the policymaking process through several political and social tactics.[4-6]

The linkage between the discipline of political science and the commercial determinants of health is, for the most part, an uncharted area of scholarly research. Although a host of public health and nutrition scientists have addressed the political involvement of major commercial food industries, their political tactics and policy influence,[7-10] research to date has fallen short of exploring the utility of political science theories and empirical approaches to explaining industry's broader political, social, and policymaking influence.

While political science's contributions to the commercial determinants of health is new and growing,[11,12] the discipline's research on industry and interest group behaviors can provide complementary approaches to further explaining the processes through which industries influence politics

Eduardo J. Gómez, *Understanding the Politics of the Commercial Determinants of Health* In: *The Commercial Determinants of Health*. Edited by: Nason Maani, Mark Petticrew, and Sandro Galea, Oxford University Press.
© Oxford University Press 2023. DOI: 10.1093/oso/9780197578742.003.0005

and policy. Given the author's pre-existing research program on the politics of noncommunicable diseases and malnutrition in developing nations, this chapter restricts its focus to the soda and ultra-processed food industry and its influence on these public health policy issues.

This chapter examines two areas of the politics of the commercial determinants of health: industry interference within and below government.[1] *Within* government, it is argued that political science's approach to industry and/or representative interest group political interference can provide alternative, more in-depth insights into how these industries influence congressional representatives' and policymakers' preferences and policy decisions. For example, the causal mechanisms introduced by political scientists can provide further insight into the clandestine versus loud and obstructive strategies used by industries to achieve these outcomes. Alternatively, political scientists may also reveal the role of formal institutions and democratic political party preferences in limiting industry policy interference. From *below*, political science research reveals how industries often mobilize community preferences in ways that can potentially incentivize national politicians to refrain from pursuing legislation threatening, for example, the food industry's policy preferences.

5.2 WITHIN GOVERNMENT

The political scientist Pepper Culpepper[13] made the important distinction between the quiet versus the loud politics of interest group activities and policy influence. According to Culpepper, quiet politics occurs under two conditions: when the policy issue is highly technical in nature and does not garner sufficient public attention (and thus low political saliency) and when government officials turn to industry for their technical expertise and guidance. Under these conditions, business groups have an opportunity to meet—often covertly, behind closed doors—with policymakers to influence their decisions.[13]

In the field of international relations, the epistemic community literature explains similar processes. In times of crisis and uncertainty, government officials often turn to international scientific experts, often fused together through similar ideological beliefs and interests, for information and policy guidance.[14] These epistemic community experts often meet with policymakers, taking advantage of the former's technical knowledge to influence public policy in their favor.[14] In Latin America, these epistemic community members have played an important role in influencing the creation of NCD policy.[15]

Alternatively, political scientists have emphasized the loud politics of lobbying behavior and the agenda-setting process. As Binderkrantz et al.[16] explain, in addition to other strategies for gaining access to different kinds of political arenas (e.g., the parliament and the bureaucracy), industries often use the media and/or nongovernmental organizations (NGOs) to voice their criticisms of proposed legislation in order to influence the agenda-setting process. West et al.[17] also show how organized private sector interests have used the media to question proposed health care legislation in the United States, in turn generating public doubt and concern about proposed health care initiatives. In this scenario, organized interest groups achieve two objectives through the use of media advertising: They alter public opinion and convince congressional representatives that there is broad-based opposition to proposed health care legislation.[17] Such was the case, West et al. contend, with the Pharmaceutical Research and Manufacturers of America and the Health Insurance Association of America's use of these loud media tactics during the William J. Clinton presidential administration and its efforts to propose an expansion of government-sponsored health care benefits. Aside from using the media to mobilize citizen and congressional opposition, Keller[18] has also alluded to the "noisy" political strategies used by interest groups; this occurs when organized interests use the media and other forms of communication to increase the political saliency of a particular issue by using frames to underscore the harm and broader consequences of reforms that went against business interests, thus in turn directly pressuring government not to pursue legislation that business deems harmful.[18]

Political scientists' insights into industry political and policy manipulation within government through the aforementioned quiet and loud lobbying tactics can provide additional insights into the study of the politics of the commercial determinants of health, especially in developing nations. For example, in countries that are seeking to introduce and/or strengthen regulatory policies, such as marketing unhealthy food products to vulnerable individuals (e.g., children and the poor), as seen in Brazil, India, and China, Culpepper's[13] approach can explain why industries continue to be so influential in undermining existing efforts and/or hampering the introduction of new ones. Indeed, it appears that marketing regulations often receive far less media coverage, and thus lower political saliency, than a controversial soda tax, due in large part to the substantially higher media attention surrounding vehement industry opposition to taxes based on their exorbitant economic costs. Industries may display less open opposition to marketing regulations due to the known complexity of enforcing such policies and the immediate economic costs involved. When these marketing regulations are less visible to the public (as opposed to a soda tax), future research may find that industry and their supportive non-state actors may have a greater opportunity and incentive to meet quietly with policymakers and strategically use the former's technical knowledge to convince the latter of the limitations to these marketing tactics. Alternatively, if industries are not in favor of stern marketing regulations, they may seek to shift the policy discussion elsewhere—for example, emphasizing the importance of advocating for physical activity in response to obesity, as seen in China.[19] To better understand the political context facilitating industry's policy influence, Culpepper's[13] approach therefore suggests that we focus on policies that are less visible and less salient to the public and, thus, also less salient to politicians, and where industry's technical expertise can be most influential—for example, marketing and sales regulation. Another fruitful area of future research is to compare these more technical policy issues with the politics of more widely controversial public health measures, such as the imposition of soda taxes; to the author's knowledge, these kinds of intersectoral comparisons have yet to be addressed from a political science perspective.

Furthermore, because researchers are examining the soda and ultra-processed food industry's use of loud lobbying strategies through usage of the media to communicate their ideas and interests,[20] West et al.'s[17] research may suggest that public health and nutrition experts should delve further into the causal mechanisms linking industry's targeting of the media and the timing of these media strategies with their impact on the public and congresses' preferences and interests. For instance, public health and nutrition policy researchers may wish to combine in-depth case study analysis, obtained through qualitative interviews with congressional members, with surveys of the general public's mood following industry's reported criticisms of proposed legislation in the media. This approach can provide further compelling evidence that industry's loud political tactics are having a direct impact on politicians' views and policy preferences.

However, it is not the effort and activities of soda and ultra-processed food industries and their supportive interest groups that always influence politicians' interests and policy views. Institutions also matter. Institutions, along with the design of congressional committees and the rules for engaging the bureaucracy and congress, in many instances serve as interest group gatekeepers. They determine if, when, and to what extent interest groups influence politicians' policy ideas and the prioritization of policy. For instance, some political scientists, such as Heitshusen,[21] maintain that the decentralization of authority to U.S. congressional subcommittees and the resulting expansion of interests and conflict over particular policies within them often force lobbying groups to engage in different types of information sharing and lobbying strategies. Heitshusen further claims that when interest groups, such as environmental lobbyists, face several supportive congressional subcommittee members, they are only required to provide limited political information to influence decisions; conversely, when facing stern opposition, as seen with labor unions, they are required to provide more technical information in order to persuade congressional members.[21] Thus, it is institutional change—that is, the decentralization and fragmentation of authority to congressional subcommittees, the fragmentation of congressional representative interests, and their degree of support for proposed policies—that determines the types of information-based strategies that interest groups pursue. This differentiates industries based on their financial and technical ability to mobilize and influence congressional policy views. Furthermore, one could also envision wealthier industries having an easier time funding the provision of additional information should congressional subcommittees oppose their policy views, compared with smaller advocacy organizations that may not have such resources and that would alternatively benefit from a more centralized committee decision-making process. Some political scientists nevertheless caution that access to institutions does not automatically translate to interest group policy influence and that it is often difficult to provide concrete evidence establishing this connection.[22]

Public health researchers would benefit from the application of this institutional theoretical approach for several reasons. First, to explain the soda and ultra-processed food industries' ongoing access and influence within congressional committees and the bureaucracy, researchers could examine the degree of decentralization and committee fragmentation present and the amount of representative support for industry within them; this can shed further light on the *institutional context* most propitious for industry's political and policy influence. If, for example, a congressional or specialized bureaucratic committee agrees with the food industry's views on the importance of particular public policy approaches to obesity reduction (e.g., physical activity), the food industry may not need to invest significant resources into persuading bureaucratic members; this offers compelling reasons for why industries may have considerable policy influence within particular institutions. As an example, in Mexico, one could investigate how congressional committees, bureaucratic agencies, or even ancillary consultative groups such as the OMENT (Observatorio Mexicano de Enfermedades no Transmisibles [Mexican Observatory on Noncommunicable Diseases]) were designed, the degree of government support for industry preferences within it, and therefore the leeway that major industries have to lobby and influence policy. Political scientists have noted that OMENT has had a consistent overrepresentation of major industry interests and influence over the design of proposed obesity legislation.[23] Nevertheless, further research is needed to examine more in-depth the decentralization of congressional and bureaucratic committees and the extent to which representation within them favors industry's interests over others.

Yet another context for challenging industry's ability to influence the policymaking process is when presidential leaders and political parties have strong policy preferences. In this situation, it is not the design of institutions but, rather, ardent presidential and/or political party preferences that create a constraining political context for industries to operate in, thus revealing how democracies can limit industry's policy influence.[24] As Paster[24] claims, when dominant political parties prefer a particular approach to health care policy, as seen in Germany, business groups are forced to either accept and adapt to political party preferences or engage in direct confrontation with them. At times, interest group strategies may shift from confrontation to adaptation and compromise based on the type of political party challenges and policy prospects interest groups confront.[24] Alternatively, history has shown that U.S. presidential interests, their personal experiences, and their passion for reform can also limit interest groups' ability to influence presidential interests in favor of health care legislation.[25] Prior to his passing, for example, Franklin Delano Roosevelt's (FDR) shifting views in support of national health care legislation overcame the American Medical Association's vehement opposition.[25] Unfortunately, FDR passed away approximately 2 weeks before his proposed legislation was to be considered in Congress. At the time, FDR held the majority in the House and Senate. In a very real sense, the United States was a heartbeat away from establishing universal health care.

5.3 FROM BELOW

Political scientists and political sociologists have also investigated major food industries' efforts to manipulate the views and interests of voters, which in turn can have an impact on the preferences of subnational and national politicians. As Walker and Rea[26] note, through a corporate mobilization process, industries have often hired professional grassroots firms to mobilize community members and to help transform society into policy allies. Moreover, Walker and Rea claim that this process can lead to the creation of "pro-corporate social movement organizations (such as Working Families for Walmart)" campaigns. By potentially influencing local community preferences through these corporate mobilization tactics, this process may in turn motivate local and national politicians to follow these community preferences and eventually vote in favor of policies that align with industry's preferences. Similarly, in the past, major tobacco industries have worked closely with the African American community and community-based organizations, such as the National Association for the Advancement of Colored People.[27] Major tobacco industries often sponsored civil rights activities to build their image and secure a market within this community.[27] In addition, major corporations, such as Philip Morris, have in the past shared with several African American newspapers an op-ed from a key leader within an influential community organization, James Hargrove, Chair of the National Black Police Association, claiming that any proposed taxes on cigarettes would be unfair for minorities.[27]

This kind of analytical approach can lead to new insights into how soda and ultra-processed food industries contract grassroots activist firms to influence the community and thus state and national political preferences. To what extent, for example, are major soda and ultra-processed food industries working through local consulting firms, NGOs, or even academic researchers to achieve these outcomes? Recent research in China and Brazil has revealed the role of the International Life Sciences Institute in infiltrating bureaucratic agencies.[11,19,28] Future work should investigate how similar contracted non-state actors are mobilizing society and shifting community and politicians' preferences in alignment with industries.

Engaging in corporate social responsibility (CSR) tactics is yet another strategy that soda and ultra-processed food industries use to persuade national politicians' policy preferences and decision-making. CSR activities emerge when industries invest in local communities through a variety of social activities, ranging from the provision of health care services to education, or when they engage in self-regulatory practices. In the area of nutrition, these voluntary CSR practices include industries deciding to restrict the marketing and sale of industry products to at-risk groups such as children. Political scientist David Vogel[12] explains how this kind of CSR tactic is used by industries to avoid ongoing criticisms from activists, potentially tarnishing an industry's reputation, with these self-regulatory tactics often being part of industry's focus, in turn providing long-term benefits. Vogel further claims that these self-regulatory practices are often used to avoid government efforts to impose stricter industry regulations. Political scientists have also argued that these CSR activities often embolden industries' efforts to influence the politics of the policymaking process because CSR activities help increase industry's political reputation.[29]

In developing nations, political scientists' focus on the usage of CSR activities to enhance industries' social and thus political legitimacy and influence can provide additional insights into the politics of the commercial determinants of health. Gómez[11] has discussed how several major soda and ultra-processed food industries have strategically invested in the provision of health, education, nutrition, and water sustainability policies in several developing nations. Gómez argues that this in part has been done to help muster community support (often among the poor) and, in the process, increase national politicians' recognition and support for these industries' contributions to society. Similar to Vogel's[12] claims, these types of CSR activities have often motivated government officials to refrain from pursuing stringent regulatory policies.

5.4 CONCLUSION

As we delve deeper and investigate the population health consequences of the commercial determinants of health, understanding and thoroughly explaining the politics of these determinants will become increasingly important. The time is ripe to explore what the scholarly community defines as the *politics of the commercial determinants of health*. This chapter argues that the existing commercial determinants and CPA literature has yet to squarely address this issue and to adequately explore what the discipline of political science has to offer in deepening our understanding of the ways in which industries contort health politics and policy in their favor. This chapter also argues that several prevailing theories and empirical approaches in political science can generate new scholarly issues, questions, and approaches to understanding this process, both from *within* and *below* government, shaping citizens' and politicians' preferences, influencing democratic processes. Going forward, public health and nutritional scientists will inevitably stand to benefit from working with political scientists to explore how the latter's approaches can lead to a more in-depth discussion of the political contexts and causal mechanisms structuring the politics of the commercial determinants of health. For political scientists concerned about these determinants, the focus should be on establishing new research programs and analytical frameworks that build upon the discipline's rich history in democratic pluralism, interest group behavior, and complex business politics.

REFERENCES

1. Madureira Lima J, Galea S. Corporate practices and health: A framework and mechanisms. *Global Health*. 2018; 14(1): 21.
2. Martino FP, Miller PG, Coomber K, Hancock L, Kypri K. Analysis of alcohol industry submissions against marketing regulation. *PLoS One*. 2017; 12(1): e0170366.
3. Kickbusch I, Allen L, Franz C. The commercial determinants of health. *Lancet Glob Health*. 2016; 4(12): e895–e896.
4. Lawton T, McGuire S, Rajwani T. Corporate political activity: A literature review and research agenda. *Int J Manage Rev*. 2013; 15(1): 86–105.
5. Savell E, Gilmore AB, Fooks G. How does the tobacco industry attempt to influence marketing regulations? A systematic review. *PLoS One*. 2014; 9(2): e87389.
6. Hillman AJ, Hitt MA. Corporate political strategy formulation: A model of approach, participation, and strategy decisions. *Acad Manage Rev*. 1999; 24(4): 825–842.
7. Fooks GJ, Williams S, Box G, Sacks G. Corporations' use and misuse of evidence to influence health policy: A case study of sugar-sweetened beverage taxation. *Global Health*. 2019; 15(1): 56.
8. Jaichuen N, Phulkerd S, Certthkrikul N, Sacks G, Tangcharoensathien V. Corporate political activity of major food companies in Thailand: An assessment and policy recommendations. *Global Health*. 2018; 14(1): 115.
9. Mialon M, Swinburn B, Allender S, Sacks G. "Maximising shareholder value": A detailed insight into the corporate political activity of the Australian food industry. *Aust N Z J Public Health*. 2017; 41(2): 165–171.

10. Williams SN. The incursion of "Big Food" in middle-income countries: A qualitative documentary case study analysis of the soft drinks industry in China and India. *Crit Public Health*. 2015; 25(4): 455–473.

11. Gómez E. *Junk Food Politics*. Johns Hopkins University Press; Forthcoming.

12. Vogel D. Private global business regulation. *Annu Rev Political Sci*. 2008; 11(1): 261–282.

13. Culpepper PD. *Quiet Politics and Business Power: Corporate Control in Europe and Japan*. Cambridge University Press; 2010.

14. Haas PM. Introduction: Epistemic communities and international policy coordination. *Int Organ*. 1992; 46(1): 1–35.

15. Gómez EJ, Méndez CA. Institutions, policy, and non-communicable diseases (NCDs) in Latin America. *J Politics Latin America*. 2021; 13(1): 114–137.

16. Binderkrantz AS, Christiansen PM, Pedersen HH. Interest group access to the bureaucracy, parliament, and the media. *Governance*. 2015; 28(1): 95–112.

17. West DM, Heith D, Goodwin C. Harry and Louise go to Washington: Political advertising and health care reform. *J Health Politics Policy Law*. 1996; 21(1): 35–68.

18. Keller E. Noisy business politics: Lobbying strategies and business influence after the financial crisis. *J Eur Public Policy*. 2018; 25(3): 287–306.

19. Greenhalgh S. Soda industry influence on obesity science and policy in China. *J Public Health Policy*. 2019; 40(1): 5–16.

20. Miller D, Harkins C. Corporate strategy, corporate capture: Food and alcohol industry lobbying and public health. *Crit Social Policy*. 2010; 30(4): 564–589.

21. Heitshusen V. Interest group lobbying and U.S. House decentralization: Linking informational focus to committee hearing appearances. *Political Res Q*. 2000; 53(1): 151–176.

22. Michalowitz I. What determines influence? Assessing conditions for decision-making influence of interest groups in the EU. *J Eur Public Policy*. 2007; 14(1): 132–151.

23. Gómez EJ. Coca-Cola's political and policy influence in Mexico: Understanding the role of institutions, interests and divided society. *Health Policy Planning*. 2019; 34(7): 520–528.

24. Paster T. How do business interest groups respond to political challenges? A study of the politics of German employers. *New Political Econ*. 2018; 23(6): 674–689.

25. Blumenthal D, Morone J. *The Heart of Power: Health and Politics in the Oval Office*. University of California Press; 2010.

26. Walker ET, Rea CM. The political mobilization of firms and industries. *Annu Rev Sociol*. 2014; 40(1): 281–304.

27. Yerger VB, Malone RE. African American leadership groups: Smoking with the enemy. *Tobacco Control*. 2002; 11(4): 336–345.

28. Maani Hessari N, Ruskin G, McKee KM, Stuckler D. Public meets private: Conversations between Coca-Cola and the CDC. *Milbank Q*. 2019; 97(1): 74–90.

29. Bernhagen P. Grooming for politics: How corporations combine lobbying with social responsibility. Paper prepared for the 73rd annual MPSA conference, April 16–19, 2015, Chicago, IL.

CHAPTER 6

The Role of Commercial Influences in Public Understanding of Harms, Causes, and Solutions

MARK PETTICREW, NASON MAANI,
AND MAY CI VAN SCHALKWYK

6.1 INTRODUCTION

A dominant focus within commercial determinants of health (CDOH) scholarship has been the strategies adopted by commercial actors to increase product consumption and expand target markets. These strategies are intended to be invisible, but many are well documented. This is particularly the case for the tobacco and infant formula industries. More recently, there has been an increasing focus on the activities of the producers of fossil fuels, food, and pesticides.[1-5]

Corporate-driven consumption involves sophisticated marketing. However, for this to be effective, the industries must put considerable effort into "preparing the ground" by influencing public and policymakers' understanding about the problems their products cause—be they risk of cancer, obesity, or global warming—and how and by whom these problems should be solved. This effort includes misleading the public about industry's role in causing the problems—such as the tobacco industry's denial that smoking causes lung cancer[6] and, in later years, the alcohol industry's misleading denials of the contribution of alcohol consumption to cancer, or the pesticide industry's denial of the contribution of neonicotinoids to the decline of bees and other pollinators.[7,8] *Explicit* denial is not the only form of denialism adopted by industry. Denialism encompasses a wide range of tactics, including undermining

Mark Petticrew, Nason Maani, and May CI van Schalkwyk, *The Role of Commercial Influences in Public Understanding of Harms, Causes, and Solutions* In: *The Commercial Determinants of Health*. Edited by: Nason Maani, Mark Petticrew, and Sandro Galea, Oxford University Press. © Oxford University Press 2023. DOI: 10.1093/oso/9780197578742.003.0006 and misrepresenting existing evidence, selectively presenting and amplifying misinformation through different channels, funding competing messages and/or research, and promoting uncertainty more generally.

Denialist strategies share a common purpose, which is the focus of this chapter. That purpose is to influence and manipulate public understanding of product harms and to deflect attention from the industry's key role in causing them. Normalization of the excessive consumption of harmful products is also a key part of the strategy. Normalization starts in childhood—for example, with the promotion of alcohol, soft drinks, gambling, and smoking to primary school children in schools.[6,9] The promotion of infant formula to new mothers begins even earlier, before the birth of the child. Similarly, the alcohol industry's denial of the harms of alcohol consumption during pregnancy involves the promotion of misinformation to pregnant women—and even occurs pre-conception.[10,11] Harmful product industries therefore take a life course approach to misinformation, as they do in promoting their products (Figure 6.1). In the case of alcohol, children are groomed from a very early age—for example, alcohol brands popular among underage drinkers are more likely to advertise in magazines with underage readerships.[12] When these children become old enough to drink legally, they are obviously of value, but the greatest value comes if they can be persuaded to drink to harmful levels. An industry evaluation of an alcohol advertising campaign stated, "If Miller Lite was to be a large profitable brand we had to attract these young heavy drinkers"[13]—or as they are known to the advertising industry experts who developed one of Stella Artois' campaigns, "Headbangers."[13] With an eye to the future, alcohol

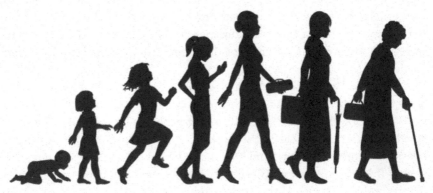

Alcohol industry
misinformation about FAS

Infant formula industry
misinformation about
breastfeeding

Tobacco industry denial
of risks of smoking in
pregnancy

Tobacco, alcohol, fossil fuel
misinformation in schools

Alcohol industry misinformation
about breast cancer

Tobacco, alcohol, fossil fuel
misinformation in universities

Tobacco, alcohol, misinformation
about CVD, stroke, COVID etc

Figure 6.1 The harmful commodity industry life course approach.

advertising must also turn the young heavy drinkers into tomorrow's heavy drinkers—in the words of a Famous Grouse whisky advertising campaign, "in the words of the advertising team who evaluated a Famous Grouse whisky advertising campaign."[13]

One might also see the alcohol industry's targeting of women from this perspective, particularly the development of spirits-based products targeted at young women. In this case, the grooming is accompanied by advertising that presents whisky drinking as empowering—for example, by launching a "women's version" of Johnnie Walker whiskey called Jane Walker "as a symbol of unity with the gender equality movement."[14] This was derided by some as being about as acceptable as "Lady Doritos," a "lady-friendly" version of the tortilla chip brand.[14]

6.2 SHAPING PUBLIC UNDERSTANDING AND ACCEPTABILITY

Shaping public opinion draws on a cross-industry playbook, part of which aims to increase and extend consumption among different sections of the public in different settings and contexts. Tobacco industry activities provide many examples—in particular, the "Torches of Freedom" march in 1929, a campaign developed by Edward Bernays for the American Tobacco Company (ATC). The ATC needed to normalize smoking in women, and to do this meant getting women to smoke outdoors. Bernays came up with the idea of a "women's equality" march, which involved 10 women walking and chain smoking openly in New York's Easter Day Parade.[15] However, modeling smoking in this way was not enough on its own to create new norms. Historian Robert Proctor notes that

> to make smoking as ordinary as, say, eating carrots or drinking orange juice . . .people also had to learn to smoke. . . . In the 1930s the American Tobacco Company organized classes for such purposes, directed principally at women. Company reps used dolls to demonstrate the proper way of holding, lighting, and smoking a cigarette.[6]

Tobacco industry "educational" anti-smoking activities in schools also have been shown to involve mixed messages and subtly promote smoking.[16] Landman et al.[16] concluded that

> the purpose of the industry's youth smoking prevention programs is not to reduce youth smoking but rather to serve the industry's political needs by preventing effective tobacco control legislation, marginalizing public health advocates, preserving the industry's access to youths, creating allies within

policymaking and regulatory bodies, defusing opposition from parents and educators, bolstering industry credibility, and preserving the industry's influence with policymakers.

It is not widely appreciated that the alcohol industry is also extremely active in schools, offering industry-funded educational materials to teachers and parents. The aims and actual content of this material—including the normalization of alcohol use—bears a close resemblance to those of the tobacco industry campaigns analyzed by Landman et al.[16] Landman et al. describe how tobacco industry youth smoking activities aim to reinforce the belief that peer pressure—not advertising—is the cause of youth smoking. Alcohol industry-funded activities, too, show the same emphasis on peer pressure, to the exclusion of the role of marketing and other industry activities.[17]

In our own analysis of three alcohol industry-funded education programs, we found that they emphasized the problem of underage drinking as located within individuals including youth, with causes of youth alcohol consumption repeatedly presented as peer pressure and "poor choices," with little or no mention of alcohol industry marketing or practices. All the education programs (from Drinkaware, the Alcohol Education Trust, and Diageo's Smashed program) promote familiarization and normalization of alcohol as a "normal" adult consumer product, which children must learn about and learn how to use "responsibly" when older.[18] Jackson and Dixon,[19] in an analysis of the use of Smashed materials in New Zealand schools, have noted that they selectively omit key health information. In particular, they selectively mention cancers of the mouth and throat as cancer-related health risks from alcohol, while more prevalent breast and bowel cancers are omitted, despite breast cancer being the leading cause of alcohol-related death in New Zealand women.[19] This has strong similarities with tobacco industry materials that avoid mentioning the risk of lung cancer.[6]

Readers can also compare these activities with those described in Chapter 12, which describes fossil fuel industry activities in schools. This is not new, of course; in *Dark Money*, Jane Mayer[20] investigated how the Koch Brothers (and other billionaires) effected a shift to the right in U.S. politics, driving corporate interests and eroding environmental and other protections. Like the Jesuits, these billionaires knew of the need to start young, in schools; Mayer describes how neoconservatives funded new foundations to shape political thinking, starting with schoolchildren; she quotes one of them (Michael Joyce) saying that "Kids in school are like bottles of wine . . . they're not worth much when they're new, but as they age they get more valuable."[20]

Industry-funded school-based materials and campaigns have similar roles: They act as a way of covertly promoting products, normalizing their use, and shaping youth values and ideas.[9] The national and international reach of such activities should not be underestimated. According to Diageo's website,

Smashed alcohol materials are now available online to more than 1 million students aged 12–14 years across 5,500 schools in the United Kingdom and have been delivered in 23 countries.

6.3 THE ECOLOGY OF INDUSTRY MISINFORMATION

6.3.1 Denialism

For corporations to be successful influencers also requires distorting facts and evidence, not just shaping opinions: If the real costs, including the harms of many products, were widely known and understood, public and policymaker support for tighter regulation, or even litigation, would likely increase. For this reason, harmful product industries frequently engage in extensive promotion of misinformation and disinformation. This includes misinformation about the causes of problems, the severity of the problems, and the most effective ways of dealing with them. In this category, we find, among many others, the tobacco industry denial that smoking causes lung cancer[21] (e.g., "Cigarette smoking has not been scientifically established as a cause of lung cancer. The cause or causes of lung cancer are unknown" [Imperial Tobacco, 2003][21]). Similarly, we observe the alcohol industry denial and omission of the role of alcohol as a cause of cancer and fetal alcohol syndrome (FAS)[10,19,22,23] (e.g., "No causal relationship has been shown between moderate drinking and breast cancer"; Educ'Alcool, a Quebec organization funded though the state-owned Quebec monopoly on alcohol sales, which has been found to disseminate alcohol industry misinformation on cancer risk and FAS[10]). The food industry has been found to foster denial of the role its products play in obesity, using complexity arguments to obscure the independent causal relationship (e.g., "We believe obesity is a complex problem which cannot be reduced to the demonization of one ingredient . . .there is no simple answer to the complex problems of obesity" [Food and Drink Federation, June 3, 2015][24]). The soft drink industry has similarly engaged in denial of the role of sugar-sweetened beverages (SSBs) in obesity, again using complexity arguments—for example,

> There's ample evidence to suggest that taxing soft drinks won't curb obesity, not least because its causes are far more complex than this simplistic approach implies. . . .Trying to blame one set of products is misguided, particularly when they comprise a mere 2% of calories in the average diet. (British Soft Drinks Association)[25]

These approaches also occur in less frequently studied harmful product industries. The gambling industry engages in denial that specific products and technologies promote addiction[24,26] (e.g., Ladbrookes' [UK gambling company] statement that "gambling related harm is complex and that simplistic approaches are not effective"[24]; see also Chapter 13). The opioid industry also engaged in denial and obfuscation of the evidence that opioids are addictive[27]—for example,

> I would cite six, seven, maybe ten different avenues of thought or avenues of evidence, none of which represented real evidence . . . what I was trying to do was to create a narrative so that the primary care audience would look at this information *in toto* and feel more comfortable about opioids in a way they hadn't before. (Prof. Russell Portenoy, opioid manufacturer consultant)[28]

6.3.2 Merchants of Misinformation

Misinformation does not emerge in a vacuum but is promoted through industry structures and bodies, usually claiming to be independent. These bodies (of which astroturfing is one manifestation) shape public opinions and perceptions, adding a veneer of authenticity to the messaging. Shaping public perceptions is also facilitated through partnerships with respected sources: charities, academics, clinicians, and others.[29] Breast cancer charities are a favored target. This has been criticized as "Pinkwashing," defined by one author as

> the practice of using the color pink and pink ribbons to indicate a company has joined the search for a breast cancer cure and to invoke breast cancer solidarity, even when the company may be using chemicals linked to cancer.[30]

This shaping of public perceptions normalizes the role of such products and their producers in daily life, as described previously.

Pharmaceutical industry funding of patient charities similarly facilitates the development of new markets and the creation of new health conditions to extend the clinical application of existing drugs. Purdue Pharma set up "pain groups" as part of a wider "pain movement" to promote the use of the opioid OxyContin to treat a wide range of conditions—from cancer and severe pain management initially to more minor conditions, and increasingly higher doses—while denying it was addictive.[27]

Industry-funded charities and other organizations are a key part of the industry misinformation infrastructure. Alcohol industry-funded organizations, some of them charities, disseminate misinformation to the public about cancer and fetal alcohol syndrome. There are at least 20 such organizations (sometimes referred to as SAPROs—social aspects public relations organizations[31]) working internationally, often benefitting from academic and medical advisors and from partnerships with legitimate health organizations, academics, clinicians, and academic institutions.

This should not be surprising, given that many prestigious universities were receiving tobacco industry money well into the 1990s (and some still are). This included funds to conduct research on health topics. Crucially, the researchers involved were not necessarily pressed by their industry funders to produce particular findings. Rather, the industry strategy was to fund research that could act as a distraction—so-called "red herring" research.[6]

Alcohol and gambling industry-funded research on "peer pressure" as a cause of consumption falls squarely into this category, as does industry-funded research on individual-level characteristics (personality and genetics) that predispose individuals to drink, gamble, or overeat. These all serve the wider purpose of deflecting attention and responsibility from the producers and marketers themselves. One example of this is food industry-funded research on personality characteristics and obesity. It is not difficult to work out why, for example, Danone might support such research[32] or why the SSB industry might fund research that underestimates the adverse effects of SSBs.[33]

6.3.3 How Irresponsible Industries Blame Individual "Irresponsibility"

It should be clear that a key part of cross-industry strategies involves the displacement of responsibility for problems (climate change, cancer, obesity, and many more) from the industry onto the individual. From an industry perspective, this helpfully restricts their obligations to solve the problem. That responsibility instead falls on the individual. From this dynamic emerges self-serving industry admonitions to "drink responsibly,"[34] "use pesticides/herbicides responsibly,"[3] and "gamble responsibly."[35] The common characteristic of these slogans is that "responsible" behavior is left strategically vague and unquantifiable.[34] Responsibility messaging from such industries has as much credibility as Philip Morris' "smoke responsibly" messages.[36]

This form of "responsibility shifting" by the alcohol and tobacco industries and others has been the focus of much analysis. It can also be seen in Purdue Pharma's response to the opioid crisis, where, after its marketing of OxyContin directly led to unprecedented levels of addiction, it blamed irresponsible consumers. Radden Keefe, who has documented the history of the opioid epidemic and the Sacker family, owners of Purdue Pharma, which developed OxyContin, explains:

> People did abuse these drugs Arthur [Sacker] conceded. But the real explanation
> for this phenomenon was not any intrinsically addictive properties of the drugs

themselves. Rather it was a reflection of the addictive personalities of the users themselves. . . .What Purdue should do, he decreed, was "hammer on the abusers in every way possible." They are "the culprits" he declared. "They are reckless criminals."[27]

In effect, this is a further example of industry normalization that we have discussed throughout this chapter. In this case, industries seek to normalize the individual nature of consumption, presenting most people as "responsible" and a minority of individuals (but not the industry itself) as irresponsible.

6.3.4 "Responsibility" Is Not a Health Outcome

Responsibility messaging often seems logical to public health practitioners and policymakers—it "just makes sense." However, it is important to remember that these are not health messages: "Responsibility" is not a health outcome. It is a public relations outcome, which simply signifies the successful deflection of responsibility from the industry to the person. Of course, it also shifts it to the taxpayer, families, their communities, and the health services or other public services that often bear the costs of this harm.

6.4 CONCLUSION: THE MULTIFUNCTIONALITY OF INDUSTRY STRATEGIES

This chapter has focused on how many industries construct meta-narratives to influence public and policy understandings of problems and restrict what are viewed as legitimate solutions. Within this, it is important to note that industry strategies usually have more than one function and/or have multiple effects. There are also many other meta-narratives not covered, such as misleading industry narratives about "illicit" product trade, about the responsibility of parents and teachers, misleading meta-narratives about science and evidence, and many others.

Internal tobacco industry documents, as so often, provide insights into how the tobacco industry thinks about this. As noted in historical R. J. Reynolds (RJR) internal documents on "How are corporate reputations created?"[37] corporate reputations are created out of corporate messaging, media, and engagement with stakeholders, including customers, and aim to change public attitudes in order to convert those who are neutral into "positive supporters" of the tobacco company. This can be done, it advises, through health campaigns and lobbying. The "responsibility campaigns" described above also fall into this category (RJR explicitly gives the example of "smoke responsibly" campaigns).

What is still lacking is evidence on the use of these meta-narratives in new industry campaigns and strategies and how to curb their use and/or impacts. To facilitate the production of this evidence, there is a pressing need for interdisciplinary collaborations between researchers working across industries. These collaborations need to extend beyond the usual health disciplines and also beyond the usual core set of research methodologies that are common in public health research.

REFERENCES

1. Michaels D. *Doubt Is Their Product: How Industry's Assault on Science Threatens Your Health*. Oxford University Press; 2008.
2. Michaels D. *The Triumph of Doubt: Dark Money and the Science of Deception*. Oxford University Press; 2020.
3. Gillam C. *Whitewash: The Story of a Weed Killer, Cancer, and the Corruption of Science*. Island Press; 2017.
4. Oreskes N, Conway E. *Merchants of Doubt: How a Handful of Scientists Obscured the Truth on Issues from Tobacco Smoke to Global Warming*. Bloomsbury; 2012.
5. Supran G, Oreskes N. Assessing ExxonMobil's climate change communications (1977–2014). *Environ Res Lett*. 2017; 12: 084019.
6. Proctor R. *Golden Holocaust: Origins of the Cigarette Catastrophe and the Case for Abolition*. University of California Press; 2011.
7. Muth F, Leonard A. A neonicotinoid pesticide impairs foraging, but not learning, in free-flying bumblebees. *Sci Rep*. 2019; 9: 4764.
8. Fang L. The playbook for poisoning the earth. *The Intercept*. January 18, 2020. Accessed December 15, 2021. https://theintercept.com/2020/01/18/bees-insec ticides-pesticides-neonicotinoids-bayer-monsanto-syngenta
9. Powell D. *Schools, Corporations and the War on Childhood Obesity: How Corporate Philanthropy Shapes Public Health and Education*. Routledge; 2020.
10. Lim A, Van Schalkwyk M, Maani Hessari N, Petticrew MP. Pregnancy, fertility, breastfeeding, and alcohol consumption: An analysis of framing and completeness of information disseminated by alcohol industry-funded organizations. *J Stud Alcohol Drugs*. 2019; 80(5): 524–533.
11. Brown A, van Tulleken C. *Breastfeeding Uncovered: Who Really Decides How We Feed Our Babies?* Pinter & Martin; 2021.
12. King C, Siegel M, Ross C, Jernigan D. Alcohol brands popular among underage drinkers are more likely than other brands to advertise in magazines with high underage readerships. *Alcoholism Clin Exp Res*. 2017; 41: 1775–1782.
13. Hessari N, Bertscher A, Critchlow N, et al. Recruiting the "heavy-using loyalists of tomorrow": An analysis of the aims, effects and mechanisms of alcohol advertising, based on advertising industry evaluations. *Int J Environ Res Public Health*. 2019; 16(21): 4092. doi:10.3390/ijerph16214092
14. Paskin B. Jane Walker backlash is a "misunderstanding." March 2, 2018. Accessed December 2, 2021. https://scotchwhisky.com/magazine/in-depth/18055/jane-walker-backlash-is-a-misunderstanding.
15. Amos A, Haglund M. From social taboo to "torch of freedom": The marketing of cigarettes to women. *Tobacco Control*. 2000; **9**: 3–8.

16. Landman A, Ling P, Glantz S. Tobacco industry youth smoking prevention programs: Protecting the industry and hurting tobacco control. *Am J Public Health*. 2002; 92(6): 917–930.

17. Petticrew M, Fitzgerald N, Durand M, Knai C, Davoren M, Perry I. Diageo's "Stop Out of Control Drinking" campaign in Ireland: An analysis. *PLoS One*. 2016; 11(9): e0160379.

18. van Schalkwyk M, Petticrew M, Maani N, et al. Distilling the curriculum: An analysis of alcohol industry-funded school-based youth education programmes. *PLoS One*. 2022; 17(1): e0259560.

19. Jackson N, Dixon R. The practice of the alcohol industry as health educator: A critique. *N Z Med J*. 2020; 133(1515): 89–96.

20. Mayer J. *Dark Money*. Anchor Books; 2017.

21. Cigarette giant to deny cancer link: Imperial uses unprecedented defence to fight claim by smoker's widow. *The Guardian*. October 5, 2003. Accessed December 3, 2021. https://www.theguardian.com/society/2003/oct/05/smoking.cancercare

22. Petticrew M, Maani Hessari N, Knai C, Weiderpass E. How alcohol industry organisations mislead the public about alcohol and cancer. *Drug Alcohol Rev*. 2017; 44: 15–17.

23. Petticrew M, Maani Hessari N, Knai C, Weiderpass E. The strategies of alcohol industry SAPROs: Inaccurate information, misleading language and the use of confounders to downplay and misrepresent the risk of cancer. *Drug Alcohol Rev*. 2018; 37(3): 313–315.

24. Petticrew M, Katikireddi S, Knai C, et al. "Nothing can be done until everything is done": The use of complexity arguments by food, beverage, alcohol and gambling industries. *J Epidemiol Community Health*. 2017; 71(11): 1078–1083.

25. Coca-Cola public statement. 2018. Accessed June 15, 2021. https://www.dw.com/en/foodwatch-germany-slams-coca-colas-denial-of-health-threat/a-43251925

26. Cassidy R. *Vicious Games*. Pluto Press; 2020.

27. Raddon Keefe P. *Empire of Pain: The Secret History of the Sackler Dynasty*. Picador; 2021.

28. Doctor who was paid by Purdue to push opioids to testify against drugmaker. *The Guardian*. April 10 2019. https://www.theguardian.com/us-news/2019/apr/10/purdue-opioids-crisis-doctor-testify-against-drugmaker. Quotes are from interview with Prof. Fortenoy on https://www.youtube.com/watch?v=Dgyu BWN9D4w.

29. Marks J. *The Perils of Partnership*. Oxford University Press; 2019.

30. Lubitow A, Davis M. Pastel injustice: The corporate use of pinkwashing for profit. *Environ Justice*. 2011; 4(2).

31. Babor TF, Robaina K. Public health, academic medicine, and the alcohol industry's corporate social responsibility activities. *Am J Public Health*. 2013; 103(2): 206–214.

32. Provenche RV, Bégin C, Gagnon-Girouard M, Tremblay A, Boivin S, Lemieux S. Personality traits in overweight and obese women: Associations with BMI and eating behaviors. *Eat Behav*. 2008; 9: 294–302.

33. Litman E, Gortmaker S, Ebbeling C, Ludwig D. Source of bias in sugar-sweetened beverage research: A systematic review. *Public Health Nutr*. 2018; 21(12): 2345–2350.

34. Maani Hessari N, Petticrew M. What does the alcohol industry mean by "responsible drinking"? A comparative analysis. *J Public Health*. 2018; 40(1): 90–97.

35. Keaton B. How to gamble responsibly (and stop when you need to). Casino.org. 2018. Accessed June 15, 2021. https://www.casino.org/blog/top-10-tips-for-responsible-gambling
36. The freedom to choose demands responsible behavior. Philip Morris records; Master Settlement Agreement. 1997. Accessed June 15, 2021. https://www.industrydocuments.ucsf.edu/tobacco/docs/#id=yqmw0088
37. Reputation management. RJ Reynolds collection. 2009 June 16. Accessed June 21, 2022. https://www.industrydocuments.ucsf.edu/tobacco/docs/#id=tyjm0222

CHAPTER 7

The Role of Corporations in Influencing Culture

NANCY TOMES

In 1987, the International Advertising Association held its third World Advertising Congress in Beijing, the capital of the People's Republic of China (PRC). The head of the PRC's State Council welcomed those attending, proclaiming that advertising "has become an indispensable element in the promotion of economic prosperity."[1] For the next 2 days, 131 speakers addressed 900 delegates from 52 countries, including nearly 600 from the PRC.[2] As they entered the Great Hall of the People to hear the talks, attendees were greeted by a robot serving Coca-Cola.[3] The spectacle of a communist nation of more than 1 billion potential consumers rolling out a "red carpet" (pun intended) to the advertising profession pointed to a significant change underway.[2] China's embrace of state-sponsored capitalism, along with economic reforms in the Soviet Union, signaled a softening of Cold War trade barriers. Nation states and corporations alike expressed enthusiasm for a new global marketplace in which transnational brands of consumer goods could flow more easily into middle- and low-income countries.

In 2013, a quarter century later, another international assembly, the 8th Global Conference on Health Promotion, met in Helsinki's Finlandia Hall. There, 650 delegates from 122 countries heard World Health Organization (WHO) Director-General Margaret Chan express concern about the health consequences of that free-flowing global marketplace.[4] "Instead of diseases vanishing as living conditions improve," she noted, "socioeconomic progress is actually creating the conditions that favor the rise of noncommunicable diseases." Trade liberalization had enabled powerful transnational corporations

Nancy Tomes, The Role of Corporations in Influencing Culture In: *The Commercial Determinants of Health*.
Edited by: Nason Maani, Mark Petticrew, and Sandro Galea, Oxford University Press. © Oxford University Press 2023.
DOI: 10.1093/oso/9780197578742.003.0007

to promote the increasing consumption of unhealthy products while using their considerable financial and political clout to evade responsibility for the consequences. And, she concluded, "It is not just Big Tobacco anymore. Public health must also contend with Big Food, Big Soda, and Big Alcohol."[5]

These two assemblies, Beijing in 1987 and Helsinki in 2013, frame the subject of this chapter, namely the *cultural* practices that transnational corporations have used to reshape global consumption patterns. Along with their direct economic and political influence, this "soft power" is hugely important yet difficult for public health policy to offset.[6] As this chapter shows, the cultural power that transnational corporations exercise over consumption patterns is difficult to counter precisely because they have become so adept at "glocalization"—that is, finding ways to embed their products' use in very diverse cultures.[7]

Transnational corporations have succeeded by linking product choice and cultural identity. As social scientists have long noted, how people choose to buy and consume products constitutes an integral part of their culture, defined by Douglas Goodman as "a system of meanings and a set of practices that constitute that system."[8] Transnational corporations based in the United States and Western Europe have excelled at promoting what Leslie Sklair terms the "culture-ideology of consumerism": a worldview in which "the meaning of life is to be found in the things that we possess" and "to consume, therefore, is to be fully alive, and to remain fully alive we must continuously consume."[9] As recent work on global cultures of consumption attests, the webs of meaning attached to products are neither monolithic nor homogeneous, either within or between countries; rather, they vary along many axes of difference, including urban/rural, regional, social status, religious affiliation, gender, and sexual orientation. Because of their diverse associations, consumption choices often become sites for intense cultural debate and conflict.[10] That is particularly true for frequently consumed products such as food, drink, and tobacco items that are associated with health and well-being.

Changing cultural patterns of consumption are tied, distally and directly, to the most urgent problems of 21st-century public health. Distally, the energy requirements needed to produce, distribute, and package those branded goods contribute to carbon footprints that are escalating global climate change.[11] More directly, transnational corporations have focused their formidable resources, including research, development, marketing, and advertising, on expanding sales of products known to increase the risk of cancer, cardiovascular disease, diabetes, alcoholism, and a host of other noncontagious diseases. This chapter focuses primarily on product categories strongly associated with negative health effects: tobacco, soft drinks, and processed foods.

Of course, the links among trade, specific products, and health risks long predate the 20th century. Trade routes from Asia to Europe created the pathway for the medieval bubonic plague[12]; the imperial quest for sugar transformed the lives of both those who consumed it and those who produced it.[13] Mercantile and industrial capitalism created the urban health conditions that gave rise to 19th-century public health.[14] But it was only in the late 19th century that large corporations based in the United States and Western Europe began to combine organizational efficiency, economies of scale, low prices, and innovative advertising in ways that allowed them to displace homemade food and local producers and gradually build national and international markets for their goods. Over the course of the 20th century, spending on both durables (vehicles and appliances) and nondurables (food, cigarettes, soft drinks, and snacks) emerged as significant drivers of economic growth first in the United States and Western Europe and then the rest of the world.[15]

This turbocharged form of consumption emerged early and robustly in the United States. In this large, resource-rich country with a short history, minimal inherited traditions, and a diverse immigrant population, American corporations developed what marketing experts would later dub a "low context" style of selling characterized by very explicit messages[16]; those messages equated consumption choices with social mobility and cultural assimilation as a "100 percent American."[17] This low context approach was crafted within a framework of light regulation, first by the U.S. Food and Drug Administration (founded in 1906) and then by the Federal Trade Commission (founded 1914), respectively charged with ensuring that products were minimally safe and that their advertising claims were minimally truthful. Their oversight convinced Americans that the products they consumed were far safer than they actually were.[18]

Although often portrayed as a natural outgrowth of prosperity and democracy, in fact, this "American way" of consumption reflected sophisticated corporate practices.[19] First, large corporations started to plow profits back into newly created research and development departments tasked with crafting product formulas that left the consumer wanting to buy more. With the exception of narcotics, which were subject to more regulation after the 1914 Harrison Act, other substances such as nicotine, caffeine, sugar, and fat could be used freely. Second, corporations invested heavily in marketing research and advertising campaigns to promote their brands. Advertising professionals developed new image-rich storytelling techniques to associate products with common aspirations to fit in, to be loved, to be healthy, and to enjoy life. Advertisements presented brand name cigarettes, soft drinks, candy, and other snacks as essential accompaniments for the enjoyment of sporting events, family gatherings, and holiday celebrations. To amplify these messages, companies bought advertising time in media outlets (newspapers, radio, and, after World War II, television) and carefully monitored how well they worked to increase sales. Due to intense competition, these advertising campaigns did not necessarily work to make one brand dominate but succeeded quite well at boosting the overall consumption of these product categories.[17,20]

Although initially focused on national markets, American corporations such as American Tobacco and Kraft Foods began to look abroad to sell their brands; their European-based counterparts, including the UK Imperial Tobacco Companies and the Swiss Nestle Company, did the same. As the ambition for international trade grew, so too did corporate investment in advertising. The first World Advertising Congress was held in Berlin in 1929[21]; by the early 1930s, the American advertising agency J. Walter Thompson had opened offices in 34 countries on five continents.[22] Although slowed down by the Great Depression and World War II, these networks created the foundation for the rapid expansion of corporate sales of tobacco, food, soft drinks, and processed foods after 1945.[23]

The history of the U.S.-based soda giant Coca-Cola illustrates how this earlier development paved the way for later expansion. In its national market, Coca-Cola excelled at promoting its caramel-colored, caffeinated soda as the "All American" drink, the "pause that refreshes," and Santa Claus's beverage of choice. At the same time, the company mastered the logistics of bottling and selling the drink almost anywhere. World War II gave Coca-Cola the chance to test that flexibility. As soon as the United States entered the war, the company created 60 overseas plants to provide the drink for 7 million American soldiers, along with their host communities. At war's end, the company expanded its production and sales in the footprint of the United States' expanding influence as a Cold War superpower.[24-26] International sales climbed dramatically in the 1950s and 1960s, albeit with complaints about "coca-colonization," a term first used by French communists in 1948.[27]

In the Cold War decades, expansion of "American"-style consumerism occurred most robustly in the United States' former allies (the United Kingdom) and occupied enemies (West Germany and Japan). In turn, the United States and its allies competed with the Soviet bloc countries to expand their markets in Latin America, Africa, and Asia. Then in the 1970s, the trade barriers between the capitalist and communist blocs began to soften. In 1979, the PRC announced its "open door" policy and began to move toward state-sponsored capitalism; in 1986, the Soviet Union embraced "glasnost" and "perestroika" in the name of economic reform. Under the "free market" ideologies championed by American President Ronald Reagan and British Prime Minister Margaret Thatcher, transnational corporations were well positioned to take advantage of that softening.[28,29]

Darker trends prompted the corporate search for new markets as well. The empirical evidence that rising rates of cancer and other noncontagious diseases were linked to rising consumption of tobacco, processed foods, and alcohol made corporate promotion of their use increasingly controversial in the United States and other high-income nations. Health concerns led to public education campaigns and regulatory restrictions on the sale and promotion of tobacco and subsequently soft drinks and processed foods. Those changes gave transnational companies even more incentive to explore new markets in developing areas of the world.

Tobacco was the bellwether of this shift. In the United States and the United Kingdom, countries in which tobacco consumption had been heavily promoted since the 1920s, large-scale epidemiological studies began to document the association between smoking and the risk of lung and other cancers. Starting in the late 1950s, an anti-tobacco movement demanded more restrictions on both products and advertisements; tobacco companies lobbied hard against both. Politicians, especially those from tobacco-producing states, were reluctant to limit consumer choices, even potentially deadly ones. They pointed to the fact that some people used tobacco products without developing cancer or coronary vascular disease as a reason for preserving the "freedom of choice," an argument that many people accepted before nicotine's addictive properties were documented in the late 1980s.[30,31]

Thus, tobacco control emerged as a variation on the "let the buyer beware" philosophy: Before purchasing, consumers needed to be fully apprised of tobacco's health risks through warning labels; advertising and promotion of tobacco products had to be limited to adults. Health advocates used new "fair use" standards to air anti-smoking advertisements—often developed pro bono by advertising agencies eager to position their industry as health conscious. Cigarette advertisements disappeared from television and radio, and restrictions on smoking in public places gradually tightened. The decline in American tobacco consumption, which peaked in the early 1970s, seemed to suggest that this approach "worked." But it also shifted blame onto people who continued to smoke; when they became sick, tobacco companies suggested, they had only themselves to blame.[32]

A similar dynamic eventually developed around food and nutrition issues as epidemiological studies established the links between new eating habits and changing disease patterns. Prospective cohort studies identified diets high in fat, sugar, salt, and alcohol as risk factors not only for many cancers but also for cardiovascular disease, diabetes, and liver failure.[33,34] Other research pointed to the addictive appeal of common ingredients used in processed foods, including sugar, fat, and salt.[35] As this evidence accumulated, calls for more regulation of their packaging and advertising increased. In the 1990s, the "consume responsibly" approach expanded to include nutritional labeling for foods and beverages along with efforts to limit the advertising of sugary products to children.[36]

As this pushback unfolded in wealthier nations, transnational corporations looked to expanding sales in middle- and low-income countries as a way to offset potential losses. Here again, tobacco companies blazed the way. While cigarette sales fell in the United States by 20% between 1975 and 1994, rates of cigarette production rose by 11%, with that product destined for new markets in the former Soviet countries, India, and the PRC. As cigarette historian Allan

Brandt notes, "Just at the moment that the cigarette was losing its glamour, sophistication, and sexual allure in the West, the companies sought to re-create these connotations of smoking in developing countries."[31] Likewise, transnational corporations selling food and beverage items expanded their sales in those same countries. By 1991, Coke derived 80% of its operating income from sales outside the United States[37]; by 1996, McDonald's had expanded its overseas business, begun with one Canadian franchise in 1967, to 100 countries.[38]

Transnational corporations often presented this expansion as a natural result of their product's desirability. Yet creating this global "supermarket" of consumer products required serious investments in research, development, marketing, and advertising. Companies had to overcome consumer ambivalence rooted in traditions of thriftiness that made spending on brand-name foods and beverages seem indulgent.[39] To that end, they calibrated both the products and their promotion to align with local tastes and traditions.[40] To oversee these efforts, transnational companies such as Coca-Cola and McDonald's increasingly recruited executive talent from outside the United States.[37]

McDonald's was a trendsetter in this regard, exporting its organizational and managerial strategies abroad while recruiting local entrepreneurs to tailor the menu to local tastes.[7,41,42] In many countries, internal development funds provided money to buy a franchise, making them an attractive means of upward mobility.[43,44] The company rewarded franchise owners for coming up with new offerings that appealed to their community; in Thailand, that meant the Samurai Pork Burger; in India, the McSpicy paneer; and in Malaysia, the Mango McFlurry.[45] McDonald's also focused on making its restaurants family friendly; in Beijing's first franchise, communist party officials reportedly rented out its space for their children's birthday parties.[46]

Snack food companies showed similar persistence and adaptability. Kraft Foods' promotion of Oreos and Tang in the PRC is a good example. One of the first American corporations to export a snack food, Kraft had early learned that "the success of Oreo is 'from the filling,'" varying its flavors to suit national tastes (for example, cocoa variations in Mexico and a combination of chocolate and strawberry in Indonesia.)[47] However, the PRC proved a particularly difficult market to crack because people were unused to eating cookies. Kraft persisted, learning through market research that Chinese consumers found the regular Oreo too sweet and preferred lower prices and smaller packages. Kraft obliged by developing a less sweet version in a smaller package, and Oreos captured 20% of the Chinese cookie market. The same tactics worked with Tang, a powdered orange drink that had lost its American market. Again, through market research, Kraft discovered that Chinese mothers wanted their children to drink more water, but the latter thought water was "boring." So Kraft promoted Tang with the promise that it "makes water more exciting."[48]

The implicit message of these campaigns was not that transnational companies meant to level local cultures but, rather, hoped to infiltrate them. They promoted the concept of global consumers as active players, choosing between the old and the new products to suit themselves. Indeed, their product appeals did *not* work for everyone. Many consumers remained wary of "American" or "Western" lifestyles and thus open to home-grown companies' appeals to "buy local." What George Ritzer terms "indigenous fast food" brands copied elements of the franchise method to compete with the international giants.[7] Also in many countries, street foods proliferated as cheaper, tastier alternatives to fast foods. Rather than one canceling out the other, corporate and local efforts interacted and intertwined.

In the early 21st century, the health implications of these changing global consumption patterns became increasingly apparent. Long fixated on infectious diseases, global health organizations now began to worry about rising rates of noncontagious diseases in middle- and low-income countries. Once again, concerns about tobacco use led the way: In 2003, WHO negotiated its first treaty, the WHO Framework Convention on Tobacco Control. Over the next decade, WHO broadened its initiatives to include "physical inactivity, unhealthy diet and the harmful use of alcohol." In 2014, it created its Global Coordination Mechanism on the Prevention and Control of NCDs to coordinate efforts to reduce unhealthy patterns of consumption. Individually, many countries have experimented with control measures, including "sin" or "fat" taxes, to discourage the consumption of tobacco, soda, and snack foods.[31,49]

Although they have resisted the more sweeping restrictions, trade associations representing tobacco, food, and beverage industries have generally been willing to pledge support for labeling and educational measures that provide information in advance of purchase. This strategy allows them to continue using ingredients (fat, sugar, and salt) that "hook" the consumer while promoting the idea of "responsible consumption."[35] The idea that consumers must learn to make "smart" choices has achieved such widespread acceptance that for many people it now has the status of common sense. Asked to comment on the value of a "fat tax" on fast food in the Indian state of Kerala, a prominent local chef echoed the prevailing sentiment: "The choice should definitely be left to the consumer. We can only educate them, and it is our responsibility to raise awareness. They should know the difference between good and bad food."[50]

But the resources available to large corporations to promote their products far exceed those of local producers. Power to compete by price, to leverage local market conditions, and to control media attention gives corporations a huge advantage. And in a world of frequent migration, the sameness of global brand experiences can deepen consumer attachment to them. In an article in *The New York Times Magazine*, Jane Hu reflected on her attachment to the McDonald's Filet-O-Fish sandwich, which she first ate as a child after moving from the PRC to Montreal, Canada. As she notes, a sandwich originally developed in 1960s America to appeal to Roman Catholics who ate fish on Fridays became a favorite of Asian immigrants and other fish-loving people as they moved into new cultural spaces. As an adult, she now sees its imperfections, but the "way it never quite lives up to the ideal, are what make the sandwich feel like home."[51]

The Internet and its expanding interactive capacities are now vastly expanding the ability of transnational corporations to make products feel like home.[52] Personal electronic devices now allow corporations to create and mine massive data sets about consumer preferences.[53] The more social or participatory Web 2.0 allows companies vast new possibilities to reach their target audience. For example, in China, Mondelez—Kraft's renamed grocery and food division—created an Oreo's feature that allowed users to combine emojis with family pictures; it generated 99 million electronic ideograms on WeChat.[54] In search of young consumers, corporations now hire "digital influencers" to boost products via their social media feeds.[55] A 2019 study by the global marketing and media agency UM outlines what it calls a "remix culture" in which global consumers mix and match product choices, choosing name brands that deliver what they promise, while valuing local brands and products as more "authentic."[56]

Accounting for cultural attachments to consumer goods poses a formidable public health challenge. Corporations broadcast their positive "binding" messages—our product is associated with "joy, laughter, sport and music" (Coke) or families enjoying togetherness (Oreos)—far more effectively that public health authorities deliver negative messages about health risks.[37,54] The complex meanings that consumers attach to their choice of brand-name products are difficult to integrate into the dominant methodologies of public health science. As Thomas Glass noted in 2006, "Culture is among a class of concepts for which there are few analogues in epidemiology," making it "the 800 pound gorilla" in the room that gets ignored.[57] Although public health research on tobacco and food products invariably acknowledges the importance of advertising and marketing, the specifics of the cultural work they do are rarely explored in-depth. In comparison, in a popular textbook on global marketing and advertising, 8 of the 11 chapters have the word "culture" in their title.[58]

The extraordinary expansion of corporate brands during the past century may make their continued cultural dominance seem inevitable. But their political and cultural influence is likely to be tested in the next 50 years. The COVID pandemic has shown the power of new viral variants to disrupt global supply chains, including those of snack foods and soft drinks,[59] while climate change heralds the end of a global intensification of consumption dependent on the availability of cheap fossil fuels.[11] Anti-consumption is a key theme of climate activist groups that do not accept corporate gestures at sustainability as sufficient and insist that "shoppers cannot ignore the climate emergency."[60] However, until the seas rise further and the hot places get hotter, the cultural attachment to these consumption patterns may be difficult to break.

REFERENCES

1. Rice MD. China's sleeping ad market wakes up. *Marketing News*. September 25, 1987; 4.
2. Admen in China get red carpet. *Advertising Age*. June 22, 1987; 89.
3. Madison Avenue invades Beijing. *The Globe and Mail*. June 22, 1987.
4. Tang K, Ståhl T, Bettcher D, De Leeuw E. The Eighth Global Conference on Health Promotion: Health in all policies: From rhetoric to action. *Health Promotion Int*. 2014; 29: i1–i8.
5. Global efforts to promote health face serious challenges from "big business." *UN News*. June 10, 2013. https://news.un.org/en/story/2013/06/441852-global-efforts-promote-health-face-serious-challenges-big-business-un-official
6. Nye J Jr. *Soft Power: The Means to Success in World Politics*. Public Affairs; 2005.
7. Ritzer G. *The McDonaldization of Society*. rev. ed. SAGE; 2005: 160–165.
8. Goodman DJ. Globalization and consumer culture. In: Ritzer G, ed. *The Blackwell Companion to Globalization*. Blackwell; 2007: 330–351. Quote on 334.
9. Sklair L. *Sociology of the Global System*. Johns Hopkins University Press; 1991. Quote on 197.
10. Ritzer G. *The Blackwell Companion to Globalization*. Blackwell; 2007.
11. Smart B. *Consumer Society: Critical Issues and Environmental Consequences*. SAGE; 2010.
12. Yue RPH, Lee HF, Wu CYH. Trade routes and plague transmission in pre-industrial Europe. *Sci Rep*. 2017; 7(1): 12973.
13. Mintz S. *Sweetness and Power*. New York, NY: Viking; 1982.
14. Berridge V, Mold A, Gorsky M, eds. *Public Health in History*. Open University Press; 2011.
15. Silla C. *The Rise of Consumer Capitalism in America, 1880–1930*. Routledge; 2018.
16. Meyer E. *The Culture Map: Breaking Through the Invisible Boundaries of Global Business*. Public Affairs; 2014: 29–59.
17. Marchand R. *Advertising the American Dream: Making Way for Modernity, 1920–1940*. University of California Press; 1985.
18. Tomes N. *Remaking the American Patient*. University of North Carolina Press; 2016: 32–37.
19. Strasser S. *Satisfaction Guaranteed: The Making of the American Mass Market*. Smithsonian Institution Press; 1989.
20. Fox S. *The Mirror Makers: A History of American Advertising and Its Creators*. University of Illinois Press; 1997.
21. Kleinert H. The World Advertising Congress 1929. *Wissenschaft-Thurm*. April 9, 2018. https://wissenschafts-thurm.de/der-weltreklamekongress-1929-eine-sternstunde-der-wirtschaftswerbung
22. Merron J. Putting foreign consumers on the map. *Business History Review*. 1999; 73(3): 465–503.
23. De Grazia V. *Irresistible Empire: America's Advance Through 20th c. Europe*. Harvard University Press; 2005.

24. Pendergrast M. *For God, Country, & Coca-Cola*. Basic Books; 2013.
25. Elmore BJ. *Citizen Coke: The Making of Coca-Cola Capitalism*. Norton; 2015.
26. Ciafone A. *Counter-Cola: A Multinational History of the Global Corporation*. University of California Press; 2019.
27. Kuisel RF. Coca-Cola and the Cold War. *French Historical Studies*. 1991; 17(1): 96–116. Reference on 101.
28. Friedman TL. *The Lexus and the Olive Tree: Understanding Globalization*. Farrar, Straus & Giroux; 1999.
29. Klein N. *No Logo: Taking Aim at the Brand Bullies*. Picador; 2000.
30. Berridge V. *Marketing Health: Smoking and the Discourse of Public Health in Britain, 1945–2000*. Oxford University Press; 2011.
31. Brandt AM. *The Cigarette Century*. Basic Books; 2007.
32. Pennock PE. *Advertising Sin and Sickness: The Politics of Alcohol and Tobacco Marketing 1950–1990*. Northern Illinois Press; 2007.
33. Levy D, Brink S. *A Change of Heart: How the People of Framingham, Massachusetts, Helped Unravel the Mysteries of Cardiovascular Disease Study*. Knopf; 2005.
34. Jayedi A, Soltani S, Abdolshahi A, Shab-Bidar S. Healthy and unhealthy dietary patterns and the risk of chronic disease: An umbrella review of meta-analyses of prospective cohort studies. *Br J Nutr*. 2020; 124: 1133–1144.
35. Moss M. *Hooked: Food, Free Will, and How the Food Giants Exploit Our Addictions*. Random House; 2021.
36. Institute of Medicine, Committee on Examination of Front-of-Package Nutrition Rating Systems and Symbols; Wartella EA, Lichtenstein AH, Boon CS, eds. *Front-of-Package Nutrition Rating Systems and Symbols: Phase I Report*. National Academies Press; 2010.
37. Cohen R. For Coke, the world is its oyster. *The New York Times*. November 21, 1991; D1.
38. James R. A brief history of McDonald's abroad. *TIME*. October 28, 2009. http://content.time.com/time/world/article/0,8599,1932839,00.html
39. Garon S, Maclachlan PL. *The Ambivalent Consumer: Questioning Consumption in East Asia and the West*. Cornell University Press; 2006.
40. Doss S, Wang Y. Acculturation and commercialization of thematic holidays in the globalization era. *Int J Business Global*. 2010; 5: 411–420.
41. Schlosser E. *Fast Food Nation: The Dark Side of the American Meal*. Houghton Mifflin; 2001.
42. Smart B, ed. *Resisting McDonaldization*. SAGE; 1999.
43. Gibson R. US franchises find opportunity to grow abroad. *Wall Street Journal*. August 11, 2009; B5.
44. Chatelain M. *Franchise: The Golden Arches in Black America*. Liveright; 2020.
45. Special McDonald's menu items from around the world. Love Food News. July 7, 2020. https://www.lovefood.com/gallerylist/60910/special-mcdonalds-menu-items-from-around-the-world
46. Carter J. The first McDonald's in Beijing was a symbol of engagement. *Sup China*. April 21, 2021. https://supchina.com/2021/04/21/the-first-mcdonalds-in-china-was-a-symbol-of-engagement
47. Racoma B. How Oreo adapts around the world. *Day Translations*. August 1, 2019. https://www.daytranslations.com/blog/oreo-adapts-globally
48. How Kraft won in China. *Forbes*. December 8, 2009.
49. Magnusson RS, Patterson D. The role of law and governance reform in the global response to non-communicable diseases. *Global Health*. 2014; 10(44): 1–18.

50. Shahani S. Is "fat tax" a new way to fight obesity in India? *Hindustan Times*. July 15, 2016.
51. Hu J. Filet-O-Fish. *The New York Times Magazine*. April 25, 2021: 20–21.
52. Kirby J. Creative that cracks the code. *Harvard Business Rev.* March 2013: 86–89.
53. Clark R. The fast machine-learners. *Campaign Asia-Pacific*. November 2016: 52–53.
54. When snack foods go digital. *Campaign Asia-Pacific*. February 2015: 11.
55. Anesha G. Food, fashion, tech: How popularity pays for India's young micro-influencers. *Hindustan Times*. September 16, 2018.
56. Four key trends shape modern consumer behavior, according to UM's Global Wave X Remix Culture Study. *PR Newswire*. July 1, 2019.
57. Glass T. Commentary: Culture in epidemiology—The 800 pound gorilla? *Int J Epidemiol*. 2006; 35: 259–261. Quote on 260.
58. De Mooij M. *Global Marketing & Advertising: Understanding Cultural Paradoxes*. 5th ed. SAGE; 2019.
59. Soft drink and ice global market report 2021: COVID 19 impact and recovery to 2030. *Global Newswire*. February 4, 2021. https://www.globenewswire.com/news-release/2021/02/04/2169700/0/en/Soft-Drink-And-Ice-Global-Market-Report-2021-COVID-19-Impact-and-Recovery-to-2030.html
60. Hauck G. Climate activists turn attention to Black Friday. *USA Today*. November 29, 2019.

CHAPTER 8

Industry Influence on Science

What Is Happening and What Can Be Done

ALICE FABBRI AND ANNA B. GILMORE

8.1 INTRODUCTION

It was January 1981 when the *BMJ* published the results of a Japanese cohort study by Dr. Takeshi Hirayama showing that non-smoking women married to smokers had an increased risk of lung cancer compared to wives of non-smokers.[1] These findings cast new light on the harmful effects of secondhand smoke and quickly became highly debated and influential. Concerned by these results, the tobacco industry launched a massive campaign to discredit the Hirayama paper, despite the fact that industry scientists had reviewed the results and found them to be correct.[2] In order to support their arguments, tobacco companies also commissioned an alternative study, the "Japanese spousal study."[3] According to internal industry documents, the tobacco industry sought to conceal the extent of their involvement in this study, whose conclusions questioned the reliability of previous research that used "marriage to a smoker" as an index of environmental tobacco exposure.[4]

This is far from a unique occurrence, as shown by the rofecoxib (Vioxx) case. Rofecoxib was introduced by Merck in 1999 as an anti-inflammatory drug to treat arthritis and was withdrawn from the market in 2004 because of safety concerns. It has been estimated that between 88,000 and 139,000 Americans suffered myocardial infarctions or strokes as a result of taking rofecoxib.[5] Despite Merck knowing, since the late 1990s, that rofecoxib might adversely affect the cardiovascular system, the pharmaceutical company misrepresented the results of clinical trials to obscure the cardiovascular toxicity

Alice Fabbri and Anna B. Gilmore, *Industry Influence on Science* In: *The Commercial Determinants of Health.* Edited by: Nason Maani, Mark Petticrew, and Sandro Galea, Oxford University Press. © Oxford University Press 2023. DOI: 10.1093/oso/9780197578742.003.0008 of Vioxx.[6] Scientific publications were often ghostwritten by Merck scientists but signed by academic investigators as first authors,[7] and the company strongly promoted Vioxx to health professionals.[8]

These are just two among many examples of how different industry sectors have strategically produced and disseminated evidence that maximizes the benefits and obscures the harmful effects of their products with the ultimate goal of minimizing regulation and increasing sales. When analyzing industry influence on science, it can be useful to break down this complex phenomenon into three main areas of influence. The first one is the influence on evidence production; this includes industry influence on the research process, from the choice of research question to the design, methods, conduct, and reporting of findings. The second one is the influence on evidence dissemination that refers to industry influence on the reach of science. The final area is the influence on evidence use, namely industry influence on the use of science in policy and practice.

In the following discussion, we analyze the strategies that corporations have used in each of the three areas, providing examples from different sectors. With these examples, we do not claim that all industry-funded research is flawed. Our aim is to present the growing body of evidence showing how industry uses science and what have been more broadly labeled "information management strategies"[9] as a key element of their corporate political activities aimed at creating a favorable environment for their business.

8.2 HOW INDUSTRY INFLUENCES SCIENCE

8.2.1 Industry Influence on Evidence Production

Considerable empirical evidence across different industry sectors has shown an association between industry funding and outcomes or conclusions favorable to the companies' products.[10,11] This "funding bias" may be due to a variety of choices that industry makes in the design, conduct, analysis, and reporting of research.[10] For example, pharmaceutical industry sponsored trials more often use placebo controls and inferior doses of active comparators, which might increase the chances that the sponsor's product will appear comparably effective.[10] Industry funding can also impose constraints on publication rights, which can lead to favorable outcomes being published while unfavorable results are withheld, creating a skewed evidence base.[12]

Although industry influence on research methods, outcomes, and reporting has been extensively studied, often less well recognized is the influence the sponsor can have at a higher level, on the research agenda itself. By "research agenda," we mean the first step in conducting research, in which the research topics are selected and framed.[13] For example, according to internal industry documents from 1959 to 1971, the sugar industry tried to deflect attention from interventions aimed at reducing sugar consumption to control tooth decay. This included strategically funding research into a vaccine against dental caries and into enzymes to break dental plaque that could reduce the harmful effects of sugar consumption without restricting intake.[14] In a more recent example, investigative journalism exposed Coca-Cola's sponsorship of research on physical activity via the Global Energy Balance Network.[15] Through sponsorships of research on physical activity, soda companies can shape obesity research and shift attention from the role of their products in obesity to the role of sedentary behaviors.[16] In conclusion, by influencing the research agenda, companies can influence the research questions that get studied and therefore the entire body of evidence available to policymakers, public health practitioners, and consumers.[13] This can consequently lead to the implementation of policies that have minimal impact on industry's profits (e.g., individual-level rather than population-based interventions).

For a more in-depth analysis of industry influence on evidence production, see Chapter 19. For discussion of gambling industry influence on evidence production, see Chapter 13.

8.2.2 Industry Influence on Evidence Dissemination

Evidence has little impact unless it is widely disseminated. In order to influence this process, industry uses two opposite techniques that we metaphorically call the megaphone effect and the silencer effect.

By *megaphone effect*, we mean the strategies that industry uses to maximize the reach of favorable research. In this regard, scientific journals represent an important vehicle. For instance, pharmaceutical companies spend large amount of money to buy reprints of favorable trials published in prestigious medical journals and then use them to market their products to physicians.[17]

Moreover, in order to ensure that the message appears scientifically credible, corporate actors recruit a range of trusted allies that help with the dissemination of industry-favorable science. In the medical sector, the use of "key opinion leaders" is a classic example of this technique. These thought leaders are usually influential doctors whose opinions have the potential to influence thousands of colleagues; they are recruited and paid by pharmaceutical companies to give lectures, present at conferences, or participate on industry advisory board committees.[18] According to a former drug company sales representative,

> Key opinion leaders were salespeople for us, and we would routinely measure the return on our investment, by tracking prescriptions before and after their

presentations. If that speaker didn't make the impact the company was looking for, then you wouldn't invite them back.[18]

Other allies include third parties such as think tanks, front groups, and astroturfing organizations that promote the corporate agenda while appearing to be independent. Given the harmful nature of its products, the tobacco industry has been a pioneer in the use of front groups to push its messages and to oppose tobacco control measures.[19] Other industries have used similar strategies. Findings from investigative journalism have shown, for example, that ExxonMobil, one of the largest oil companies, heavily funded think tanks and several other organizations in the Unites States that tried to undermine the scientific evidence on climate change "employing 'reports' designed to look like a counterbalance to peer-reviewed studies, [and] skeptic propaganda masquerading as journalism."[20]

Another effective strategy is the dissemination of information via the organization or sponsorship of conferences and "educational events." This strategy has been documented for several industries (e.g., the alcohol industry[21]), and it has been extensively studied in the pharmaceutical sector. Internal pharmaceutical industry documents have shown that continuing medical education events have been effectively used to deliver promotional messages.[22] Moreover, a recent analysis of the Open Payments database (the national transparency program in the United States) has shown that receiving industry payments for educational training is associated with increased prescribing of promoted, brand-name medications instead of low-cost generics.[23]

The opposite phenomenon is the *silencer effect*, namely the strategies that industry uses to suppress unfavorable science. For decades, the asbestos industry funded research on the hazards of asbestos and then systematically suppressed its findings.[24] The withholding of this information led to millions of workers being exposed to this carcinogen. An internal industry memo from 1979 perfectly summarizes the asbestos industry behavior for almost half a century, stating "I can easily see why we have members of the Congress calling us 'liars.'"[24] The tobacco industry offers another example of suppression of research. Internal industry documents revealed that by the 1980s, British American Tobacco was conducting internal research on the harmful effects of secondhand smoke. The company suppressed the dissemination of its internal research findings and continued to deny the health hazards of passive smoking.[25]

Attacks on researchers are another example of industry obstructing the dissemination of knowledge and silencing unfavorable voices. Since the mid-1960s, the asbestos industry orchestrated a campaign to discredit Dr. Irving J. Selikoff, one of the most prominent experts on asbestos-related diseases, questioning his medical qualifications and the motives behind his work. He was also accused of distorting the science and misleading the public about the hazards of asbestos; interestingly, these are the same accusations that asbestos companies have been found guilty of.[26] More recently, climate scientists have become targets of similar attacks.[27]

8.2.3 Industry Influence on Evidence Use

Apart from influencing the production and dissemination of evidence, another important area of corporate influence is on how evidence is evaluated and used. There is evidence that corporations have influenced this process in order to create industry-friendly scientific and policymaking environments that in turn make it easier to use industry-favorable evidence and more difficult to use unfavorable evidence in policy and regulatory settings.

Going somehow beyond the previously described efforts to create doubts around the harmful effects of smoke, in the 1990s the tobacco industry launched public relations campaigns about "sound science" and "good epidemiology practices" for the conduct of epidemiological studies. With these campaigns, industry tried "to fix epidemiology proactively" proposing scientific standards of proof that placed the bar so high that a large body of research on harms would be automatically invalidated.[28] Such standards would make it increasingly more difficult to demonstrate that passive smoking, as well as other environmental factors, posed serious risks to human health.

Commercial actors have also altered the mechanisms though which evidence is used in policymaking by shaping regulatory frameworks. According to internal industry documents, from the 1990s corporations played an instrumental role in the adoption across the European Union of a set of reforms called "Better Regulation" which require that the policymaking process includes a stakeholder consultation and an impact assessment (using a cost–benefit analysis approach) of all new policy proposals.[29,30] British American Tobacco led this campaign for policy change because it predicted it would make it easier to prevent the implementation of public health policies that would negatively impact their business.[30] Corporations have successfully used these tools to ensure they are consulted and to feed industry-favorable science into the consultation and impact assessment processes, as a key part of their attempts to weaken, delay, or prevent public health policies.[31,32]

8.3 TAKE-HOME MESSAGES

The examples described in this chapter illustrate just some of the multifaceted strategies that industry uses to control evidence production, dissemination, and use. For a more comprehensive picture of this phenomenon, we refer readers to a recent evidence-based typology of industry influence on science.[33]

Two important take-home messages can be drawn. First, the previously mentioned strategies should not be considered as standalone but, rather, as part of a comprehensive corporate approach to science. All these strategies work synergistically and allow corporations to increase the production, dissemination, and use of favorable science and to minimize the same aspects of unfavorable science.[33] This promotes the consumption of industry products and undermines the adoption of public health policies that could threaten industry profitability. Second, remarkable similarities can be detected in the behaviors of different industry sectors, and this highlights the need to develop comprehensive solutions as discussed next.

8.4 WHAT CAN BE DONE

The best antidote to industry influence on science would be to change the current funding model of science. For example, the Italian Medicines Agency (Agenzia Italiana del Farmaco) has set up a program to support independent research on pharmaceuticals by requiring pharmaceutical manufacturers to contribute 5% of their yearly marketing expenditure.[34] Moreover, California and Thailand have shown that it is possible to fund research through a dedicated tax on tobacco and alcohol.[35] These innovative funding models based on legally mandated contributions or dedicated manufacturer taxes could be implemented in several areas to allow independent research on chemicals, nutrition, alcohol, etc.[35] Such models would also have advantages for the corporate sector, enabling them to fund the best researchers who increasingly reject funding from such sectors. Criteria have been developed on which such a tax-based model of funding could be administered to ensure independence.[36]

These solutions would require an urgently needed paradigm change, but meanwhile, short-term solutions—although partial and insufficient—could be implemented. The easiest first step would be to increase transparency. Despite the policy consensus on the importance of transparency, disclosures of funding source and conflict of interest are still inconsistent and incomplete.[37] These shortcomings could be overcome by the creation of a publicly accessible and author-centric registry of financial interests.[38] However, it is important to note that transparency is not a panacea, and it may actually have "adverse effects."[39]

In the current era in which research partnerships between academia and the commercial sector are increasingly encouraged as a tool to accelerate innovation with apparently little concern for or safeguards against possible detrimental impacts, another solution could be for universities to enforce robust mechanisms for reviewing industry funding. A useful framework for this assessment could be represented by the five PERIL indicators that focus on purpose (degree to which the purposes of the donor and of the recipient organization diverge), extent (degree to which the recipient organization is dependent on that specific funding source), relevant harm (level of harm generated by the product of the sponsor, identifiers (extent to which the donor is visibly associated with the recipient organization, for example, via logos), and link (whether the funding is received directly from the industry or via an independent intermediary body).[40] Applying the PERIL criteria could help research organizations break down risks when considering whether to accept industry funding.

Universities and research institutes should also develop strict institutional conflict of interest policies for their investigators. A clear institutional policy would provide researchers with a road map to follow and would free them from deciding on their own what is appropriate and what is not when they interact with commercial sponsors. In the area of pharmaceutical promotion, the introduction of institutional policies on acceptance of gifts from pharmaceutical representatives has been associated with reduced prescribing of newly approved psychotropic drugs.[41] It would be important for future studies to investigate the impact that policies on investigators' conflict of interest have on research outputs.

Finally, the previously mentioned top-down solutions need to be coupled with bottom-up approaches. Training on research integrity and industry influence on science should become part of the mandatory curriculum of academic programs because most students are currently not exposed to these topics during their pre- and postgraduate training. Top-down solutions can never replace the attention that researchers should have for their own integrity and independence.

REFERENCES

1. Hirayama T. Non-smoking wives of heavy smokers have a higher risk of lung cancer: A study from Japan. *BMJ*. 1981; 282(6259): 183–185.
2. Ong E, Glantz SA. Hirayama's work has stood the test of time. *Bull World Health Organ*. 2000; 78(7): 938–939.
3. Lee PN. "Marriage to a smoker" may not be a valid marker of exposure in studies relating environmental tobacco smoke to risk of lung cancer in Japanese non-smoking women. *Int Arch Occup Environ Health*. 1995; 67(5): 287–294.
4. Hong M-K, Bero LA. How the tobacco industry responded to an influential study of the health effects of secondhand smoke. *BMJ*. 2002; 325(7377): 1413–1416.
5. Lenzer J. FDA is incapable of protecting US "against another Vioxx." *BMJ*. 2004; 329(7477): 1253.
6. Krumholz HM, Ross JS, Presler AH, Egilman DS. What have we learnt from Vioxx? *BMJ*. 2007; 334(7585): 120–123.
7. Ross JS, Hill KP, Egilman DS, Krumholz HM. Guest authorship and ghostwriting in publications related to rofecoxib: A case study of industry documents from rofecoxib litigation. *JAMA*. 2008; 299(15): 1800–1812.

8. Waxman H. Re: The marketing of Vioxx to physicians. Memorandum to Democratic Members of the Government Reform Committee Congress of the United States. May 5, 2005.

9. Ulucanlar S, Fooks GJ, Gilmore AB. The policy dystopia model: An interpretive analysis of tobacco industry political activity. *PLoS Med*. 2016; 13(9): e1002125.

10. Lundh A, Lexchin J, Mintzes B, Schroll JB, Bero L. Industry sponsorship and research outcome. *Cochrane Database Syst Rev*. 2017; 2(2). doi:10.1002/14651858. MR000033.pub3.

11. Adekunle L, Chen R, Morrison L, et al. Association between financial links to indoor tanning industry and conclusions of published studies on indoor tanning: Systematic review. *BMJ*. 2020; 368: m7.

12. Gøtzsche PC, Hróbjartsson A, Johansen HK, Haahr MT, Altman DG, Chan A-W. Constraints on publication rights in industry-initiated clinical trials. *JAMA*. 2006; 295(14): 1645–1646.

13. Fabbri A, Lai A, Grundy Q, Bero LA. The influence of industry sponsorship on the research agenda: A scoping review. *Am J Public Health*. 2018; 108(11): e9–e16.

14. Kearns CE, Glantz SA, Schmidt LA. Sugar industry influence on the scientific agenda of the National Institute of Dental Research's 1971 National Caries Program: A historical analysis of internal documents. *PLoS Med*. 2015; 12(3): e1001798.

15. O'Connor A. Coca-Cola funds scientists who shift blame for obesity away from bad diets. *The New York Times*. August 9, 2015. https://well.blogs.nyti mes.com/2015/08/09/coca-cola-funds-scientists-who-shift-blame-for-obes ity-away-from-bad-diets

16. Nestle M. *Soda Politics: Taking on Big Soda (and Winning)*. Oxford University Press; 2015.

17. Smith R. Medical journals and pharmaceutical companies: Uneasy bedfellows. *BMJ*. 2003; 326(7400): 1202–1205.

18. Moynihan R. Key opinion leaders: Independent experts or drug representatives in disguise? *BMJ*. 2008; 336(7658): 1402–1403.

19. Apollonio DE, Bero LA. The creation of industry front groups: The tobacco industry and "Get Government Off Our Back." *Am J Public Health*. 2007; 97(3): 419–427.

20. Mooney C. Some like it hot. *Mother Jones*. 2005. https://www.motherjones.com/environment/2005/05/some-it-hot

21. Babor TF. Alcohol research and the alcoholic beverage industry: Issues, concerns and conflicts of interest. *Addiction*. 2009; 104(Suppl 1): 34–47.

22. Steinman MA, Bero LA, Chren M-M. Landefeld CS. Narrative review: The promotion of gabapentin: An analysis of internal industry documents. *Ann Intern Med*. 2006; 145(4): 284–293.

23. Yeh JS, Franklin JM, Avorn J, Landon J, Kesselheim AS. Association of industry payments to physicians with the prescribing of brand-name statins in Massachusetts. *JAMA Intern Med*. 2016; 176(6): 763–768.

24. Lilienfeld DE. The silence: The asbestos industry and early occupational cancer research—A case study. *Am J Public Health*. 1991; 81(6): 791–800.

25. Bero L. Implications of the tobacco industry documents for public health and policy. *Annu Rev Public Health*. 2003; 24: 267–288.

26. McCulloch J, Tweedale G. Shooting the messenger: The vilification of Irving J. Selikoff. *Int J Health Serv*. 2007; 37(4): 619–634.

27. Union of Concerned Scientists. Heads they win, tails we lose: How corporations corrupt science at the public's expense. February 17, 2012. https://www.ucsusa.org/resources/heads-they-win-tails-we-lose

28. Ong EK, Glantz SA. Constructing "sound science" and "good epidemiology": Tobacco, lawyers, and public relations firms. *Am J Public Health*. 2001; 91(11): 1749–1757.

29. Smith KE, Fooks G, Collin J, Weishaar H, Mandal S, Gilmore AB. "Working the system"—British American Tobacco's influence on the European Union treaty and its implications for policy: An analysis of internal tobacco industry documents. *PLoS Med*. 2010; 7(1): e1000202.

30. Smith KE, Fooks G, Gilmore AB, Collin J, Weishaar H. Corporate coalitions and policy making in the European Union: How and why British American Tobacco promoted "Better Regulation." *J Health Polit Policy Law*. 2015; 40(2): 325–372.

31. Evans-Reeves KA, Hatchard JL, Gilmore AB. "It will harm business and increase illicit trade": An evaluation of the relevance, quality and transparency of evidence submitted by transnational tobacco companies to the UK consultation on standardised packaging 2012. *Tobacco Control*. 2015; 24(e2): e168–e177.

32. Ulucanlar S, Fooks GJ, Hatchard JL, Gilmore AB. Representation and misrepresentation of scientific evidence in contemporary tobacco regulation: A review of tobacco industry submissions to the UK government consultation on standardised packaging. *PLoS Med*. 2014; 11(3): e1001629.

33. Legg T, Hatchard J, Gilmore AB. The science for profit model—How and why corporations influence science and the use of science in policy and practice. *PLoS One*. 2021; 16(6): e0253272.

34. Agenzia Italiana del Farmaco. Independent research on drugs funded by the Italian Medicines Agency. n.d. http://www.agenziafarmaco.gov.it/wscs_render_attachment_by_id/tipo_file0109.pdf?

35. Gilmore AB, Capewell S. Should we welcome food industry funding of public health research? No. *BMJ*. 2016; 353: i2161.

36. Cohen JE, Zeller M, Eissenberg T, et al. Criteria for evaluating tobacco control research funding programs and their application to models that include financial support from the tobacco industry. *Tobacco Control*. 2009; 18(3): 228–234.

37. Grundy Q, Dunn AG, Bero L. Improving researchers' conflict of interest declarations. *BMJ*. 2020; 368: m422.

38. Dunn AG, Coiera E, Mandl KD, Bourgeois FT. Conflict of interest disclosure in biomedical research: A review of current practices, biases, and the role of public registries in improving transparency. *Res Integr Peer Rev*. 2016; 1(1): 1.

39. Cain D, Loewenstein G, Moore D. The dirt on coming clean: Perverse effects of disclosing conflicts of interest. *J Legal Stud*. 2005; 34: 1–25.

40. Adams PJ. Assessing whether to receive funding support from tobacco, alcohol, gambling and other dangerous consumption industries. *Addiction*. 2007; 102(7): 1027–1033.

41. King M, Essick C, Bearman P, Ross JS. Medical school gift restriction policies and physician prescribing of newly marketed psychotropic medications: Difference-in-differences analysis. *BMJ*. 2013; 346: f264.

CHAPTER 9

Role in Trade Deals and Investment

PEPITA BARLOW AND ERIC CROSBIE

9.1 INTRODUCTION

The reintegration of national economies after World War II was arguably one of
the most significant developments of the 20th century. Global trade increased
27-fold between 1950 and 2008, and although trade growth has slowed in
recent years, trade remains a major source of income, accounting for 60% of
global gross domestic product in 2019.[1] The lives and livelihoods of the world's
inhabitants were undoubtedly transformed as a consequence. Trade integration created jobs and raised wages by creating demand for exported goods,
thereby lifting households out of poverty.[2] At the same time, trade promoted
peace and political cooperation between countries.[3]

Yet trade also has downsides. The menu of goods on offer through trade,
and the actions of their purveyors, can be detrimental to health. Today, global
trade is dominated by transnational corporations (TNCs). According to one
estimate, TNCs account for as much as two-thirds of global trade.[4] TNCs' expansion into new markets was facilitated by reductions in trade and investment costs due, in part, to intercountry trade deals. Coca-Cola, McDonald's,
and Nestle are among the many companies that benefitted from these deals
and whose brands are archetypal symbols of contemporary globalization, including in low- and middle-income countries (LMICs). As TNCs expanded
into new markets, they exported and aggressively marketed a feast of calorie-
dense ultra-processed foods and sugary drinks.[5] In so doing, they contributed
to a widespread rise of diseases caused by unhealthy diets, including obesity
and diabetes.[6] Once dubbed "diseases of affluence," these illnesses are now increasingly common in the world's poorest countries, many of which still suffer
from high rates of undernutrition.[7,8]

Pepita Barlow and Eric Crosbie, *Role in Trade Deals and Investment* In: *The Commercial Determinants of Health.*
Edited by: Nason Maani, Mark Petticrew, and Sandro Galea, Oxford University Press. © Oxford University Press 2023.
DOI: 10.1093/oso/9780197578742.003.0009

As set out in this chapter, the role of trade deals in facilitating corporate influence on the quantity, nutritional quality, and diversity of foods we import and eat is but one example of the many ways in which corporate actors impact peoples' opportunities for living long and healthy lives through trade. The following sections describe free trade agreements (FTAs) in further detail and how they affect health via impacts on regulatory environments and consumption of health-damaging and health-promoting products, employment, production, the environment, medicines, health care, and policy.[9]

9.2 TRADE REGIMES IN THE 20TH AND 21ST CENTURIES

Since the early 1990s, governments worldwide have increasingly sought to promote international trade and investment by negotiating FTAs. These treaties are designed to reduce barriers to cross-border trade and investment. They are sometimes known as regional trade agreements, when signed by several members in a geographic region, or preferential trade agreements, because they grant preferential market access to signatories. In the early 1990s, there were 22 FTAs globally; as of June 17, 2022, there were 355 in force.[10] One example is the recently renegotiated United States–Mexico–Canada Agreement, which became effective in July 2020 and replaced the North American Free Trade Agreement, established in 1994.

FTAs incorporate rules that many governments sign as members of the World Trade Organization (WTO), a multilateral organization established in 1995. WTO members commit to reducing trade taxes and tariffs and to further rules designed to prevent regulatory differences between states ("nontariff" trade barriers). Such commitments are made when members sign a suite of agreements on accession. The agreements cover goods, via the General Agreement on Trade and Tariffs; services, via the General Agreement on Trade in Services; and intellectual property (e.g., trademarks, patents, and copyright), via the Agreement on Trade-Related Aspects of Intellectual Property Rights (TRIPS). These accompany a suite of additional agreements, rules, and procedures for resolving disputes between states ("state–state disputes"). Such disputes arise when a member government believes another member government is violating an agreement or a commitment that it has made in the WTO—including through policies designed to protect health but that have a detrimental impact on trade.

FTAs go a step further than WTO rules via "TRIPS-plus" measures that extend the intellectual property provisions in TRIPS, and additional measures that avoid "behind the border" trade barriers through, for example, the harmonization of existing regulations.[3] Clauses that set investor protections and investor–state dispute settlement (ISDS) procedures are particularly controversial. These allow TNCs to directly sue a government, including where public health policy affects a TNC's future profits, and they were first incorporated in U.S. FTAs following aggressive lobbying from TNCs. Additional clauses in FTAs relate to Good Regulatory Practices (GRPs), which can include requirements for industry consultation during regulatory discussions. GRP principles can provide a right for industry stakeholders to contest policy choices early in the policy development process[11] rather than ISDS, which only occurs after a policy has been enacted.

9.3 IMPACTS ON UPSTREAM DETERMINANTS OF HEALTH

Proponents of FTAs have argued that they promote well-being through their beneficial economic impacts.[12] Although economic gains from FTAs may well foster improvements in human welfare, such benefits are not guaranteed, are distributed unevenly, and can accompany substantial harms. In short, FTAs can have both beneficial and deleterious impacts on the upstream determinants of health. By facilitating both commercial and political activities by TNCs in new jurisdictions, FTAs influence the consumption of health-promoting and health-damaging products, working conditions and employment, and the environment.[9] Furthermore, the creation of new policy and dispute-resolution rules enables TNCs to exert political pressure on governments seeking to introduce new health regulations, thereby constraining government policy.

9.3.1 Consumption of Health-Damaging and Health-Promoting Products

Increased exports and foreign investment by TNCs as a result of FTAs can alter the quantity, quality, and price of health-promoting and health-damaging goods, as well as the extent to which consumers are exposed to marketing and advertising of these products. For example, by expanding trade, FTAs can impact the consumption of unhealthy commodities and their ingredients, including ultra-processed and calorie-dense foods, sugar and sugary drinks, tobacco, and alcohol.[12] This happens where tariff barriers are reduced and imports of these products rise as TNCs expand investment for local production and sale, leading to lower prices. Both foreign and domestic producers of these products respond to rising competition as a result of trade by lowering their prices or expanding their marketing efforts.

The association between trade liberalization, market entry by TNCs, and unhealthy commodity consumption has been widely documented. For example, one study reported that per capita cigarette consumption increased by 10% in Taiwan, Japan, South Korea, and Thailand after they implemented tariff reductions via trade agreements with the United States in the early

1990s.[13] Several studies have documented increases in the quantity of processed snack foods, sugar, sugary drinks, and total calories consumed after countries ratified FTAs, especially with the United States.[14,15] For example, Canada's trade deals with the United States in 1989 and 1994 led to a threefold increase in the amount of high-fructose corn syrup used in food production and a 170 kcal per person per day increase in the number of calories that Canadians are estimated to have consumed.[16,17] There is comparatively little research documenting increases in alcohol consumption, although transnational alcohol companies are quickly expanding their market share, sales, and marketing efforts in LMICs. For example, Anheuser-Busch InBev, the world's largest alcohol beverage company, sells its products in more than 150 countries.[18] Their expansion was likely aided by FTAs.

Trade and investment also promote consumption of health-promoting products. By raising wages and employment, FTAs can increase access to health-sustaining public services such as health care and education, as well as other goods and services that are essential to good health, such as housing.[19] Furthermore, it has long been argued that trade promotes food security. By increasing food imports, lowering food prices, smoothing supply during weather shocks, and fostering income gains that enable households to afford food, trade enables households to purchase sufficient food, on a consistent basis, throughout the year.[20] One study of almost half a million households in 132 countries reported that food insecurity was indeed lowest in the most liberalized developed economies.[21] However, for many low-income households, these benefits failed to materialize, especially in the poorest countries. This underscores how the impacts of trade vary substantially both within and between countries. These distributional differences can be far more pronounced than aggregate effects, as has been demonstrated in studies examining the effects of trade on health outcomes that are heavily influenced by nutrition, such as child mortality, and research on the employment-related effects of FTAs, as discussed below.[19,22]

9.3.2 Production, Work, and the Environment

Free trade agreements alter the quantity, scope, and intensity of commercial production, thereby influencing employment, wages, job insecurity, and working conditions—all of which affect physical and mental health.[23,24] For example, FTAs can impact health via changing employment and wages, as illustrated in a study of U.S. mortality.[25] Pierce and Schott[25] analyzed whether import competition from China as a result of U.S. trade legislation affected deaths from causes linked to unemployment and financial insecurity—so-called deaths of despair. There was substantial variation in the extent to which local businesses were affected by import competition following the bill's passage. The counties with the highest concentrations of businesses that were exposed to import competition experienced rising unemployment and wage stagnation. The authors found that deaths of despair increased substantially in these counties. Moving from the 25th to 75th percentile of exposure to import competition was associated with an increase in the mortality rate from drug overdoses by 2 or 3 deaths per 100,000 people each year after the policy.

Another consequence arises from intensified production, work injuries, stress, and illnesses as a result of rising export demand following tariff declines. One study assessed these outcomes in China after it joined the WTO and found a 7.6% increase in the probability that an individual experienced an illness or injury for every one standard deviation increase in exposure to tariff declines.[26] These findings applied only to the least-skilled workers. For high-skilled workers and those with the highest levels of educational attainment, tariff exposure correlated with reduced illness or injury rates.

Changes to commercial production as a result of FTAs also have implications for health via their impacts on the environment. Some effects are beneficial. Many FTAs contain provisions seeking to enhance environmental protections; participation in these agreements is associated with reduced air pollution.[27] However, much depends on whether production is reallocated toward more environment-damaging activities or to countries with lower environmental standards. Furthermore, import demand in one country can have environmental and health impacts elsewhere. One study estimated that international trade in 2007 alone caused a shift of more than 700,000 global pollution-related deaths away from regions that import goods to those that produce and export them.[28] High-income countries are also major exporters of hazardous materials to low-income countries.[29] In addition, deforestation is partially driven by trade and can increase the spread of infectious diseases by exposing local and global populations to novel pathogens.[30]

9.3.3 Medicines, Health Care, and Policy

Free trade agreements facilitate the impact of TNCs on upstream determinants of access to medicines, health services, and policy. Trade in pharmaceutical goods accounted for 3.2% of total world merchandise trade in 2019, and trade in medical instruments, appliances, and diagnostic apparatus is rising rapidly.[31] Trade by TNCs can increase access to medical products and treatments, leading to better quality care and improved clinical outcomes. However, FTAs can also create pressures on health systems due to clauses that impact the availability, affordability, and access to medicines. Clauses that expand on the intellectual property provisions in TRIPS are contested. Extensions to patent protections and data exclusivity in these TRIPS-plus clauses are said to inflate medicine prices, delay the manufacture of generic medicines, and reduce their affordability and access to them.[32] Transnational pharmaceutical corporations support these clauses, arguing that they facilitate research and development. However, studies conducted in the Dominican Republic, Costa Rica, Colombia, and Jordan reported that public spending on medicines was hundreds of millions of dollars higher due to the increased proportion of active pharmaceutical ingredients subject to exclusive rights in their respective FTAs with the United States.[33(p261)]

Impacts on health systems extend beyond the pharmaceutical sector. FTAs also contain clauses or "legal weapons" that TNCs use to exert political pressure on governments to alter, abandon, or delay effective health regulations. For example, WTO members are obliged to design new regulations and policies that avoid "unnecessary trade costs" because the stated objective of the measure could be achieved with a less costly alternative. Research indicates that WTO members often cite WTO rules to dispute or challenge a health policy that introduces trade costs at a TNC's request.[34] TNCs can further invoke ISDS clauses (and other FTA rules) to initiate a trade dispute where new regulations are considered to be an "expropriation" of the value of their investment. This often includes "indirect expropriation," which can be said to arise where government measures could affect the value of an investment—including anticipated future profitability.[3] ISDS provisions enable TNCs to challenge and potentially block, weaken, and delay health policies that could protect health by disputing the measure in international courts or pre-dispute meetings. A prominent example occurred in 2011 when the international tobacco firm Philip Morris brought an ISDS case against the Australian Government to seek compensation for the impact of its tobacco plain packaging law.[35] Tobacco companies also lobbied and paid Cuba, the Dominican Republic, Honduras, Indonesia, and Ukraine to challenge Australia's plain packaging law at the WTO.[36]

Although the courts ruled in favor of Australia, the legal battle was costly: It was reported that Australia spent $40 million defending its world-first plain packaging laws in these international courts. Fear of such costs is an important mechanism through which the use of FTAs by TNCs can impact policy decisions. TNCs can influence policy by using trade rules to threaten a dispute. This in turn can have a "chilling effect" on policy, whereupon governments delay, alter, or abandon a health regulation in order to avoid a dispute and associated costs. These pre-dispute challenges or legal threats appear to be far more common than formal trade disputes.[37] For example, a range of health policies, including noncommunicable disease prevention measures, have been challenged at WTO and were followed by policy change without escalating to a dispute. One recent example occurred in 2019 when Saudi Arabia proposed an upper limit on the amount of sugar in snack foods: Saudi Arabia abandoned the policy after several WTO members argued (in a pre-dispute challenge) that the measure was inconsistent with WTO commitments.[38]

9.4 TRADE, FREE TRADE AGREEMENTS, AND CORPORATE POWER

The pathways discussed in this chapter demonstrate how FTAs influence the upstream determinants of health. By facilitating corporations' commercial and political activities, FTAs can subsequently constrain governments' ability to regulate and can impact consumption of health-promoting or health-damaging products, employment and working conditions, the environment, health care and access to medicines, and policy.

To the extent any form of influence implies the exercise of power, FTAs are a vehicle for the exercise of corporate power on health. This is enabled by specific clauses within these deals—reflecting the disproportionate power of corporations. Trade negotiations often privilege the consideration of corporate interests because corporate representatives occupy positions on governmental trade committees and large corporations have considerable financial resources to lobby trade negotiators. By comparison, health officials often lack such resources and are seldom given a "seat at the table" in trade committee discussions.[39] Furthermore, governments in LMICs typically have fewer resources to devote to legal disputes and are therefore more likely to be targeted by wealthy corporations and nations and also more likely to acquiesce to their demands.[37] As such, the design of FTAs, and the health damages that arise as a result, reflects this wider power imbalance.

In order to develop healthier trade policies in the future, it will be necessary to re-balance the structure of trade negotiations and trade governance to ensure that opportunities for health protection are realized. Several steps can be taken in this regard. First, any doubt about whether health policies are allowable within trade agreements can be addressed when they are negotiated and written. Second, the use of ISDS and GRP can be removed or severely restricted to not allow TNCs to intimidate and directly challenge progressive public health policies, especially in LMICs with few financial resources to devote to legal disputes. Third, existing trade agreements with ISDS and GRP could be renegotiated to remove these clauses. Finally, trade negotiations and disputes should be more transparent, enabling civil society and public health advocates to analyze their impacts. Transparency also enables the public to hold governments accountable when they fail to protect populations from harm—as has often happened as a result of past FTAs and must be avoided in the future.

REFERENCES

1. World Bank. *World Development Indicators*. World Bank Group; 2018.
2. Winters LA. Trade liberalisation and poverty: What are the links? *World Econ.* 2002; 25(9): 1339–1367. doi:10.1111/1467-9701.00495
3. Dür A, Baccini L, Elsig M. The design of international trade agreements: Introducing a new dataset. *Rev Int Organ.* 2014; 9(3): 353–375. doi:10.1007/s11558-013-9179-8

4. United Nations Conference on Trade and Development. *World investment report 2018*. United Nations; 2018.

5. Stuckler D, Nestle M. Big food, food systems, and global health. *PLoS Med*. 2012; 9(6): 7. doi:10.1371/journal.pmed.1001242

6. Baker P, Machado P, Santos T, et al. Ultra-processed foods and the nutrition transition: Global, regional and national trends, food systems transformations and political economy drivers. *Obes Rev*. 2020; 21(12): e13126. https://doi.org/10.1111/obr.13126

7. McKeown T. *The Origins of Human Disease Continued*. Basil Blackwell; 1988.

8. Hooper L, Bartlett C, Davey SG, Ebrahim S. Advice to reduce dietary salt for prevention of cardiovascular disease. *Cochrane Database Syst Rev*. 2004; 2004(1): CD003656. doi:10.1002/14651858.CD003656.pub2

9. Barlow P, McKee M, Basu S, Stuckler D. The health impact of trade and investment agreements: A quantitative systematic review and network co-citation analysis. *Global Health*. 2017; 13(1): 13.

10. World Trade Organization. Regional trade agreements database. 2021. Accessed March 17, 2021. https://rtais.wto.org/UI/charts.aspx

11. Labonté R, Crosbie E, Gleeson D, McNamara C. USMCA (NAFTA 2.0): Tightening the constraints on the right to regulate for public health. *Global Health*. 2019; 15(1): 1–15.

12. Friel S, Hattersley L, Townsend R. Trade policy and public health. *Annu Rev Public Health*. 2015; 36(1): 325–344. doi:10.1146/annurev-publhealth-031914-122739

13. Chaloupka FJ, Laixuthai A. U.S trade policy and cigarette smoking in Asia. NBER Working Paper No. 5543. April 1996. doi:10.3386/w5543

14. Cowling K, Stuart EA, Neff RA, Vernick J, Magraw D, Pollack Porter K. The relationship between joining a US free trade agreement and processed food sales, 2002–2016: A comparative interrupted time-series analysis. *Public Health Nutr*. 2020; 23(9): 1609–1617. doi:10.1017/S1368980019003999

15. Barlow P, Sanap R, Garde A, Winters LA, Mabhala MA, Thow AM. Reassessing the health impacts of trade and investment agreements: A systematic review of quantitative studies, 2016–20. *Lancet Planet Health*. 2022; 6(5): e431–e438.

16. Barlow P, McKee M, Stuckler D. The impact of U.S. free trade agreements on calorie availability and obesity: A natural experiment in Canada. *Am J Prev Med*. 2018; 54(5): 637–643.

17. Barlow P, McKee M, Basu S, Stuckler D. Impact of the North American Free Trade Agreement on high-fructose corn syrup supply in Canada: A natural experiment using synthetic control methods. *CMAJ*. 2017; 189(26): E881–E887. doi:10.1503/cmaj.161152

18. ABInBev. Anheuser-Busch InBev reports fourth quarter and full year 2020 results. 2021. Accessed March 18, 2021. https://www.ab-inbev.com/content/dam/abinbev/news-media/press-releases/2021/02/AB%20InBev_Press%20Release_EN_FY20_FINAL.pdf

19. Barlow P. Does trade liberalization reduce child mortality in low- and middle-income countries? A synthetic control analysis of 36 policy experiments, 1963–2005. *Soc Sci Med*. 2018; 205: 107–115.

20. Clapp J. *Food Security and International Trade: Unpacking Disputed Narratives*. United Nations Food and Agricultural Organisation; 2015.

21. Barlow P, Loopstra R, Tarasuk V, Reeves A. Liberal trade policy and food insecurity across the income distribution: An observational analysis in 132 countries, 2014–17. *Lancet Glob Health*. 2020; 8(8): e1090–e1097.

22. Panda P. Does trade reduce infant mortality? Evidence from sub-Saharan Africa. *World Dev*. 2020; 128: 104851.

23. Paul KI, Moser K. Unemployment impairs mental health: Meta-analyses. *J Vocat Behav*. 2009; 74(3): 264–282. doi:10.1016/j.jvb.2009.01.001

24. Benavides FG, Benach J, Diez-Roux AV, Roman C. How do types of employment relate to health indicators? Findings from the second European survey on working conditions. *J Epidemiol Community Health*. 2000; 54(7): 494–501. doi:10.1136/jech.54.7.494

25. Pierce JR, Schott PK. Trade liberalization and mortality: Evidence from US counties. *Am Econ Rev Insights*. 2020; 2(1): 47–64.

26. Fan H, Lin F, Lin S. The hidden cost of trade liberalization: Input tariff shocks and worker health in China. *J Int Econ*. 2020: 103349.

27. Brandi C, Schwab J, Berger A, Morin J-F. Do environmental provisions in trade agreements make exports from developing countries greener? *World Dev*. 2020; 129: 104899. https://doi.org/10.1016/j.worlddev.2020.104899

28. Zhang Q, Jiang X, Tong D, et al. Transboundary health impacts of transported global air pollution and international trade. *Nature*. 2017; 543(7647): 705–709. doi:10.1038/nature21712

29. Ogunseitan OA, Schoenung JM, Saphores J-DM, Shapiro AA. The electronics revolution: From e-wonderland to e-wasteland. *Science*. 2009; 326(5953): 670–671.

30. DeFries RS, Rudel T, Uriarte M, Hansen M. Deforestation driven by urban population growth and agricultural trade in the twenty-first century. *Nat Geosci*. 2010; 3(3): 178–181.

31. IHS Markit. Trade in pharmaceuticals and medical goods in 2019 and COVID-19 implications for 2020. 2021. Accessed March 17, 2021. https://ihsmarkit.com/resea rch-analysis/trade-in-pharmaceuticals-and-medical-goods-in-2019-and-covid19.html

32. Gleeson D, Lexchin J, Labonté R, et al. Analyzing the impact of trade and investment agreements on pharmaceutical policy: Provisions, pathways and potential impacts. *Global Health*. 2019; 15(1): 78.

33. World Health Organization. *Promoting Access to Medical Technologies and Innovation: Intersections Between Public Health, Intellectual Property and Trade*. World Health Organization; 2020.

34. Barlow P, Gleeson D, O'Brien P, Labonte R. Industry influence over global alcohol policies via the World Trade Organization: A qualitative analysis of discussions on alcohol health warning labelling, 2010–19. *Lancet Glob Health*. 2022; 10(3): e429–e437.

35. Knaus C. Philip Morris cigarettes charged millions after losing plain packaging case against Australia. *The Guardian*. 2017. Accessed July 10, 2017. https://www.theguardian.com/business/2017/jul/10/philip-morris-cigarettes-charged-milli ons-after-losing-plain-packaging-case-against-australia

36. Jarman H. Attack on Australia: Tobacco industry challenges to plain packaging. *J Public Health Policy*. 2013; 34(3): 375–387. doi:10.1057/jphp.2013.18

37. Barlow P, Labonte R, McKee M, Stuckler D. Trade challenges at the World Trade Organization to national noncommunicable disease prevention policies: A thematic document analysis of trade and health policy space. *PLoS Med*. 2018; 15(6): e1002590.

38. World Trade Organization. Addendum to technical regulation (G/TBT/N/SAU/1108/Add.2).

39. Jarman H. Trade policy governance: What health policymakers and advocates need to know. *Health Policy*. 2017; 121(11): 1105–1112.

SECTION 3

Case Studies by Industry

CHAPTER 10

Hidden from View

Alcohol Industry Efforts to Keep the Epidemic of
Alcohol-Related Harm from Public Awareness

TIM STOCKWELL AND ERIN HOBIN

10.1 INTRODUCTION

Alcohol is perhaps the most ancient of psychoactive substances, with evidence of its manufacture and use dating back to Neolithic times, some 8,000 years or more in the past.[1] Alcohol can be manufactured from almost any plant, fruit, or seed, and it even occurs naturally without active cultivation. In the modern world, global and hugely profitable commercial operations efficiently cultivate the necessary plant ingredients and then manufacture, store, distribute, market, and retail alcoholic beverages to suit every taste, every occasion, and every budget. Alcohol is now more available, affordable, and acceptable to more people on the planet than ever before. Its use, however, has been causally linked by scientists to several hundred varieties of acute and chronic health problems.[2] Despite the global burden caused by alcohol, the great majority of the world's population is unaware of either the scope or the scale of alcohol's risk to health. In this chapter, we discuss the ways in which commercial vested interests in the production and sale of alcohol maintain their huge global markets, thereby helping sustain its burden on health, safety, and well-being. We also highlight public policies that can improve public health and safety outcomes while having less impact on the profitability of alcohol producers and retailers, such as minimum unit pricing (MUP).[3]

Tim Stockwell and Erin Hobin, Hidden from View In: *The Commercial Determinants of Health*. Edited by: Nason Maani, Mark Petticrew, and Sandro Galea, Oxford University Press. © Oxford University Press 2023. DOI: 10.1093/oso/9780197578742.003.0010

10.2 THE SCALE OF ALCOHOL'S BURDEN ON HEALTH AND WELL-BEING

The World Health Organization's Global Burden of Disease project has for some decades placed alcohol in the top 10 leading risk factors for premature death and preventable disease, injury, and disability. Precise methods and underlying assumptions for estimation have varied throughout the years, but the scale of alcohol-attributable harm globally is estimated to be 3 million preventable deaths annually and 90 million disability-adjusted life years.[4] This is a slightly higher level of harm globally than that from the COVID-19 pandemic in its first year[5] and three times greater than the extent of harm attributable to all other psychoactive substances combined, with the exception of tobacco.[4]

Alcohol has a special status in many modern societies as a widely used substance that accompanies most social occasions and celebrations; is heavily marketed across traditional and new digital media; and can be purchased alongside grocery items, and increasingly, even delivered to one's doorstep. Popular demand for and the wide use of alcohol in many societies appear to have blinded consumers to its risks.[6] An example of a real but underappreciated health consequence of alcohol is cancer. A recent UK study found that only 13% of survey respondents identified alcohol as a carcinogen without prompting,[7] despite recent estimates of more than 740,000 alcohol-attributable deaths per year globally or 4.1% of all cancer deaths. Multinational drink companies and governments of countries with high alcohol production have worked hard to ensure the general public is unaware of the cancer risk, or indeed most risks, from alcohol use. This has included working through the World Trade Organization to successfully oppose cancer warning labels in Thailand,[8] for example, and the use of legal threats to obstruct publicly funded research examining the effectiveness of cancer warning labels on alcohol containers in a remote northern territory in Canada.[9]

10.3 THE COMMERCIAL VESTED INTEREST IN HAZARDOUS ALCOHOL CONSUMPTION

Alcohol industry advocates often maintain that the great majority of consumers use its product "responsibly" and that only a very small number of people misuse it and experience problems. This point of view is easier to defend when analyses are conducted of average consumption levels in a population as estimated from self-report surveys and when conservative criteria are applied.

The International Alcohol Control (IAC) study group recently estimated the proportion of alcohol consumed in different countries on high-risk drinking occasions, defined as consuming five or more drinks.[10] Across multiple countries, it was estimated that between 50% and 60% of alcohol purchased was consumed by people on high-risk drinking occasions. It is notable that the IAC alcohol survey methodology involves detailed questions on precise typical quantities drunk across multiple drinking contexts and does not suffer from the same degree of underreporting that plagues most national self-report surveys.

Other studies of self-report data have made direct adjustments for underreporting, principally by comparing total self-reported per capita consumption against estimates based on official alcohol sales. Typically, self-report surveys only account for between one-third and one-half of the alcohol known to have been sold in a country.[11] Zhao et al.[12] used a large national Canadian survey to estimate the proportion of alcohol consumed above the then generous national Low Risk Drinking Guidelines (LRDGs) after adjustment for underreporting. Two significant results emerged. First, unadjusted estimates showed that only 7% of respondents reported exceeding Canada's LRDGs but that, in fact, after adjustment for underreporting, 27% exceeded guidelines for minimizing long-term health risks and 39% exceeded guidelines for short-term risks. Second, as with the IAC study, it was also shown that the great majority of alcoholic drinks consumed in a year by Canadians were drunk on occasions when LRDGs were exceeded: 68% of drinks were consumed in a pattern that consistently exceeded risk levels for long-term harm, and as many as 81% were consumed on risky drinking occasions.[12]

These data starkly highlight the extreme conflict of interest that applies to all commercial operators who profit from the production, retail, and marketing of alcoholic beverages with regard to public health and safety issues: The great majority of their profits rely on the hazardous consumption of their product.

10.4 IMPLICATIONS OF THE TOTAL CONSUMPTION MODEL OF ALCOHOL-RELATED HARM

The idea that the total alcohol consumption of a population directly predicts the resulting amount of alcohol-related harm is relatively new. Kettil Bruun and colleagues[13] first proposed this idea in 1975 in their controversial book, *Alcohol Control Policies in Public Health Perspective*, providing evidence mainly from Scandinavia and North America that adverse outcomes such as deaths from liver cirrhosis and cases of violent crime rise and fall with the total amount of alcohol consumed in a society. Although it is definitely the case that drinking patterns and contexts contribute to the risk from drinking in addition to the total volume consumed, strong associations have been demonstrated across scores of different countries between total per capita alcohol consumption and the number of hazardous drinkers in a population. Kehoe and colleagues[14] were able to demonstrate that alcohol consumption in a population follows a *gamma* distribution in countries from all continents—that is, the average consumption of a population reliably predicts its proportion of hazardous and harmful drinkers. This clear, mathematical relationship between total alcohol consumption and rates of harm is now widely used as the basis for estimating the burden of alcohol-related harm in a population. In the International Model for Alcohol Harm and Policy,[2] for example, it is used for estimating alcohol-attributable morbidity and mortality in a population and how these change when policies are introduced to either increase or decrease sales and consumption. The broad relationships between alcohol consumption, policies, and related harms are illustrated in Figure 10.1.

The close relationship between total population consumption and total harm from alcohol should not be surprising given the evidence described above. It is also the reason why the World Health Organization[15] has repeatedly identified reductions in per capita alcohol consumption as a primary objective for strategies to reduce alcohol-related harm, despite strong efforts by multinational alcohol producers to lobby against the use of this indicator.

The centrality of total alcohol consumption as a predictor of harm and hence as an indicator used to assess the success of public health strategies highlights the acute conflict between commercial actors and public health interests. Stated simply, when the alcohol industry collectively increases its sales and profits, public health and safety almost inevitably lose out. A few exceptions, however, of policies that allow some industry sectors to maintain or even increase their profits while selling less ethanol are discussed later in this chapter.

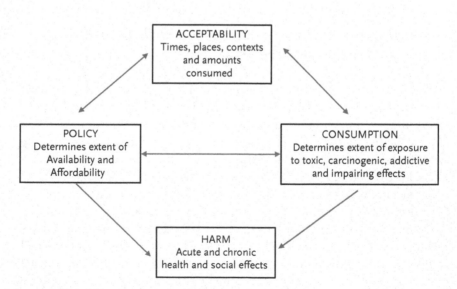

Figure 10.1 Drivers of alcohol consumption and related harm.

10.5 THE CASE FOR REGULATION OF ALCOHOL MARKETS IN THE INTEREST OF PUBLIC HEALTH

In the late 19th and early 20th centuries, principally in North America and Scandinavia, alcohol distribution and retail monopolies were introduced to regulate alcohol markets in the interests of public health and safety. Mostly diluted versions of these monopolies still exist in 17 U.S. states for sales of spirits and/or wine, in all Canadian provinces and territories, and in several Nordic countries. The Finnish (Alko) and Swedish (Systembolaget) alcohol monopolies are noteworthy for being located within Ministries for Health and Social Affairs rather than the North American approach of having these operations located usually within departments of finance, reflecting a concern with revenue collection rather than public health and safety.[16] Specifically, both Alko and Systembolaget have limits set on the profits they can make, consistent with the purpose of reducing commercial interest in the sale and distribution of alcohol. Government alcohol control systems can facilitate ready access to the key policy levers of pricing and availability, but they also need a special mandate to do so in the interests of public health and safety rather than simple free-market economics.

Government-owned distribution and retail systems result in lower alcohol consumption and related harms than do privately owned systems. In other words, removing or reducing the profit incentive from these operations is associated with improved health and safety outcomes. A systematic review of the effects of alcohol monopoly privatization events[17] estimated a median increase in per capita sales of alcoholic beverages affected by the privatization of 44.4% across 12 studies, with a range of effect sizes from 0% to 305%. Following that review, a series of studies of the effects of a gradual privatization of the retail sale of alcohol in British Columbia, Canada, was conducted. Across 89 local areas of the province, it was possible to link increases in the number of private liquor stores with increases in per capita alcohol consumption,[18] alcohol-attributable deaths,[19] and alcohol-attributable hospitalizations.[20]

10.6 COUNTERING AND REGULATING THE COMMERCIAL DETERMINANTS OF ALCOHOL-RELATED HARM

It has been well documented that during the COVID-19 pandemic, alcohol industry groups worldwide successfully lobbied to reduce restrictions on their trade in order to support the viability of constituent businesses (e.g., see Andreasson and colleagues[21]). For improved public health outcomes, the evidence points to the need for higher prices, fewer outlets, reduced hours of sale, heavily restricted marketing and advertising, higher legal drinking ages, and stronger enforcement of both liquor licensing and impaired driving laws.[22] Collectively, such measures reduce harm but also shrink alcohol markets and reduce profitability, and so are fiercely opposed by alcohol industry groups that instead advocate for lower taxes, increased availability, and fewer restrictions on marketing.

Collectively, alcohol industries engage in a variety of strategies to influence governments and protect their market against policies that would improve public health and safety outcomes. Globally, this includes the use of international trade agreements and the World Trade Organization (see Chapter 9) to restrict the power of governments to use key policies such as taxation and product labeling.[23] Multinational drink companies have also partnered with tech media giants such as Facebook and Google to create additional opportunities for marketing their products while resisting efforts to restrict these.[24] High-profile attempts have been used to create an appearance of good corporate citizenship while at the same time promoting the consumption of alcohol and nullifying public health messages. The widespread practice of promoting alcohol alongside breast cancer awareness campaigns without identifying that alcohol itself is carcinogenic is an example of such an attempt.[25] Alcohol producers and retail groups also strive to be represented on regional, national, and international alcohol strategy initiatives, including through the World Health Organization.[26] Room and colleagues[27] made a persuasive case that such efforts to subvert public health in the interests of international trade of a hazardous product make an international treaty on alcohol desirable, similar in scope and authority as those designed to place restrictions on international trade in tobacco and other psychotropic drugs, such as cannabis.

As many societies are beginning to open up social and commercial life and look to a recovery in the post-COVID-19 pandemic period, it is important that alcohol policies are not further eroded and that deregulations to support alcohol-related businesses (e.g., home delivery, longer hours, and lower wholesale prices) are not maintained indefinitely. There are a few examples of specific policies and policy mixes that can reduce harms from alcohol use and support businesses to make profits while selling less alcohol. A prime example is MUP, whereby governments enforce floor or minimum prices for a unit of alcohol (e.g., in Scotland, 50p for a "unit" or 8 g of ethanol).[28] MUP targets cheap alcohol that is favored by hazardous and harmful drinkers. Minimum pricing has been shown to reduce alcohol consumption, crime, and alcohol-related deaths.[3,29,30] By reducing price competition, it also increases profits for producers and retailers. Minimum prices have mostly been applied for off-premise liquor sales, but in Canada they are also applied in many provinces to sales from bars and restaurants. Whereas in many countries off-premise liquor sales have increased during the COVID-19 lockdowns,[31] sales from on-premise outlets (bars and restaurants) have been heavily hit. On-premise minimum prices would reduce price competition between bars and restaurants and enable operators to make more money from selling less alcohol. Although some have criticized MUP as a means of creating additional profits for the industry sector, this also presents an opportunity for those profits to be shared with government, which could also be achieved by increasing alcohol excise taxes.[9] Another virtue of MUP is its demonstrated ability to reduce health inequalities as a result of the disproportionate reductions in alcohol-related harms experienced by low-income groups.[29]

10.7 CONCLUSION

Free market economics will not work to minimize health risks in a situation where adverse consequences often occur many years after consumption of a product, and especially when harms are only partly attributable to this consumption and not usually identified as such in hospital records or on death certificates. The public health movement to reduce alcohol-related harm is needed to counter alcohol industry influence that serves to protect alcohol markets from evidence-based policies that would restrict alcohol markets and profits of producers, distributors, marketers, and retailers. The collective effects of alcohol industry lobbying have resulted in customers globally being uninformed and also misinformed about health risks of its products (e.g., carcinogenicity). This has helped create public apathy or outright opposition to effective policies that would reduce their consumption by reducing alcohol's affordability and convenience of access. There is no evidence of self-correcting behaviors among consumers who are kept in the dark about the risk of adverse consequences that may not occur for some decades.

To reduce the adverse effects of the alcohol industry on public health and safety, it is essential to minimize their influence in regional, national, and international policymaking by ensuring they play little or no part in the development of strategies to reduce alcohol-related harm.[22,32]

REFERENCES

1. Liu L, Li Y, Hou J. Making beer with malted cereals and qu starter in the Neolithic Yangshao culture, China. *J Archaeol Sci Rep.* 2020; 29: 102134.
2. Sherk A, Stockwell T, Rehm J, Dorocicz J, Shield KD. *The International Model of Alcohol Harms and Policies (InterMAHP).* Canadian Institute for Substance Use Research; 2017.
3. Taylor N, Miller P, Coomber K, et al. The impact of a minimum unit price on wholesale alcohol supply trends in the Northern Territory, Australia. *Aust N Z J Public Health.* 2021; 45(1): 26–33.
4. Peacock A, Leung J, Larney S, et al. Global statistics on alcohol, tobacco and illicit drug use: 2017 status report. *Addiction.* 2018; 113(10): 1905–1926.

5. World Health Organization. COVID-19 weekly epidemiological update data as received by WHO from national authorities, as of 7 March 2021. 2021. Accessed July 19, 2021. https://apps.who.int/iris/bitstream/handle/10665/340087/nCoV-weekly-sitrep9Mar21-eng.pdf?sequence=1

6. Madden M, McCambridge J. Alcohol marketing versus public health: David and Goliath? *Global Health*. 2021; 17(1): 45.

7. Bates S, Holmes J, Gavens L, et al. Awareness of alcohol as a risk factor for cancer is associated with public support for alcohol policies. *BMC Public Health*. 2018; 18(1): 688.

8. O'Brien P, Stockwell T, Vallance K, Room R. WHO should not support alcohol industry co-regulation of public health labelling. *Addiction*. 2021; 116(7): 1619–1621.

9. Stockwell T, Solomon R, O'Brien P, Vallance K, Hobin E. Cancer warning labels on alcohol containers: A consumer's right to know, a government's responsibility to inform, and an industry's power to thwart. *J Stud Alcohol Drugs*. 2020; 81(2): 284–292.

10. Viet Cuong P, Casswell S, Parker K, et al. Cross-country comparison of proportion of alcohol consumed in harmful drinking occasions using the International Alcohol Control Study. *Drug Alcohol Rev*. 2018; 37(Suppl 2): S45–S52.

11. Stockwell T, Zhao J, Greenfield T, Li J, Livingston M, Meng Y. Estimating under- and over-reporting of drinking in national surveys of alcohol consumption: Identification of consistent biases across four English-speaking countries. *Addiction*. 2016; 111(7): 1203–1213.

12. Zhao J, Stockwell T, Thomas G. An adaptation of the Yesterday Method to correct for under-reporting of alcohol consumption and estimate compliance with Canadian low-risk drinking guidelines. *Can J Public Health*. 2015; 106(4): e204–e209.

13. Bruun K, Edwards G, Lumui M, et al. *Alcohol Control Policies in Public Health Perspective*. Finnish Foundation for Alcohol Studies; 1975.

14. Kehoe T, Gmel G, Shield KD, Gmel G, Rehm J. Determining the best population-level alcohol consumption model and its impact on estimates of alcohol-attributable harms. *Popul Health Metrics*. 2012; 10: 6.

15. World Health Organization. *Global Strategy to Reduce the Harmful Use of Alcohol*. World Health Organization; 2010.

16. Stockwell T, Sherk A, Norström T, et al. Estimating the public health impact of disbanding a government alcohol monopoly: Application of new methods to the case of Sweden. *BMC Public Health*. 2018; 18(1): 1400.

17. Hahn RA, Middleton JC, Elder R, et al. Effects of alcohol retail privatization on excessive alcohol consumption and related harms: A community guide systematic review. *Am J Prev Med*. 2012; 42(4): 418–427.

18. Stockwell T, Zhao J, Macdonald S, Pakula B, Gruenewald P, Holder H. Changes in per capita alcohol sales during the partial privatization of British Columbia's retail alcohol monopoly 2003–2008: A multi-level local area analysis. *Addiction*. 2009; 104(11): 1827–1836.

19. Stockwell T, Zhao J, Macdonald S, et al. Impact on alcohol-related mortality of a rapid rise in the density of private liquor outlets in British Columbia: A local area multi-level analysis. *Addiction*. 2011; 106(4): 768–776.

20. Stockwell T, Zhao J, Martin G, et al. Minimum alcohol prices and outlet densities in British Columbia, Canada: Estimated impacts on alcohol-attributable hospital admissions. *Am J Public Health*. 2013; 103(11): 2014–2020.

21. Andreasson S, Chikritzhs T, Dangardt F, et al. *Alcohol and Society 2021: Alcohol and the Coronavirus Pandemic: Individual, Societal and Policy Perspectives*. Swedish Society of Nursing, SFAM, SAFF, CERA, Swedish Society of Addiction Medicine, SIGHT, Movendi International & IOGT-NTO; 2021.

22. Vallance K, Stockwell T, Wettlaufer A, et al. The Canadian Alcohol Policy Evaluation project: Findings from a review of provincial and territorial alcohol policies. *Drug Alcohol Rev*. 2021; 40(6): 937–945.

23. Diamond NJ. Trade agreements and public health: A primer for health policy makers, researchers and advocates. *ICSID Rev Foreign Investment Law J*. 2020; 35(3): 646–650.

24. Room R, O'Brien P. Alcohol marketing and social media: A challenge for public health control. *Drug Alcohol Rev*. 2021; 40(3): 420–422.

25. Mart S, Giesbrecht N. Red flags on pinkwashed drinks: Contradictions and dangers in marketing alcohol to prevent cancer. *Addiction*. 2015; 110(10): 1541–1548.

26. Anderson P. Global alcohol policy and the alcohol industry. *Curr Opin Psychiatry*. 2009; 22(3): 253–257.

27. Room R, Schmidt L, Rehm J, Mäkelä P. International regulation of alcohol. *BMJ*. 2008; 337: a2364.

28. Scottish Government. Alcohol and drugs: Minimum unit pricing. 2018. Accessed January 19, 2021. https://www.gov.scot/policies/alcohol-and-drugs/minimum-unit-pricing

29. Holmes J, Meng Y, Meier PS, et al. Effects of minimum unit pricing for alcohol on different income and socioeconomic groups: A modelling study. *Lancet*. 2014; 383(9929): 1655–1664.

30. Zhao J, Stockwell T, Martin G, et al. The relationship between minimum alcohol prices, outlet densities and alcohol-attributable deaths in British Columbia, 2002–09. *Addiction*. 2013; 108(6): 1059–1069.

31. Stockwell T, Zhao J, Alam F, Churchill S, Naimi T, Shi Y. Alcohol sales in Canadian liquor outlets as a predictor of subsequent COVID-19 infection rates: A time series analysis. Forthcoming.

32. Anderson P, Chisholm D, Fuhr DC. Effectiveness and cost-effectiveness of policies and programmes to reduce the harm caused by alcohol. *Lancet*. 2009; 373(9682): 2234–2246.

CHAPTER 11

Learning from 70 Years
of Tobacco Control

Winning the War and Not Just the Battles

ANNA B. GILMORE AND SARAH DANCE

11.1 INTRODUCTION

Tobacco control is often held up as the poster child for the commercial determinants of health because significant progress has been made in addressing
both the epidemic and its corporate vector, the tobacco industry (TI). Notably,
the world's first public health treaty, the World Health Organization (WHO)
Framework Convention on Tobacco Control (FCTC), contains a specific
article—Article 5.3—that requires countries to protect their policies from the
vested interests of the TI. A key stimulus for the FCTC, negotiations for which
began in 1996, was the publication in 1995 of the first "vector research" that
critically examined the TI's role in driving the tobacco epidemic.[1] Prompted
initially by the release of previously secret internal documents via whistleblowers, this area of research later received further impetus when additional
documentation was released through congressional hearings and litigation.[2,3]

The FCTC has undoubtedly advanced implementation of tobacco control
policies worldwide,[4] with approximately 65% of the global population now
covered by at least one key measure.[5] Yet progress against the world's leading
cause of preventable mortality remains shockingly slow. Despite Article 5.3,
the now overwhelming evidence of TI malfeasance, its consequent and extensive denormalization, blame for this slow progress lies almost entirely at the
door of the TI.[6]

Anna B. Gilmore and Sarah Dance, *Learning from 70 Years of Tobacco Control* In: *The Commercial Determinants of Health*. Edited by: Nason Maani, Mark Petticrew, and Sandro Galea, Oxford University Press. © Oxford University Press 2023. DOI: 10.1093/oso/9780197578742.003.0011

The purpose of this chapter, therefore, is to learn from this. Tobacco may be uniquely deadly: It is the only legal product that kills between one-half[7] and two-thirds[8] of its long-term users when used precisely as its manufacturers intend—but its manufacturers otherwise have much in common with the commercial disease vectors featured in other chapters of this volume. We therefore review what has been learned about TI practices and what types of research and advocacy have helped, and we critically review progress so that lessons can be learned for addressing the commercial determinants of health more broadly.

11.2 WHAT HAVE WE LEARNED ABOUT TOBACCO INDUSTRY PRACTICES?

We now possess extensive knowledge of the diverse TI practices that influence health. These range from its legal and scientific strategies to hide the harms of smoking to its poor treatment of tobacco farmers and retailers juxtaposed with strategically using them as the acceptable face of its influence strategies, involvement in illegal activities including bribery[9] and tobacco smuggling[10] (Box 11.1), and on–off claims of commitment to "harm reduction" each time the industry is seriously threatened and which signal a corporate transformation that has yet to occur.[1-3,11] In short, the evidence is clear that there is little that major tobacco companies will not do to expand sales and maximize profits.

Box 11.1 TOBACCO INDUSTRY INVOLVEMENT IN TOBACCO SMUGGLING AND ITS RESPONSE TO EFFORTS TO ADDRESS THIS

Extensive research reveals the TI's large-scale involvement in tobacco smuggling. In the 1990s, one-third of exported cigarettes ended up on the illicit market. This was a core part of the TI's global business strategy, and in some markets the majority of its cigarettes were smuggled. It brought the TI a number of advantages—for example, it avoided excise duties, meaning cigarettes could be sold more cheaply (at no less profit to the industry) and thus more were sold; and it avoided import duties, enabling the TI to import to closed markets such as the former Soviet Union to establish a demand for cigarettes. Tobacco companies then used the presence of illicit tobacco to argue for market opening and to argue against tobacco control policies (e.g., claiming high taxes or other legislation drove the illegal trade while the industry was ultimately responsible).

These revelations prompted multiple legal challenges and investigations, which led to guilty pleas, fines, and even imprisonments. The industry's reputation was heavily damaged. Various countries implemented legal agreements attempting to hold the TI to account, and the Illicit Trade Protocol was developed as part of the FCTC. This included requirements for a global "track and trace" system in which tobacco products would be marked so they could be tracked through their supply chain and traced back to determine how they ended up on the illicit market.[10]

In response, the industry claimed to have changed—to now be the victim of and the solution to the illicit trade in cigarettes. Yet, now it can be seen that such claims remain false. TI involvement in the illicit trade continues, and the majority of smuggled cigarettes still originate from the TI's own supply chain. What has changed now is that the TI has used its resource advantage to control every aspect of the debate and create confusion. Tobacco companies control the data on tobacco smuggling to claim others are responsible. They have developed their own technology for track and trace, which would put them in charge of the global system meant to prevent their involvement in smuggling, and are promoting it to governments via third parties to hide their links. They are funding major accountancy firms to publish reports and represent them at conferences. They are providing training and equipment or funding (sometimes through third parties) for customs officials and agencies such as Interpol and the World Customs Organization meant to hold them to account. They have set up significant research funding on illicit trade, which works to buy allies, credibility, and, if it works like previous TI research funding, favorable findings.

In short, major advances were made in identifying and addressing industry involvement in tobacco smuggling, but the TI has used its significant resource advantage to fight back. The fight has got dirtier, involving increasingly complex and hidden webs of funding and third parties such that progress is now threatened.

11.2.1 Practices That Cause Harm Primarily by Increasing Sales

Because of the uniquely deadly nature of cigarettes, TI practices with most relevance to health are those that primarily work, both directly and indirectly, to increase tobacco sales. These practices can be categorized into four main groups:

1. Corporate political activity (its policy influence strategies[12])

2. Scientific activity (comprising both product research and development and the other strategic ways in which the TI uses science, including to hide the harms of active and passive smoking or create confusion about the impacts of regulations of proven effectiveness[13])[1]
3. Marketing (the ways in which it promotes its products, broadly understood as the four Ps—price, place, promotion, and product. This includes marketing even where advertising is restricted,[14] reshaping norms to nullify cultural barriers to smoking, and manipulation of product design to increase addictiveness[6])
4. Reputation management and legitimation techniques, often referred to as corporate social responsibility (CSR). CSR in this case is a misnomer—there is nothing responsible about the TI's use of such practices; rather, they are used to shape policy outcomes that work against public welfare.[15,16] Ultimately, corporations with such appalling track records have to engage extensively in reputation management to legitimate their involvement in every sphere, and CSR is therefore a key part of TI political, scientific, and marketing activity.[13,15] Recently leaked Phillip Morris International documents covering the period 2014–2024 make this clear, identifying "denormalization and demonization" as key threats and "normalization" as the first strategic objective in a 10-year corporate affairs plan.[17]

Using the above practices, major tobacco companies have worked assiduously to expand sales throughout the world, pushing for and taking advantage of growing trade and investment liberalization, now clearly documented to significantly increase tobacco use.[18] They promoted privatization of state-owned tobacco industries, arguing this would solve the tobacco smuggling problem they had created (see Box 11.1); and avoided competitive tenders, thus underpaying for assets while negotiating lengthy tax holidays as a quid pro quo for investment. Their aggressive marketing that targeted population subgroups with low levels of smoking (women and children) while simultaneously claiming marketing simply encourages existing users to switch brands, negotiation of favorable policies as a condition of investment, and aggressive lobbying against further regulation worked collectively to drive up smoking rates. The International Monetary Fund promoted TI privatization as part of loan conditionality despite clear evidence of harm.[18]

11.2.2 Other Core Business Practices

In addition to the previously discussed practices, there are other core business practices that all corporations engage in and which also impact on health, albeit not directly through consumption of tobacco. These include supply chain management, employment practices, and financial and tax strategies.

Examples of each, respectively, include deforestation to grow and cure tobacco leaf; poor treatment of tobacco farmers and factory workers; engagement in extensive tax evasion (see Box 11.1); and avoidance, including profit shifting, such that highly profitable transnational tobacco companies pay very little tax.[19,20]

As the previous examples illustrate, industry actions in most of these categories can vary from legal to illegal, with many in a "gray zone" between the two. Power and the limited liability and personhood afforded to corporations lie at the heart of the industry's ability to act in these ways with little fear of retribution. Simultaneously, many of the practices documented above result in the costs of tobacco being increasingly externalized from tobacco companies to individuals and the state, thereby further increasing the industry's wealth relative to those left to bear those costs. Due to space limitations, we focus hereinafter on its policy influence strategies.

11.2.3 Downstream Policy Influence

There is overwhelming evidence that the TI seeks to block, weaken, or delay any policy that counters its interests, and it is particularly aggressive in efforts to oppose the most effective (e.g., tax increases) or globally groundbreaking policies (e.g., plain packaging when first introduced). If, despite its efforts, a policy is legislated, the TI seeks to overturn it through litigation and, if finally implemented, to circumvent it and manufacture "evidence" the policy has been ineffective, which in turn is used to counter the policy elsewhere.

Systematic reviews of the extensive evidence on TI policy influence strategies, largely in the form of country case studies, show the TI consistently uses the same strategies across time and place,[21,22] enabling the development of an evidence-based taxonomy of TI corporate political activity (CPA).[12] This has been used to predict and counter the TI's influence strategies and to show that alcohol, food, and gambling companies use very similar practices[23-25]— findings in line with evidence of their financial,[2] operational,[26] and board-level ties.[27] The taxonomy shows that the TI's overarching argument-based strategy is to claim that each policy will lead to vast negative social and economic consequences, while denying any potential for benefit.[12] Such arguments are then widely disseminated through a variety of "instrumental strategies" or actions.

Although the industry's overall CPA "toolbox" remains the same, contextual variations occur in the specific "tools" used. For example, whereas in the 1990s the industry was, almost without fail, able to directly access policymakers, with the advent of Article 5.3 and growing industry denormalization, that became virtually impossible in many jurisdictions. Consequently, there was a large increase in the use of "constituency management"—the funding and creation of third parties and front groups that operate as the more acceptable voice of the TI. More recently, there have been an increase in the complexity of third party funding to further disguise industry links (see Box 11.1[28]); growing attempts to attack and fragment the public health community, a strategy first outlined decades ago; and increasingly lavishly funded "reputation management" initiatives to polish the TI's tarnished image.[28] By contrast, in some countries, where the TI has not yet reached pariah status, it is still able to predominantly use direct influence strategies and simply works to maintain rather than having to rehabilitate its image.[29]

11.2.4 Upstream Policy Influence

While the public health community focuses predominantly on securing downstream public health policies, the TI, often working with other corporations whose products are damaging to health, has deliberately, and often successfully, attempted to influence "upstream" policies—the rules under which downstream policies are made.

The TI has done this in three main ways that work to make it more difficult to pass and easier to challenge public health policies. First, it attempts to establish rules on the way science is used in policy by, for example, promoting what it calls a "risk-based" or "science-based" approach to policymaking.[13] This is intended to prevent a more precautionary approach and to preclude the regulation of, for example, secondhand smoke, which, despite often ubiquitous exposure and significant population-level impacts, has low relative risk.[13] Second, it establishes systems of policymaking that enable corporate influence and embed corporate power. For example, requiring each policy undergoes a business-oriented impact assessment and stakeholder consultation gives corporations threatened by regulation a specific role in commenting on and supplying evidence for regulation,[26] despite the clear conflict of interest. In the European Union, British American Tobacco pushed for such rules anticipating they would make it more difficult to pass public health policies,[30] and tobacco companies have gone on to use them in this way, overwhelming public consultations with third party responses and highly misleading evidence they have funded.[31,32] Such systems have been labeled a threat to democracy because they bring policymaking under an unprecedented level of corporate control yet are widely promoted as making regulation "better" and more evidence based, and increasingly underpin policymaking in much of the world.[33] Third, it attempts to influence the content of trade and investment agreements[6] by, for example, pushing for the right for corporations to directly challenge legislation and for enhanced and intellectual property rights to make it more difficult to pass policies regulating product packaging and branding.[6]

11.3 WHAT HAVE WE LEARNED ABOUT MONITORING, RESEARCH, AND ADVOCACY TO ADDRESS TOBACCO INDUSTRY INTERFERENCE AND ADVANCE TOBACCO CONTROL?

11.3.1 Approaches and Data Sources

Tobacco industry monitoring, first recommended in the 2001 World Health Assembly resolution "Transparency in Tobacco Control"[34] and later in the Article 5.3 guidelines,[35] can play a key role in advancing tobacco control but is often misunderstood in other sectors. Workshops and expert groups have been convened, and technical resources on this topic outline diverse foci and sources for "monitoring."[36-38] The reality, however, is that monitoring all these sources in a timely enough manner to take action is impossible within resource constraints, and the return on investment would be small. Yet practical information on applied monitoring is rarely published because of fear the TI will adapt. This has limited opportunities for learning as monitoring begins to be applied to other corporate vectors.

At the University of Bath, we believe monitoring, which simply means to keep under systematic review, should be integrated with research and accountability in a dynamic model we call TI monitoring, research, and accountability (Figure 11.1). In this way, important observations emerging from monitoring can be rapidly investigated so that timely action can be taken or, where appropriate, more in-depth research instigated. For example, monitoring of industry materials highlighted that despite a trend toward cheaper cigarettes in high-income countries, TI profitability was increasing, prompting in-depth research on TI pricing.[39,40] This showed tobacco companies were absorbing the tax increases on the cheapest products, leading to ever larger price differentials between cheap and expensive cigarettes, thereby minimizing the intended impact of tobacco tax increases and driving inequalities in smoking.[39] This led to the implementation of a minimum excise tax in the United Kingdom in 2017.[41] A few elements are key to making this model practical and impactful. First, monitoring must be as automated, dynamic, and responsive as possible so that resources can be continuously refocused on areas of high policy relevance. Second, it must be ensured that findings can be rapidly communicated and acted on. To that end, we created a knowledge exchange platform (see https://tobaccotactics.org) that has become a globally used resource. Third, informal personal networks are essential for both information gathering and dissemination and accountability. Finally, rather than bearing the burden of seeking data, the public health community should aim to ensure the industry is statutorily required to provide such data.

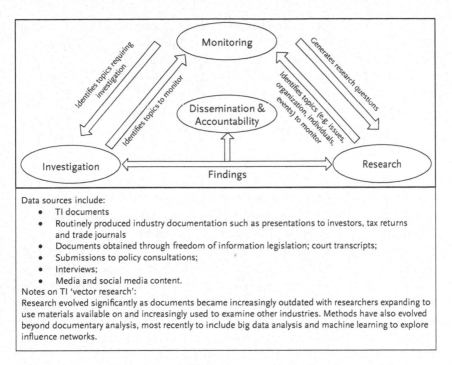

Data sources include:
- TI documents
- Routinely produced industry documentation such as presentations to investors, tax returns and trade journals
- Documents obtained through freedom of information legislation; court transcripts;
- Submissions to policy consultations;
- Interviews;
- Media and social media content.

Notes on TI 'vector research':

Research evolved significantly as documents became increasingly outdated with researchers expanding to use materials available on and increasingly used to examine other industries. Methods have also evolved beyond documentary analysis, most recently to include big data analysis and machine learning to explore influence networks.

Figure 11.1 University of Bath model of TI monitoring, research, and accountability.

11.3.2 Effectiveness

There is no doubt that vector research (including monitoring) has played a key role in advancing tobacco control.[2,3,42] The first vector research[1,43] changed attitudes regarding the TI and influenced politicians, in the United States at least, to take action while also stimulating further litigation and document discovery.[2,3,42] The subsequently released documents helped further denormalize smoking and the TI and prompted seminal WHO reports, the 2001 World Health Assembly resolution on "Transparency in Tobacco Control" and ultimately the FCTC.[2]

Despite these early reviews[2,3] and subsequent observations that the countries (in all income groups) with the most successful tobacco control policies also have the most active programs of industry monitoring and research (e.g., Thailand, Brazil, the United Kingdom, and Australia),[6] there has been remarkably little empirical research on *how* vector research leads to policy change, nor on the elements of such research that help ensure it is impactful. Yet three key ways this research leads policy impacts are worth highlighting. First, it identifies and provides evidence for policies needed to address industry behavior—both new policies and adaptations to existing policies that the industry has learned to circumvent. Second, when undertaken during the acute policy window, it has proven essential to ensuring passage of legislation and countering the legal challenges against it. Third, by revealing unpalatable truths,[2] vector research leads to TI denormalization.[44]

11.4 CRITICAL REVIEW OF PROGRESS AND LESSONS LEARNED: THE NEED TO WIN THE WAR AND NOT JUST THE BATTLES

As detailed previously, significant advances have been made in tobacco control. Above all downstream, largely national policy "wins" are increasingly secured in part due to the expanded knowledge of and capacity to address TI interference. Yet progress is slow. Every policy requires a resource-intensive David and Goliath battle to implementation, and many countries still struggle to advance or enforce basic policies.[6,14] Article 5.3 is not a panacea. Instead, as outlined above, industry influence strategies have adapted and become more difficult and time-consuming to reveal. Finally, the major tobacco companies are now fighting back harder than ever, driven by the threat to their bottom line as a result of tobacco control's successes[11,28] and enabled to do so because we have not sufficiently addressed the systems drivers.

As a result, history is repeating itself,[11,28] and in key policy areas major advances made following revelations of industry misconduct are now being threatened (see Box 11.1). Consequently, although tobacco control has driven down global cigarette sales, the rate of decline in smoking prevalence is now stalling.[45] Tobacco control may have been winning the battles, but up against a better resourced global opponent, it may be in danger of losing the war.

It is essential that those focused on tobacco control and other areas of public health involving corporate vectors learn from this experience. To secure short-term policy wins, monitoring, exposing, and countering the industry's policy influence strategies are essential, but the public health community must simultaneously do five other things. First, it must understand and address the industry's longer term influence strategies, including persistent attempts to reshape norms, beliefs, and attitudes in its interests. Second, it must look upstream to identify and address the ways in which tobacco and other unhealthy commodity industries are attempting to reshape politics, trade, and governance (and specific "upstream" policies therein) in order to prevent these from constraining the options for public interest policymaking. Third, it must work to counter industry across multiple jurisdictional levels—from global to local—engaging the diverse sectors beyond health that the industry assiduously targets and ensuring that the right organizational structures and coordinating mechanisms are available to do this. For example, despite the FCTC, tobacco control is operationalized largely at the national level which makes it hard to counter global corporations which carefully coordinate their strategies and messaging from global to local level. Fourth, it must understand which research leads to policy change and why, and ensure that research is undertaken. Fifth and finally, it must move from repeatedly identifying the problems to focus on solutions; and, most importantly, recognize the need for more radical solutions.

The primary lesson from this chapter is that operating within the existing system will only get us so far. To date, we have not sufficiently addressed the underlying structural drivers—the TI's excess profitability[40] and the inequalities in power and resources between transnational tobacco companies, on the one hand, and nation states and civil society, on the other hand, both driven by TI's ability to externalize the costs of the harm it causes to state and society. As a result, the TI remains able and incentivized to oppose every policy that threatens its profits, and the more it is pushed, the greater the resistance. More radical structural and systems change will be needed to address the commercial determinants of health. This might include removing the profit incentive from selling harmful products, ensuring the costs of the harm caused are factored into the corporation's bottom line, changing the rules on corporate regulation and limited liability, and/or pushing to change the global political and economic system that underpins these problems.

NOTE

1. We have now developed detailed taxonomies of industry corporate political activity and scientific activity that enable these activities to be better understood and addressed.

REFERENCES

1. Glantz SA, Barnes DE, Bero L, Hanauer P, Slade J. Looking through a keyhole at the tobacco industry: The Brown and Williamson documents. *JAMA*. 1995; 274(3): 219–224.
2. Hurt RD, Ebbert JO, Muggli ME, Lockhart NJ, Robertson CR. Open doorway to truth: Legacy of the Minnesota tobacco trial. *Mayo Clin Proc*. 2009; 84(5): 446–456.
3. Bero L. Implications of the tobacco industry documents for public health and policy. *Annu Rev Public Health*. 2003; 24(1): 267–288.
4. Chung-Hall J, Craig L, Gravely S, Sansone N, Fong GT. Impact of the WHO FCTC over the first decade: A global evidence review prepared for the Impact Assessment Expert Group. *Tobacco Control*. 2019; 28(Suppl 2): s119–s128.
5. World Health Organization. *WHO Report on the Global Tobacco Epidemic, 2019: Offer Help to Quit Tobacco Use*. World Health Organization; 2019.
6. Gilmore AB, Fooks G, Drope J, Bialous SA, Jackson RR. Exposing and addressing tobacco industry conduct in low-income and middle-income countries. *Lancet*. 2015; 385(9972): 1029–1043.

7. World Health Organization. *WHO Report on the Global Tobacco Epidemic, 2011: Warning About the Dangers of Tobacco*. World Health Organization; 2011.

8. Pirie K, Peto R, Reeves GK, Green J, Beral V. The 21st century hazards of smoking and benefits of stopping: A prospective study of one million women in the UK. *Lancet*. 2013; 381(9861): 133–141.

9. Jackson RR, Rowell A, Gilmore AB. "Unlawful bribes?": A documentary analysis showing British American Tobacco's use of payments to secure policy and competitive advantage in Africa. UCSF Center for Tobacco Control Research and Education. 2021. https://escholarship.org/uc/item/4qs8m106

10. Gilmore AB, Gallagher AWA, Rowell A. Tobacco industry's elaborate attempts to control a global track and trace system and fundamentally undermine the Illicit Trade Protocol. *Tobacco Control*. 2019; 28(2): 127.

11. Evans-Reeves K, Gilmore A. Addiction at any cost. Philip Morris International Uncovered. 2020. https://exposetobacco.org/pmi-uncovered

12. Ulucanlar S, Fooks GJ, Gilmore AB. The policy dystopia model: An interpretive analysis of tobacco industry political activity. *PLOS Med*. 2016; 13(9): e1002125.

13. Legg T, Hatchard J, Gilmore AB. The science for profit model—How and why corporations influence science and the use of science in policy and practice. *PLoS One*. 2021; 16(6): e0253272.

14. Savell E, Gilmore AB, Sims M, et al. The environmental profile of a community's health: A cross-sectional study on tobacco marketing in 16 countries. *Bull World Health Organ*. 2015; 93(12): 851–861G.

15. Fooks GJ, Gilmore AB, Smith KE, Collin J, Holden C, Lee K. Corporate social responsibility and access to policy élites: An analysis of tobacco industry documents. *PLoS Med*. 2011; 8(8): e1001076.

16. Fooks G, Gilmore A, Collin J, Holden C, Lee K. The limits of corporate social responsibility: Techniques of neutralization, stakeholder management and political CSR. *J Business Ethics*. 2013; 112(2): 283–299.

17. Philip Morris International. 10 year corporate affairs objective and strategies. 2014. https://www.documentcloud.org/documents/4333395-10-Year-Corporate-Affairs-Objectives-and.html

18. Gilmore AB, Fooks G, McKee M. A review of the impacts of tobacco industry privatisation: Implications for policy. *Global Public Health*. 2011; 6(6): 621–642.

19. Vermuelen SD, Dillen M, Branston J. R. Big tobacco, big avoidance. The Investigative Desk. 2020. https://www.bath.ac.uk/publications/big-tobacco-big-avoidance/attachments/Big_Tobacco_Big_Avoidance.pdf

20. Branston JR, Gilmore AB. The failure of the UK to tax adequately tobacco company profits. *J Public Health*. 2020; 42(1): 69–76.

21. Savell E, Gilmore AB, Fooks G. How does the tobacco industry attempt to influence marketing regulations? A systematic review. *PLoS One*. 2014; 9(2): e87389.

22. Smith KE, Savell E, Gilmore AB. What is known about tobacco industry efforts to influence tobacco tax? A systematic review of empirical studies. *Tobacco Control*. 2013; 22(2): e1.

23. Paixão MM, Mialon M. Help or hindrance? The alcohol industry and alcohol control in Portugal. *Int J Environ Res Public Health*. 2019; **16**(22): 4554.

24. Lauber K, Rutter H, Gilmore AB. Big food and the World Health Organization: A qualitative study of industry attempts to influence global-level non-communicable disease policy. *BMJ Global Health*. 2021; 6(6): e005216.

25. Hancock L, Ralph N, Martino FP. Applying corporate political activity (CPA) analysis to Australian gambling industry submissions against regulation of television sports betting advertising. *PLoS One*. 2018; 13(10): e0205654.

26. Smith KE, Fooks G, Gilmore AB, Collin J, Weishaar H. Corporate coalitions and policy making in the European Union: How and why British American Tobacco promoted "Better Regulation." *J Health Polit Policy Law*. 2015; 40(2): 325–372.

27. Collin J, Plotnikova E, Hill S. One unhealthy commodities industry? Understanding links across tobacco, alcohol and ultra-processed food manufacturers and their implications for tobacco control and the SDGS. *Tobacco Induced Dis*. 2018; 16(1): A80.

28. Hird T, Gallagher A, Evans-Reeves K, et al. Understanding the long-term policy influence strategies of the tobacco industry: Two contemporary case studies. *Tobacco Control*. 2022; 31: 297–307.

29. Matthes BK, Robertson L, Gilmore AB. Needs of LMIC-based tobacco control advocates to counter tobacco industry policy interference: Insights from semi-structured interviews. *BMJ Open*. 2020; 10(11): e044710.

30. Smith KE, Fooks G, Collin J, Weishaar H, Mandal S, Gilmore AB. "Working the system"—British American Tobacco's influence on the European Union treaty and its implications for policy: An analysis of internal tobacco industry documents. *PLoS Med*. 2010; 7(1): e1000202.

31. Ulucanlar S, Fooks GJ, Hatchard JL, Gilmore AB. Representation and misrepresentation of scientific evidence in contemporary tobacco regulation: A review of tobacco industry submissions to the UK Government Consultation on Standardised Packaging. *PLoS Med*. 2014; 11(3): e1001629.

32. Peeters S, Costa H, Stuckler D, McKee M, Gilmore AB. The revision of the 2014 European tobacco products directive: An analysis of the tobacco industry's attempts to "break the health silo." *Tobacco Control*. 2016; 25(1): 108–117.

33. Berry C, Devlin, S. Threat to democracy: The impact of "Better Regulation" in the UK. New Economics Foundation. October 12, 2015. https://neweconomics.org/2015/10/threat-to-democracy

34. World Health Organization. Fifty-fourth World Health Assembly. 2001. https://apps.who.int/iris/handle/10665/260183

35. World Health Organization. Guidelines for implementation of Article 5.3. 2008. https://fctc.who.int/publications/m/item/guidelines-for-implementation-of-article-5.3

36. Cruz TB. Monitoring the tobacco use epidemic IV. The vector: Tobacco industry data sources and recommendations for research and evaluation. *Prev Med*. 2009; 48(1, Suppl 1): S24–S34.

37. World Health Organization. *WHO Report on the Global Tobacco Epidemic, 2017: Monitoring Tobacco Use and Prevention Policies*. World Health Organization; 2017.

38. World Health Organization. Technical resource for country implementation of the WHO Framework Convention on Tobacco Control Article 5.3. 2012. https://www.who.int/publications/i/item/9789241503730

39. Gilmore AB, Tavakoly B, Taylor G, Reed H. Understanding tobacco industry pricing strategy and whether it undermines tobacco tax policy: The example of the UK cigarette market. *Addiction*. 2013; 108(7): 1317–1326.

40. Hiscock R, Branston JR, McNeill A, Hitchman SC, Partos TR, Gilmore AB. Tobacco industry strategies undermine government tax policy: Evidence from commercial data. *Tobacco Control*. 2018; 27(5): 488.

41. Tobacco Control Research Group. The introduction of a minimum excise tax (MET) on cigarettes. 2021. https://www.bath.ac.uk/case-studies/the-introduct ion-of-a-minimum-excise-tax-met-on-cigarettes

42. Cummings KM, Pollay RW. Exposing Mr. Butts' tricks of the trade. *Tobacco Control*. 2002; 11(Suppl 1): i1–i4.

43. Glantz S, Slade J, Bero LA, Hanauer P, Barnes DE. *The Cigarette Papers*. University of California Press; 1998.

44. Malone RE, Grundy Q, Bero LA. Tobacco industry denormalisation as a tobacco control intervention: A review. *Tobacco Control*. 2012; 21(2): 162.

45. Reitsma MB, Kendrick PJ, Ababneh E, et al. Spatial, temporal, and demographic patterns in prevalence of smoking tobacco use and attributable disease burden in 204 countries and territories, 1990–2019: A systematic analysis from the Global Burden of Disease Study 2019. *Lancet*. 2021; 397(10292): 2337–2360.

CHAPTER 12

The Fossil Fuel Industry

Fueling Doubt and Navigating Contradiction

MAY CI VAN SCHALKWYK, NASON MAANI,
AND MARK PETTICREW

As is well known, BP responded early to the issue of climate change.
> —Carl-Henric Svanberg, BP Chairman (2010)

The Gulf of Mexico is a very big ocean. The amount of volume of oil and dispersant we are putting into it is tiny in relation to the total water volume.
> —BP Chief Executive Tony Hayward, in the wake
> of the Gulf of Mexico oil spill (2010)

12.1 THE FOSSIL FUEL INDUSTRY IN CONTEXT

Fossil fuels are woven into the fabric of social and political systems the world over, rendering the fossil fuel industry almost unique in its economic, social, cultural, and political positioning. Indeed, Timothy Mitchell's historical analysis, *Carbon Democracy*, proposes that fossil fuels have both enabled and constrained the emergence and form of modern democracies.[1] In particular, these developments shaped the oil industry and the power it holds. Oil companies have at times been enabled to control the supply of oil and access to other forms of energy, to exploit political crises to obtain tax exemptions and subsidies and to justify raising oil prices, and to create dependencies for their products.[1] Furthermore, although advances in fossil fuel production and use have, for some, enabled once unimaginable ways of living, indiscriminate extraction and burning of fossil fuels have led to global warming and the devastation of

May Ci van Schalkwyk, Nason Maani, and Mark Petticrew, *The Fossil Fuel Industry* In: *The Commercial Determinants of Health*. Edited by: Nason Maani, Mark Petticrew, and Sandro Galea, Oxford University Press. © Oxford University Press 2023. DOI: 10.1093/oso/9780197578742.003.0012 ecosystems, threatening the sustainability of the systems upon which life on earth relies.

While recognizing the vast literature on the fossil fuel industry, this chapter aims to introduce some of the research documenting the strategies adopted by the industry that undermine public health and environmental protection. The intention is to demonstrate the value of studying the activities of the fossil fuel industry through a commercial determinants of health (CDOH) lens. Here, the term *fossil fuel industry* is used to refer to corporate entities engaged in the extraction, transport, refinement, and sale of oil, coal, and gas, and their derivative products, as well as their owners, trade bodies, and those entities acting on their behalf while in receipt of their funding, such as think tanks, public relations, and legal firms. The chapter focuses on publicly listed companies, without intending to minimize the role of state-owned fossil fuel firms. Furthermore, it is important to recognize that many of the industry's strategies detailed herein have, at times, been enabled by other segments of society, including governments, the press, academics and academic journals, and professional associations.[2-5]

12.2 THE FOSSIL FUEL INDUSTRY AS A COMMERCIAL DETERMINANT OF HEALTH

The climate crisis cannot be fully conceptualized without considering the role of the fossil fuel industry.[6] As with asbestos, lead, tobacco, and opioids, for example, to understand and address the impacts of fossil fuels, the actions and interests of the industry, well-documented in literatures predominantly outside of the public health field, should be seen as core aspects of the climate emergency confronting the world. By adopting a CDOH lens, we can start to reveal why this is the case and begin to address this gap in the health narrative on climate change. Reflecting an understanding that corporate strategies and business practices have important implications for public health, the field of CDOH seeks to, in part, understand efforts by corporations to "manage" crises in ways that prioritize their interests at the expense of human health and the environment. Indeed, this book details how industries respond to external threats in ways undermining of public health and the advancement of knowledge—the fossil fuel industry is no exception.

The fossil fuel industry has had to navigate substantial crises that threaten to disrupt its business model, from accumulating awareness of the impacts of lead gasoline and oil spills to smog and poor management of extraction sights and, finally climate change.[6] At its core, maximizing the profits of this industry through the production, sale, and use of its products is contributing to anthropogenic global warming (AGW) and its many ecological, health, and equity consequences.[4] The business interests of the fossil fuel industry thus conflict with advancing the public good. Indeed, despite intensifying warnings that the use of their products was having likely damaging and potentially irreversible effects,[6-9] elements within the fossil fuel industry have pursued decades-long dynamic and multifaceted public and political strategies to protect their interests. A striking feature is the breadth and sophisticated nature of their strategies—much like fossil fuel extraction, numerous techniques and settings have been exploited, irrespective of the consequences. Their corporate strategies have centered on (a) casting doubt on the evidence documenting the causes and impacts of global warming and creating the illusion of debate to mask the presence of scientific consensus[2-4]; (b) mobilizing others in the pursuit of influencing public debate; and (c) efforts to construct a constrained public understanding, structured around the inevitability and desirability of a fossil fuel–saturated world in which industry's and society's interests are in alignment, and the industry is part of the solution.[2-5,10-13]

12.3 MANUFACTURERS OF DOUBT

The creation of doubt represents a critical element of the fossil fuel industry's efforts to protect its interests and has contributed to decades of division and delay.[2-4,10,12,14] This is particularly evident in the United States, where a group of prominent scientists in collaboration with a network of think tanks and private corporations with financial backing from tobacco and fossil fuel interests played critical roles in the manufacturing of doubt about the evidence documenting the threat posed by acid rain, tobacco, chlorofluorocarbons, and, finally, global warming.[4] This was largely achieved by adopting several denialist tactics: promotion of false experts, cherry-picking of the data, undermining of independent scientists and their work, creating the illusion of an established scientific debate despite the existence of a mounting consensus among climate experts, distortion of the literature through the funding of biased research, and strategic exploitation of the scientific process and the concepts of proof and uncertainty.[4] As Oreskes and Conway explain, a central logic to these pursuits was to "attempt to convince the public, through mass media campaigns, to accept an interpretation well outside the mainstream of professional science."[15] Mastering doubt was part of globally coordinated efforts by major fossil fuel giants to ward off or weaken potential regulation and threats to unhindered fossil fuel extraction and use.[6] These tactics and corporate positions were strategically adapted with time toward efforts to control the narrative about climate change risks and solutions, as doubt and denial become untenable (and potentially litigious) positions to hold.[2,6,9] This is captured well by Bonneuil et al.'s description of Total's shift toward recognizing the legitimacy of the Intergovernmental Panel on Climate Change and effort to reframe its own role: "Climate change was to be theoretically diagnosed by science but practically solved by business, without the two spheres interfering with one another."[6]

Focused analyses of industry documents have provided additional important insights into the nature of the industry's propaganda. For example, ExxonMobil adopted a strategy through which it moderated the content of its communications depending on the intended audience, with the use of doubt rhetoric increasing as the materials become more publicly facing in nature.[8] Over the period spanning 1977–2014, ExxonMobil acknowledged that climate change was both real and caused by human activity in internal documents and peer-reviewed literature, using the latter to portray itself as a knowledgeable expert when interacting with government officials. Simultaneously, advertorials commissioned by ExxonMobil in *The New York Times* were used to communicate messages of doubt by emphasizing uncertainty about the existence of AGW, as well as its causes, seriousness, and solvability.[8] ExxonMobil was not only contributing to the pollution of the planet but also polluting public discourse and understanding.

Another important example of the manipulation of doubt is the coal industry's efforts to question evidence linking black lung, a disabling and potentially fatal disease, with exposure to coal dust. The coal industry mastered its approach to manufacturing doubt in the courtroom, exploiting the legal system where the burden of proof can be placed on employees who lack the recourses and knowledge required to prove that harms incurred resulted from workplace exposure.[11] As observed in many legal proceedings involving corporate entities, manipulation of scientific concepts such as confounding, causation, and biological inconsistency was repeatedly employed by the industry and its legal defense.[11] Industry-funded physicians helped reframe the disease by labeling it as "miner's asthma" to downplay the seriousness of the condition and conspired to promote potential confounders that would cloud the link between coal dust exposure and black lung. Industry-funded legal teams were also found to have manipulated and withheld evidence, even to the extent of legal misconduct.[11]

12.4 CONSTRAINING IDEAS AND MASTERING CONTRADICTION

The manufacture of doubt represents only one of the fossil fuel industry's diverse strategies to influence public discourse and policy debates. Other activities serve to constrain how environmental issues are conceptualized, what responses are possible and legitimate, and to portray the industry as the solution. The rhetorical strategies of the coal industry are instructive in understanding the elaborate ways in which corporate advocacy has been used to shape public discourse and the substantial resources dedicated to this pursuit.[5] Schneider and colleagues have described a number of rhetorical strategies based on in-depth analyses of coal industry advocacy campaigns.[5] The term *industrial apocalyptic* describes a set of rhetorical strategies adopted by the industry to construct narratives that conflate the demise of the coal industry as a threat to entire economic, political, or cultural systems. These rhetorical appeals rest on foretelling catastrophic outcomes and calling upon audiences to act swiftly to avoid such outcomes, thereby conflating industry and societal interests. Those who seek to regulate or ban certain industry practices become rhetorically portrayed as villainous, and their actions are equated to treason. The concept of *corporate ventriloquism* seeks to demonstrate how the use of front groups and other similar entities can be conceptualized as rhetorical processes that position the voice of the industry as the voice of citizenship. *Technological shell game* describes another rhetorical process through which the industry deflects attention from environmental and health impacts by the deployment of strategic ambiguity in relation to the feasibility, expense, and effectiveness of technological interventions. This strategy helps the industry navigate the contradiction that arises from its demands for minimal government regulation while arguing for increases in government research and development funding. For example, the coal industry sought to portray its efforts to promote clean coal as evidence that the industry was driven by market forces to act voluntarily, while justifying public funding of the initiative by adopting aspirational and ambiguous narratives to inspire confidence in the benefits. Conversely, to undermine the position of those who critique the coal industry as producers of harmful technologies or goods, the industry would lay what is referred to as the *hypocrite's trap*, whereby a critic's credibility is called into question by highlighting their own use of, or dependence on, those very products. Last, *energy utopia* captures another set of rhetorical devices that serve to cast access to coal as critical to realizing prosperity, "the good life," and the expansion of coal markets as the answer to global poverty. Their framework can enable analysis of the activities of other industries similarly "under pressure." This is particularly likely to be the case as other fossil fuel elements, namely oil and gas, are confronted with the same pressures and dwindling legitimacy experienced by the coal industry.[5]

Analysis of ExxonMobil's rhetorical strategies similarly reveals the use of a technological shell game discourse to dampen public and political concern by trivializing the gravity and solvability of AGW.[9] This strategy is complemented by the construction of certain framings that portray society's use of, and dependence on, fossil fuels as inevitable and "supply" as an innocuous response to consumer demand. By mobilizing the concepts of risk and individual responsibility, ExxonMobil has constructed a public narrative that disproportionately portrays climate change as a potential risk (as opposed to a harmful reality), the benefits of fossil fuels as real, and their use as inevitable answers to the world's energy demands. This logic enabled the industry to locate the problem as emerging from demand, place the blame on individuals and the onus for action on consumers and governments, thereby distancing attention away from industry supply.[9] As noted by Supran and Oreskes, these rhetorical strategies are reminiscent of those adopted by the tobacco industry, which sought to appear to have warned about the "risks," thereby shifting responsibility for harms arising onto consumers while keeping the controversy about causation alive.[16,17]

12.5 "GREENWASHING" AS STRATEGY

When faced with the threat of impending regulations and declining legitimacy, corporations that produce dangerous products often embrace corporate social responsibility (CSR) programs as a form of issue management. The activities of the fossil fuel industry are particularly instructive in revealing how CSR is employed in such a way as to give the appearance of change and commitment to reform while advancing the industry's interests and preserving the status quo. Reflecting their duplicitous nature, fossil fuel industry CSR efforts are often referred to as "greenwashing" or "green speak."[13]

Several scholars have explored the ways in which fossil fuel industry CSR campaigns serve to portray the industry as part of the solution and as legitimate partners in the quest to transition away from unsustainable energy systems. These studies help expose how corporations align their image with sustainability and environmental stewardship while simultaneously placing the onus on individual consumers to act, constraining what are perceived as legitimate answers to issues such as AGW, and maintaining damaging business practices.[13,18]

BP's Helios Power media campaign serves as an important case study through which to appreciate the harmful nature of these campaigns. Rhetorical analysis demonstrates how the Helios Power campaign enabled BP to create a "green" image and assert its position as being part of the green solution.[13] The campaign promoted individualized tools and technological solutions while marginalizing notions of collective agency and non-market solutions, foreclosing alternative ideas and public engagement with other ways of creating sustainable societies.[13] ExxonMobil adopted similar strategies in the company's green advertising.[18] ExxonMobil's "Energy Solutions" campaign constructed a greenwashed narrative by exploiting the credentials and social meanings associated with scientists and technological solutions. Again, this served to frame the problem and the solutions in ways favorable to the corporation while downplaying the role of public agency and avoiding stimulating any critique of unsustainable lifestyles and levels of resource use.[18]

Broadly, the sustainability agenda and responses to climate change are being appropriated by the fossil fuel industry and their allies, subsuming these concepts into the logic of the market, and in turn promoting market-driven solutions and adopting the image of sustainability and "going green" as a means of advancing the corporate image.[19] As Wright and Nyberg explain, "Businesses have argued that the cure for the environmental ills within corporate capitalism is more corporate capitalism and that the problem, as if by magic, is therefore actually the solution."[19]

12.6 PETRO PEDAGOGY

The fossil fuel industry has a long history of seeking to influence education on fossil fuels and global warming, and education policy more broadly.[5,14,20–23] These activities extend back at least as far as the 1940s and were at times executed with the support of organizations that have become renowned for providing their services to harmful industries, such as the public relations firm Hill & Knowlton.[22] This arm of fossil fuel corporate strategy encompasses the provision of biased resources that (a) promote the virtues of fossil fuels and stimulate doubt about the causes and seriousness of climates change and/or (b) adopt narrow individualizing discourses that blame consumers and promote individual responsibility as the basis for action, hindering critique of the industry and the hegemony of neoliberal rationalities.[14,20,21] Eaton and Day have coined these practices as "neoliberal petro-pedagogy," which constitute the pedagogical arm of the fossil fuel industry's "regime of obstruction."[20]

Influencing ideas and understandings through the dissemination of misinformation and corporate-sanctioned viewpoints through sponsored resources represents one aspect of the industry's activities. Another channel of influence has been to acquire key positions within education policy networks. For example, as Tannock explains, "Rather than limiting itself to the narrow promotion of pro-petroleum rhetoric, BP has long seen its interests as being best served by the general promotion of pro-business practices and values throughout UK public education."[21] BP has positioned itself within UK education policy networks to advance a neoliberal and uncritical approach to science, technology, engineering, and mathematics (STEM) education that aligns with industry interests, with similar approaches promoted by other oil giants in the United States.[21,24] This form of STEM leaves unsustainable and unjust practices and futures unquestioned and "poses a significant threat to our collective efforts to tackle the global climate crisis."[21]

12.7 COUNTERING CORPORATE INFLUENCE

Recognition of the fossil fuel industry as an important threat to addressing AGW is key to making meaningful progress in the interests of public health and environmental sustainability.[25] Concerningly, however, broad recognition of the fossil fuel industry as representing a commercial determinant of health is yet to emerge. Engagement with the industry remains largely the norm, and fossil fuel corporations and their representatives are granted frequent access to policymakers and political elites. Indeed, it is remarkable to consider the extent to which the fossil fuel industry has been enabled to engage with the scientific, educational, political, and public fora within which global warming debates take place.

More debate about the role of the industry in policymaking and in communicating to the public is needed. In this regard, Marteau and colleagues stress the need to implement stronger measures to protect the policymaking process from corporate influence, including exclusion of the industry, as prescribed for the tobacco industry under Article 5.3 of the Framework Convention on Tobacco Control, and using regulations and criminal law to curb corporate environmental destruction and misleading of the public.[25] Research on effective ways of managing conflicts of interests and engagement with corporate actors will be instrumental in this respect. The literature documenting the industry's strategies to create doubt and distort understanding can inform the design of denormalization interventions.

12.8 CONCLUSION

The fossil fuel industry wields considerable power, which it has used to influence scientific debate, public knowledge and opinion, and policy across time and space. Faced with mounting evidence on the damage and harms associated with the burning of fossil fuels, the industry mobilized to generate doubt and marshal denialist campaigns. This led to the pervasive spread of doubt about the evidence and to policy inertia. The industry has used diverse strategies to draw the boundaries around what is possible and legitimate, encircling only ideas and norms that align with its worldviews and business interests. The industry has cast itself as part of the solution, as a fellow citizen, while marginalizing and vilifying other actors and perspectives as delegitimate and, at worst, dangerous. Exploitation of the logics of risk and personal responsibility has enabled the shifting of blame to consumers, while strategically avoiding explicitly denying the dangers of global warming. These strategies need to be challenged and new ways of thinking and living enabled to flourish absent undue industry influence—moving beyond a pipeline of corporate ideas to a flowing river of possibility.

REFERENCES

1. Mitchell T. *Carbon Democracy: Political Power in the Age of Oil*. Verso; 2011.

2. Mann ME. *The New Climate War: The Fight to Take Back Our Planet*. Scribe; 2021.

3. Michaels D. *The Triumph of Doubt: Dark Money and the Science of Deception*. Oxford University Press; 2020.

4. Oreskes N, Conway EM. *Merchants of Doubt: How a Handful of Scientists Obscured the Truth on Issues from Tobacco Smoke to Global Warming*. Bloomsbury; 2011.

5. Schneider J, Schwarze S, Bsumek PK, Peeples J. *Under Pressure: Coal Industry Rhetoric and Neoliberalism*. Palgrave Macmillan; 2016.

6. Bonneuil C, Choquet P-L, Franta B. Early warnings and emerging accountability: Total's responses to global warming, 1971–2021. *Global Environ Change*. 2021: 102386.

7. Franta B. Early oil industry knowledge of CO_2 and global warming. *Nat Clim Change*. 2018; 8(12): 1024–1025.

8. Supran G, Oreskes N. Assessing ExxonMobil's climate change communications (1977–2014). *Environ Res Lett*. 2017; 12(8): 084019.

9. Supran G, Oreskes N. Rhetoric and frame analysis of ExxonMobil's climate change communications. *One Earth*. 2021; 4(5): 696–719.

10. Farrell J. Corporate funding and ideological polarization about climate change. *Proc Natl Acad Sci USA*. 2016; 113(1): 92–97.

11. Goldberg RF, Vandenberg LN. Distract, delay, disrupt: Examples of manufactured doubt from five industries. *Rev Environ Health*. 2019; 34(4): 349–363.

12. Mayer J. *Dark Money: How a Secretive Group of Billionaires Is Trying to Buy Political Control in the US*. Scribe; 2016.

13. Smerecnik KR, Renegar VR. Capitalistic agency: The rhetoric of BP's Helios Power campaign. *Environ Commun*. 2010; 4(2): 152–171.

14. Saltman K, Goodman R. Rivers of fire: BPAmaco's iMPACT on education. In: Saltman K, Gabbard D, eds. *Education as Enforcement: The Militarization and Corporatization of Schools*. 2nd ed. Routledge; 2011: 36–56.

15. Orestes N, Conway EM. Challenging knowledge: How climate science became a victim of the Cold War. In: Proctor R, Schiebinger L, eds. *Agnotology: The Making and Unmaking of Ignorance*. Stanford, CA: Stanford University Press; 2008.

16. Brandt AM. *The Cigarette Century: The Rise, Fall, and Deadly Persistence of the Product That Defined America*. Basic Books; 2009.

17. Proctor RN. *Golden Holocaust: Origins of the Cigarette Catastrophe and the Case for Abolition*. University of California Press; 2011.

18. Plec E, Pettenger M. Greenwashing consumption: The didactic framing of ExxonMobil's energy solutions. *Environ Commun*. 2012; 6(4): 459–476.

19. Wright C, Nyberg D. *Climate Change, Capitalism, and Corporations*. Cambridge University Press; 2015.

20. Eaton EM, Day NA. Petro-pedagogy: Fossil fuel interests and the obstruction of climate justice in public education. *Environm Educ Res*. 2020; 26(4): 457–473.

21. Tannock S. The oil industry in our schools: From Petro Pete to science capital in the age of climate crisis. *Environ Educ Res*. 2020; 26(4): 474–490.

22. Zou JJ. *Oil's pipeline to America's schools: Inside the fossil-fuel industry's not-so-subtle push into K–12 education*. Center for Public Integrity; 2017.

23. Huber M. Refined politics: Petroleum products, neoliberalism, and the ecology of entrepreneurial life. *J Am Stud*. 2012; 46(2): 295–312.

24. Coles G. *Miseducating for the Global Economy: How Corporate Power Damages Education and Subverts Students' Futures*. Monthly Review Press; 2018.

25. Marteau TM, Chater N, Garnett EE. Changing behaviour for net zero 2050. *BMJ*. 2021; 375: n2293.

CHAPTER 13

The Gambling Industry

Harmful Products, Predatory Practices, and the Politics of Knowledge

MAY CI VAN SCHALKWYK AND REBECCA CASSIDY

13.1 INTRODUCTION

The modern transformation of gambling into a highly profitable commercial activity supplied by major corporations has been profound. In an increasing number of places (with some important exceptions, including India, China, and Qatar), gambling is promoted as a harmless and sociable leisure activity that is best governed by market forces.[1] At the same time, evidence of the harms associated with gambling, which range from individual health impacts, addiction, debt, job loss, or homelessness to relationship breakdown, suicide, violence, crime, and wider social costs, is growing.[2-4]

Expansion of availability and participation has been associated with a rise in gambling harms, including gambling disorder and related morbidities. Initial attempts to estimate disease burden suggest that the burden of harm related to gambling exceeds that attributable to drug dependence and several common chronic diseases, and a growing body of literature indicates that the greatest burden of harm falls on the most vulnerable and disadvantaged, serving to exacerbate and entrench inequities.[3,5]

Regulation has often failed to keep pace with advances in the strategies used by the industry to design and promote their products.[3] Policy responses have largely emphasized what is referred to as "responsible gambling," placing the onus on individuals to exercise self-control in their use of dangerous products that are presented as safe for most.[1,6,7] This framing creates a "minority"

May Ci van Schalkwyk and Rebecca Cassidy, *The Gambling Industry* In: *The Commercial Determinants of Health*. Edited by: Nason Maani, Mark Petticrew, and Sandro Galea, Oxford University Press. © Oxford University Press 2023. DOI: 10.1093/oso/9780197578742.003.0013 of pathologized "problem gamblers," shifts the burden of responsibility from the industry and the government to the individual consumer,[1,6-8] elides the spectrum of harms, and ignores the fact that for every problem gambler an average of between 6 and 17 others may be harmed.[3]

In this chapter, we explore how the industry has shaped this context through the employment of strategies well documented in the literature on other harmful industries, arguing that examining the gambling industry through the commercial determinants of harm (CDOH) lens will both improve policy and support public health. Throughout, we refer to "the gambling industry," recognizing however that "the industry" is not monolithic and constitutes many different forms and venues (e.g., betting shops, casinos, bingo halls, online products, and convenience gambling in pubs, supermarkets) and actors (e.g., bookmakers, online operators, trade bodies, broadcasters, and advertisers).[1] During the past 40 years, the United Kingdom has embraced an agenda of gambling liberalization, making it an important case study for exploring the conduct of the industry and other actors when responding to these changes. The chapter draws primarily on insights gained from these developments, which are likely to be instructive for other contexts.

13.2 THE GAMBLING INDUSTRY AND THE COMMERCIAL DETERMINANTS OF HEALTH

Although the act of gambling and games of chance can be traced back thousands of years and adopt different meanings and form depending on the time, culture, and context, it is the recent expansion of gambling into a multibillion-dollar commercial activity, provided in many locations by transnational corporations, that represents a threat to public health. This step change in the supply of gambling, not unlike the rise of the tobacco and other industries in the 20th century, makes it a strong candidate for a CDOH approach.

A CDOH approach provides a logic through which to conceptualize the impacts of corporate practices and products on health.[9] Like the tobacco industry,[10] the gambling industry, enabled by conducive policy environments, political narratives, and high profit margins, has acted to normalize and popularize gambling as a "legitimate" and "harmless" leisure activity.[1] This has included engineering the social conditions that promote consumption, drawing on advances in communication, marketing strategies, and public relations. This process has often taken place under the auspices of "free market" politics, in opposition to public opinion, with little or no evidence of a growth in public demand for the expansion of gambling opportunities.[11,12] This development is driven by beneficiaries of the growth of gambling, including governments (through taxation, political donations, and revolving doors), corporations, shareholders, consultants, and other financial and legal providers of services to the industry. The extreme profits that can be made in the industry serve to quickly build and maintain its economic and political power, simultaneously creating financial dependencies and conflicts of interest.

In his analysis of this expansion, Adams has described the gambling industry as an "extractive industry."[13] This conceptualization is useful from a CDOH research perspective for several reasons. First, it helps reveal the ways in which gambling extracts wealth from individuals and communities through the exploitation of pre-existing systems and vulnerable communities, while ensuring the cooperation of allies gained through selective contributions to academia, treatment, education facilities, and other "good causes."[14,15] The recent expansion of betting companies into Africa using infrastructure designed to support financial inclusion (smartphones, broadband, and mobile money services) provides a clear illustration of this extractive logic.[16,17] Second, it enables researchers to learn from examples of other extractive industries in finding solutions to the problems posed by the expansion of commercial gambling. Third, it disrupts the insularity that industry funding and an attendant lack of openness and interdisciplinarity have created in the field of gambling research.

The gambling industry draws on a well-established corporate "playbook" to vindicate expansion as a socially and economically responsible process and to block, delay, or weaken regulation that could threaten profits (Box 13.1).[2,1,7,14,18,19] This playbook is reflected in and reproduced by the deep and extensive nexus of relationships and shared interests that exist between the industry, regulators, policymakers, and governments. This network extends into the research community, with academia, the regulators, and the industry working closely together—with important implications for the evolution and direction of the research agenda. These networks, described by Hancock as the "elite Reno policy network," have emerged in many Western countries alongside the growing influence and profits of the industry.[6] Writing primarily about Australia, Markham and Young have referred to these phenomena as the "rise of the global industry–state gambling complex,"[20] with Orford referring to the "gambling establishment" in the UK context.[12] The gambling industry uses established corporate political activities previously identified by analyses of the alcohol and tobacco industries to counter efforts to advance policies that would improve public health, including strategic use of evidence and arguments that rest on particular ideas and framings of gambling harms and responsibility.[21]

13.3 OWNING THE EVIDENCE

It is conventional for UK politicians tasked with assessing the impact of gambling regulation or drafting new policies to bemoan the lack of evidence

Box 13.1 TACTICS USED BY THE GAMBLING INDUSTRY TO MAINTAIN THE STATUS QUO AND RESIST CHANGE

1. Delaying changes to policy by insisting on perfect evidence of causal relationships between products and problems, interventions and outcomes, while at the same time introducing unproven and ineffective interventions that are less likely to affect profits
2. Emphasizing the findings of population-level prevalence studies that do not provide any information about levels or volumes of gambling harm and their distribution across society, including among non-gamblers and the families of gamblers
3. Presenting opposition to interventions that will reduce profits as a way to protect the freedom of individual consumers and misrepresenting this position as apolitical and "evidence-based"
4. Misusing arguments about the complexity of gambling harm in order to undermine support for interventions that are based on the best available knowledge

available to inform their thinking.[1] This is partly accurate—gambling research has not received sufficient investment, nor has it been conducted independently of industry influence, resulting in an international evidence base that is limited in terms of both scope and quality.[7,14,22,23] Indeed, gambling research has been described as "unimaginative, conceptually bereft and theoretically vacuous."[24] However, an equally profound problem is that policymakers have tended to adopt, promote, and defend a particular understanding of what constitutes "evidence" and how it should be used to inform action. This understanding aligns with industry interests and those who benefit from industry profits, often at the expense of public health.[18] As a result of this contentious understanding of "evidence," changes to policy that are likely to impact profits are strongly resisted and rarely introduced on the basis that it is not possible to provide incontrovertible proof of a causal relationship between gambling products or practices and harms or that proposed policies will achieve their goal without any unintended consequences.[1,18]

The clearest illustration of this framing of "evidence" can be found in the arguments used to delay changes that would restrict the maximum stakes of fixed odds betting terminals (FOBTs), the name given to electronic gambling machines (EGMs) in the United Kingdom (similar products are known as "pokies" in Australia, "video lottery terminals" in Canada, and EGMs in the United States).[1,7] UK-based trade bodies and corporate representatives have consistently repeated variations on the argument that "there is no empirical evidence of a causal link between gaming machines and problem gambling" (ABB 2013), distracting attention from the international literature and, indeed, the evidence provided by those in the United Kingdom who had themselves experienced harm as a result of using FOBTs.[1] Although it might sound reasonable to ask for evidence of a "causal relationship" between a particular product and particular behavior, in practice, given the range of products available to gamblers in the United Kingdom, the complexity of a behavior such as "problem gambling," and the social context in which gambling occurs, to obtain unquestionable proof is infeasible as well as potentially unethical. The repeated insistence upon perfect evidence of a one-to-one causal relationship between a particular product, in this case FOBTs, and a particular behavior, "problem gambling," has misled policymakers and detracted from the overwhelming international evidence which suggests that high-speed, continuous forms of gambling, such as FOBTs, are associated with increased harm.[3]

Direct, causal linear relationships are rarely sought or established in public health due to the complexity of the systems in which behaviors, processes, and products are embedded, a point discussed in greater depth in Chapter 2. The demand for causal evidence both conceals the complex system from which harms arise and delays changes to policy based on the balance of knowledge about products and harms, broadly conceived. This strategy mirrors the activities of the tobacco and other industries in their efforts to set unattainable levels of proof as the standard that must be reached before action is justified, and it misrepresents scientific uncertainty, either as evidence of no harm or as sufficient cause for doubt and therefore delay.[25,26] It is also indicative of the industry's and its allies' tendency to efface the critical difference between the levels of evidence at hand to inform policy and the political decision to act based on any given evidence of potential harm.[26] The former is often asserted as objectively dictating when action is justified. However, as Schrecker explains, deciding when to act to prevent harm is a value judgment, and "no algorithm will provide a correct answer, and the choice of how much evidence is enough should be addressed as an issue of public health ethics."[26]

Changes to policy that are likely to impact profits are resisted on the basis of a lack of evidence of the existence of the problem they are designed to solve. On the other hand, interventions that are less likely to impact profits are routinely introduced by the gambling industry, without any evidence of their efficacy. This double standard has been noted in Australia as well as the United Kingdom, and it generates an ad hoc ecosystem consisting of various unaccountable schemes, conceived and maintained by the industry, often with the endorsement of government, with a focus on "responsible gambling" or, more recently, "safer gambling," including educational programs for gamblers that emphasize self-control.[6,20,21,27]

13.4 OWNING THE DISCOURSE

The unprecedented expansion of the gambling industry and the normalization of gambling have been enabled by the coalescence of multiple cultural, social, economic, and political changes that can be described as the rise of neoliberalism. The shifting of risk from the state to the individual, the rise of the responsible and rational individual consumer as the logic through which citizenship has come to be defined, and normalization of risk (epitomized by the deregulation of financial markets) have all aligned with the interests of an industry that relies heavily on the notions of consumer freedom, self-regulation, and risk-taking.

These wider changes have aided the industry in its efforts to build and normalize a discourse structured around certain understandings and ideas about gambling harms and responsibility. The gambling industry recognized at an early stage the merits of promoting ideas about gambling addiction as arising from an inherent flaw within an individual's neuropsychology.[7] Advancing such understanding could absolve the industry; its products and gambling environments as problems arising from a person's gambling could be assigned to a "brain" pathology.[7,23]

By establishing and continually restating this position, ignoring or attacking alternatives, and funding research that aligned with this position, "problematic" or "pathological" gambling came to be known through the neurosciences, siphoning off a category of faulty individuals into which the problem would be located, creating a legitimate object of study for gambling research, and placing every other aspect of gambling, including the industry, outside its purview. Through these efforts, measuring and monitoring the size of this "minority" population became the legitimate way to study gambling. The emphasis on within-country prevalence studies fundamentally shifted the focus away from problematizing the industry or the impacts of liberalizing policies.[28] For the remainder of the "normal" population, the industry pursues an agenda of promoting "responsible gambling" that reinforces a discourse of personal responsibility and self-control based on the consumption of information and behavior-based tools.[7] Notions of personal responsibility are thus embedded in gambling industry corporate social responsibility discourses that present the industry as responsible corporate actors delivering enjoyment to the masses while taking action to "educate" consumers who have failed to consume "responsibly." Addiction is portrayed as the fault of the individual and not the result of policies, products, or their providers.[29]

13.5 PERFECTING THE PRODUCTS

The industry has also benefitted from light-touch regulatory systems that encouraged it to pursue product and marketing strategy development to stimulate demand and consumption.[1,7] In a similar way to the firearms industry in the United States,[30] commercial secrecy surrounds product design and development within the gambling industry, hindering understanding of the public health implications posed by new products and how technologies are mobilized to extend length and intensity of play and to maximize profit. Systems for measuring and monitoring harm are often nonexistent or, if they do exist, categorically removed from the product, relocated in a health or treatment context, framed as a societal problem rather than one associated with particular products or places.

Gambling industries have benefitted from and accelerated technological advancements without scrutiny. Indeed, we are only just beginning to understand the technological capabilities of the gambling industry, mostly due to recent legal action that reveals how the gambling industry uses behavioral data to track customers.[31] It is in this space that the synergies between the rise of the gambling industry, advances in product design and player tracking as described by Schüll,[7] and surveillance capitalism as documented by Zuboff[32] become apparent. Zuboff has detailed the ways in which major technology corporations such as Google and Facebook are able to harvest behavioral data generated from interactions between people and products with online capability—data which provide lucrative insights into consumer markets that can be used as means to meet commercial ends. As Zuboff explains, "Big Tech" benefited from the early progress made by the gambling industry in tracking its players to analyze, predict, and influence consumer behavior. Major tech industries have advanced these early developments, harvesting the "behavioral surplus" data that are produced through continuous interaction with online technologies, in turn selling the insights these data contain to corporate clients, including online betting firms. The gambling industry is benefiting from the advances made by Big Tech by maximizing the profit potential of knowledge about the behavior of individuals.[32] These advancements in corporate conduct warrant much greater scrutiny from a public health perspective and open up spaces for CDOH researchers to critique concepts of self-control and consumer freedom that are promoted by the industry.

13.6 POTENTIAL RESEARCH AND TRANSLATIONAL GOALS

There are promising developments in the field of gambling research, with more independent analyses being conducted using novel methods to study gambling harms.[2,4] Other research efforts are directed at exploring the effects of product features,[33,34] including high-profit complex live-odds bets heavily promoted by the industry.[35,36] Cross-discipline collaborations are facilitating the sharing of knowledge, drawing parallels with other industries and their strategies.[3,18,19,37]

The gambling industry and its academic and political allies have generally been spared the scrutiny afforded to other areas involving corporate actors. Research that problematizes the *how* and *why* of the gambling policymaking process is urgently needed. Compared to other industries, there is limited research into gambling policymaking processes and how industry influences take shape and are exercised. The barriers that prevent this work from taking place, including access to industry and political elites and to the shadowy world of policy creation, must be highlighted and overcome. This area of work can learn from research conducted on industries such as tobacco and fossil fuels, employing a range of complementary methods, including stakeholder interviews, qualitative and quantitative document analyses, freedom of information requests, media studies, and network analyses. Casting a CDOH perspective on the gambling industry helps build the case for conducting systematic analyses of industry practices, with the aim of understanding how the industry builds and sediments favored ideas and policy regimes, and the implications such activities have for public health. How the industry responds to policy change and seeks to exploit new and emerging markets warrants further exploration.

As occurred with legal action taken against tobacco[38] and pharmaceutical companies,[39] research into legal proceedings involving the gambling industry could provide important insights into how the industry orchestrated the widespread use and acceptance of its products and also into arguments formulated to deflect blame away from corporate products and practices onto the consumer.

13.7 CONCLUSION

Adopting a CDOH perspective advances the field of gambling research by problematizing, from a public health perspective, the ways in which the gambling industry, often in partnership with other allies, has established and maintained policy and research paradigms favorable to its interests. Ways of understanding have emerged that deflect from the negative impacts of policies, industry practices, and products and have enabled the expansion and advancement of what is conceptualized as a socially desirable and enjoyable leisure industry provided by responsible corporate actors that inform consumers and fund good causes. Harms are construed as being experienced by a static pathologized minority, who became the focus of inventions, research, and surveillance. Such ideas have been maintained through sustained

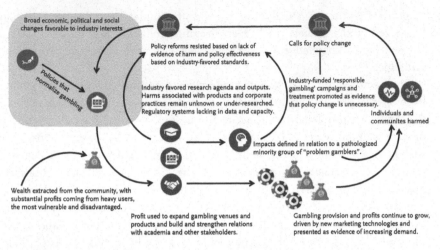

Figure 13.1 The cycle of resistance to change and (re)producing the void of knowledge.

assertions about the lack of evidence (maintained by industry influence) as to the *cause* and *extent* of harms, how to address them, and by demands for unattainable levels of proof of causation before action is taken, creating a vicious cycle that reproduces a void of knowledge and inertia (Figure 13.1). The gambling industry continues to benefit from the normalization of these discourses, which provide the basis for further liberalization and expansion globally. Viewing gambling through a CDOH lens not only subjects gambling policy to scrutiny that it has thus far avoided but also opens up broader questions, showing that the methods we use to create and distribute wealth are choices for us to make, rather than inevitabilities that we are obliged to accept.

NOTES

1. For comprehensive accounts on the consistent use of terms by ministers and members of industry trade associations, see Cassidy[1] and Schüll.[7]
2. For more discussion on gambling industry arguments and alignment with other harmful industries, see van Schalkwyk et al.[18]

REFERENCES

1. Cassidy R. *Vicious Games: Capitalism and Gambling.* Pluto Press; 2020.
2. Browne M, Rawat V, Newall P, Begg S, Rockloff M, Hing N. A framework for in-direct elicitation of the public health impact of gambling problems. *BMC Public Health.* 2020; 20(1): 1717.

3. Sulkunen P, Babor TF, Egerer M, et al. *Setting Limits: Gambling, Science and Public Policy*: Oxford University Press; 2019.

4. Muggleton N, Parpart P, Newall P, Leake D, Gathergood J, Stewart N. The association between gambling and financial, social and health outcomes in big financial data. *Nat Hum Behav*. 2021; 5(3): 319–326.

5. Abbott MW. Gambling and gambling-related harm: Recent World Health Organization initiatives. *Public Health*. 2020; 184: 56–59.

6. Hancock L, Smith G. Critiquing the Reno Model I–IV international influence on regulators and governments (2004–2015)—The distorted reality of "responsible gambling." *Int J Mental Health Addict*. 2017; 15(6): 1151–1176.

7. Schüll ND. *Addiction by Design: Machine Gambling in Las Vegas*: Princeton University Press; 2014.

8. Borrell J. A thematic analysis identifying concepts of problem gambling agency: With preliminary exploration of discourses in selected industry and research documents. *J Gambling Issues*. 2008; 22: 195–218.

9. Maani N, McKee M, Petticrew M, Galea S. Corporate practices and the health of populations: A research and translational agenda. *Lancet Public Health*. 2020; 5(2): e80–e81.

10. Brandt AM. *The Cigarette Century: The Rise, Fall, and Deadly Persistence of the Product That Defined America*. Basic Books; 2009.

11. Goodman R. *The Luck Business*. Touchstone; 1996.

12. Orford J. *The Gambling Establishment: Challenging the Power of the Modern Gambling Industry and Its Allies*: Taylor & Francis; 2019.

13. Adams PJ. *Gambling, Freedom and Democracy*. Routledge; 2008.

14. Adams PJ. *Moral Jeopardy: Risks of Accepting Money from the Alcohol, Tobacco and Gambling Industries*. Cambridge University Press; 2016.

15. Adams PJ. Gambling and democracy. In: Bowden-Jones H, Dickson C, Dunand C, Simon O, eds. *Harm Reduction for Gambling A Public Health Approach*. Routledge; 2019: 5–12.

16. Owuor VO. Why smartphone gambling is on the up among African millennials. *The Conversation*. November 24, 2019.

17. Owuor VO. The uneasy relationship between online betting and mobile money transactions. *The Conversation*. April 23, 2018.

18. van Schalkwyk MCI, Petticrew M, Cassidy R, et al. A public health approach to gambling regulation: Countering powerful influences. *Lancet Public Health*. 2021; 6(8): e614–e619.

19. Petticrew M, Katikireddi SV, Knai C, et al. "Nothing can be done until everything is done": The use of complexity arguments by food, beverage, alcohol and gambling industries. *J Epidemiol Community Health*. 2017; 71(11): 1078–1083.

20. Markham F, Young M. "Big Gambling": The rise of the global industry–state gambling complex. *Addict Res Theory*. 2015; 23(1): 1–4.

21. Hancock L, Ralph N, Martino FP. Applying corporate political activity (CPA) analysis to Australian gambling industry submissions against regulation of television sports betting advertising. *PLoS One*. 2018; 13(10): e0205654.

22. Cassidy R, Loussouarn C, Pisac A. *Fair Game: Producing Gambling Research*. Project Report. European Research Council, Goldsmiths University of London;, 2014.

23. Vrecko S. Capital ventures into biology: Biosocial dynamics in the industry and science of gambling. *Econ Society*. 2008; 37(1): 50–67.

24. Young M, Markham F. Beyond disclosure: Gambling research, political economy, and incremental reform. *Int Gambling Stud*. 2015; 15(1): 6–9.

25. Oreskes N. The fact of uncertainty, the uncertainty of facts and the cultural resonance of doubt. *Philos Trans A Math Phys Eng Sci.* 2015; 373(2055); 20140455.

26. Schrecker T. Can health equity survive epidemiology? Standards of proof and social determinants of health. *Prev Med.* 2013; 57(6): 741–744.

27. Livingstone C, Rintoul A. Moving on from responsible gambling: A new discourse is needed to prevent and minimise harm from gambling. *Public Health.* 2020; 184: 107–112.

28. Young M. Statistics, scapegoats and social control: A critique of pathological gambling prevalence research. *Addict Res Theory.* 2013; 21(1): 1–11.

29. Geiger BB, Cuzzocrea V. Corporate social responsibility and conflicts of interest in the alcohol and gambling industries: A post-political discourse? *Br J Sociol.* 2017; **68**(2): 254–272.

30. Diaz T. *Making a Killing: The Business of Guns in America*: New Press; 2000.

31. Satariano A. What a gambling app knows about you. *The New York Times.* March 24, 2021.

32. Zuboff S. *The Age of Surveillance Capitalism: The Fight for the Future at the New Frontier of Power.* Profile Books; 2018.

33. Barton KR, Yazdani A, Ayer N, et al. The effect of losses disguised as wins and near misses in electronic gaming machines: A systematic review. *J Gambling Stud.* 2017; 33(4): 1241–1260.

34. Graydon C, Dixon MJ, Stange M, Fugelsang JA. Gambling despite financial loss—The role of losses disguised as wins in multi-line slots. *Addiction.* 2019; 114(1): 119–124.

35. Newall PWS. Behavioral complexity of British gambling advertising. *Addict Res Theory.* 2017; 25(6): 505–511.

36. Newall PWS, Thobhani A, Walasek L, Meyer C. Live-odds gambling advertising and consumer protection. *PLoS One.* 2019; 14(6): e0216876.

37. Knai C, Petticrew M, Capewell S, et al. The case for developing a cohesive systems approach to research across unhealthy commodity industries. *BMJ Global Health.* 2021; 6(2): e003543.

38. Friedman LC, Cheyne A, Givelber D, Gottlieb MA, Daynard RA. Tobacco industry use of personal responsibility rhetoric in public relations and litigation: Disguising freedom to blame as freedom of choice. *Am J Public Health.* 2015; 105(2): 250–260.

39. Michaels D. *The Triumph of Doubt: Dark Money and the Science of Deception.* Oxford University Press; 2020.

CHAPTER 14

Sugar-Sweetened Beverages

ERIC CROSBIE, LAURA SCHMIDT, JIM KRIEGER, AND
MARION NESTLE

14.1 INTRODUCTION

Between 1990 and 2019, the share of the global burden of disease associated
with noncommunicable diseases (NCDs), including cardiovascular diseases,
diabetes, cancers, and chronic respiratory diseases, increased from 43% to
54%.[1] NCDs now account for 71% of deaths globally, and this proportion is
expected to rise to more than 85% by 2030.[2] Among NCD deaths, two-thirds
are related to modifiable risk factors: tobacco use, alcohol use, physical inactivity, and unhealthy dietary intake.[3] With respect to dietary intake, sugar-
sweetened beverages (SSBs), such as sodas, fruit drinks, sweetened teas and
coffees, and sports and energy drinks, are of particular concern. Their overconsumption is strongly associated with weight gain, obesity, an increased incidence of NCDs, and overall mortality.[4]

These effects are due to the large amounts of SSBs consumed, the calories
and direct metabolic effects of the sugars they deliver, the rapid absorption
of those sugars in liquid form, and the displacement of calories from more
nutritious sources.[4] SSB products comprise the largest source of added sugars
in the diet in some countries and provide few or no other nutrients.[4] Higher
SSB consumption and its associated illnesses are more common among low-
income groups and those experiencing income disparities, systemic racism,
and discrimination; the effects of COVID-19 are also more severe among these
groups.[5]

Nutrition scientists, health scholars, public health practitioners, and
policymakers have for decades focused on *proximal determinants* of health,
meaning individual biological and behavioral risk factors that influence health

Eric Crosbie, Laura Schmidt, Jim Krieger, and Marion Nestle, *Sugar-Sweetened Beverages* In: *The Commercial
Determinants of Health*. Edited by: Nason Maani, Mark Petticrew, and Sandro Galea, Oxford University Press.
© Oxford University Press 2023. DOI: 10.1093/oso/9780197578742.003.0014

outcomes. From a public health perspective, these are downstream factors. The focus on proximal determinants has led to a bias toward encouraging individuals to improve their health by modifying use of tobacco, alcohol, and drugs, as well as their diets. This approach has generated criticism for its focus on individuals and its limited effect in curbing NCDs.[2] This focus on individual risk is reinforced by the wide availability of behavioral health data, dominant biomedical paradigms of health education and practice, disease intervention research funding, and the medicalization of health.[6]

In recent decades, an emphasis on the *distal determinants* of health has emerged with a focus on the socioeconomic and environmental causes of health problems—the upstream factors that shape proximal determinants.[7] This chapter examines one distal determinant—the role of the SSB industry as a commercial vector of disease. It reviews the strategies of this industry and provides examples of best practices to address commercial determinants of health to combat the NCD epidemic and its consequences.

14.2 EXAMINING THE VECTOR: THE SSB INDUSTRY

Epidemiologists who study communicable diseases such as malaria, tuberculosis, HIV/AIDS, and COVID-19 focus on the vector of the disease, whether animal, insect, or viral. In the case of diet-influenced NCDs, the food and beverage industries must be considered as disease vectors. They help facilitate the spread of NCDs by producing and marketing calorie-dense, ultra-processed foods and by influencing science and public policy to protect their profits. For the remainder of this chapter, we focus on the SSB industry vector.

The SSB industry was globally valued at $1.55 trillion in 2018 and is expected to be worth $1.885 trillion in 2023. Although this industry's supply chain includes many producers, manufacturers, and distributors, it is dominated by two transnational beverage corporations—Coca-Cola and PepsiCo. As of April 2021, these two companies reported a net worth of $229.17 billion and $196.75 billion, respectively, and in 2020, they reported revenues of $33.01 billion and $25.83 billion, respectively.[8] Both have more than doubled their net worth since 2009.[8] Both companies produce a wide range of beverage products varying in colors, flavors, and sugar levels. Both rely on low-cost municipal water supplies to procure a key product ingredient.

The SSB industry is a member of notable business groups and trade associations, including the American Beverage Association, the International Chamber of Commerce, and the International Council of Beverage Associations. These organizations represent the interests of member companies during policy discussions, trade negotiations, and the development of dietary guidelines and other government regulations. They often act on behalf of the companies— seen most prominently in their efforts opposing SSB tax initiatives.[9]

14.3 SSB INDUSTRY MARKETING

From 2014 to 2020, Coca-Cola and PepsiCo spent on average a combined $4 billion annually on advertising their products worldwide.[10] In 2019, Coca-Cola and PepsiCo spent $283 million and $224 million respectively on advertising their products in the United States.[10] Even so, per capita consumption of SSBs (primarily sodas) in the United States began declining in 2000 but then leveled off (2010–2013), except for a small uptick during the COVID-19 pandemic.[11] Increased sales of energy and sports drinks and other non-soda beverages have compensated for some of these losses.[12]

The SSB industry has aggressively advertised, promoted, and sponsored its products globally and used discriminatory, racialized marketing tactics to drive sales among disproportionally affected populations, including youth, people of color, and low-income communities and countries.[13,14] This industry historically has advertised on traditional media such as television, radio, and print. However, given the expense of advertising on these medium and their limited reach, the SSB industry has increasingly turned to the internet and social media. SSB companies have recruited popular celebrities to endorse their products in all media; these include sports athletes (e.g., Lebron James and Cristiano Renaldo), musicians (e.g., Michael Jackson, Taylor Swift, and Beyoncé), and movie stars (e.g., Penelope Cruz and Courtney Cox). The industry also employs promotional giveaways, discounts, and buy-one-get-one-free promotions. It sponsors sports events, musical concerts, and festivals in many countries to promote its image and products. These companies sponsor global sporting events such as the Olympics or the World Cup, watched by millions of viewers.[15]

14.4 SSB INDUSTRY STRATEGIES TO BLOCK, WEAKEN, AND DELAY GOVERNMENT REGULATIONS

Similar to the tactics of the tobacco and alcohol industries, the SSB industry has developed structural, discursive, and instrumental strategies to promote sales and prevent product regulation.[16] The SSB industry seeks to shape global trade agreements and conventions to block adoption of national policies it opposes. For example, the SSB industry has lobbied trade negotiators to remove barriers (e.g., tariffs and capital controls), thereby allowing global market entry and expansion, and permitting global advertising.[17] In many low- and middle-income countries, such trade agreements have resulted in a dietary transition away from traditional diets and toward those containing a larger proportion of ultra-processed foods and drinks.[18] It has lobbied and helped draft investment protections such as intellectual property rights (e.g., trademarks) and dispute settlement mechanisms in trade agreements, effectively altering trade rules to constrain policymakers seeking to implement public health policies.[19,20] Even when trade rules do not apply, the SSB industry still exaggerates the interpretation and application of these rules and threatens governments in an attempt to block, weaken, and delay public health proposals.[21,22] Although these actions may target a particular country, often the intent is to create a "chilling effect" by preventing the diffusion of best public health practices regionally and globally.[21,23]

Other forms of global preemption (limiting national and subnational authority) include lobbying governments during ongoing Codex Alimentarius negotiations,[24] which establish international standards and guidelines relating to food production and food safety. Although Codex is not a trade agreement, this collection of international standards is recognized by trade agreements and is referenced by governments during trade disputes at the World Trade Organization. Thus, the SSB industry's attempts to alter Codex standards are a key pillar in its strategy to obtain favorable trade agreements that preempt national public health policies.[24]

In addition to global preemption, the SSB industry has used subnational state preemption in the United States to prevent localities from enacting municipal SSB taxes. This has had a chilling effect on other localities seeking to enact similar taxes, diminishing discussion and policy actions.[9,25] Once preemption policies are in place, they are extremely difficult to repeal.[26]

The SSB industry also uses discursive, or argument-based, strategies that have helped drive NCD epidemics. Similar to the tobacco and alcohol industry, the SSB industry has attempted to frame rising rates of NCDs as a personal or parental responsibility, thereby shifting the blame to individuals (downstream) and away from the unhealthy products they produce (upstream). Coca-Cola, for example, sponsored a global campaign called the Global Energy Balance Network, which recruited nutrition and physical activity scholars to argue that the solution to the obesity crisis lies in individuals balancing diet with physical activity, with a stronger emphasis on the latter.[27] The SSB industry has also sponsored research to spread misinformation and create doubt about the harmfulness of its products. The industry takes the position that SSB taxes are regressive in that they disproportionally affect low-income populations, drive the loss of jobs in beverage-related businesses, and increase costs to consumers with no improvement in public health.[28] These arguments, however, have largely been refuted by research (see the next section).

The SSB industry has also used a wide range of instrumental, or action-based, strategies to pursue its interests. These include more traditional strategies such as lobbying and providing political donations to policymakers and positioning industry executives in government regulatory agencies (a practice known as the "revolving door") that allow SSB companies to participate in—and weaken—policy negotiations.[29] Companies create corporate social responsibility initiatives to position themselves as good corporate citizens, protect the industry's image and credibility, and avoid government regulations. Companies also consult with experts in public think tanks, and recruit academics and professional associations, to create the illusion of "independent" research and obtain favorable reports.[30] Much of the research funded by SSB companies is aimed at demonstrating that SSBs are harmless, discrediting research to the contrary, and staving off unfavorable regulation.[31]

The industry actively engages in public–private partnerships that give companies a seat at the governmental policymaking table, enhance their legitimacy, and make them appear to be part of the solution—rather than the cause—of health problems.[32] To further carry out these strategies, the industry uses front groups, such as the International Life Sciences Institute, to work with governments throughout the world to focus anti-obesity efforts on increased physical activity rather than dietary changes.[31]

14.5 BEST PRACTICES FOR MINIMIZING COMMERCIAL VECTOR INFLUENCE AND REGULATING SSBS

Reducing SSB consumption and its associated NCD burden requires minimizing commercial vector influence by exposing industry deception and its funding of research and political campaigns and by requiring full disclosure of conflicts of interest and political activities. Countering commercial vector influence also requires communication campaigns to debunk common industry arguments. These approaches can be supported with published research from previously secret internal food industry documents, which have recently revealed the SSB industry's relationships with the tobacco industry,[33] its targeted marketing of ethnic groups,[34] and its efforts to control and privatize public water supplies in countries that face water scarcity.[35]

Legislative and regulatory policies are a powerful tool for modifying corporate behaviors. Current public health policies that affect SSB companies include licensing requirements, sales bans in public schools, marketing restrictions, labeling, and, more recently, taxation. A growing body of research demonstrates that SSB taxes are effective in reducing sales of taxed products,[36] in increasing awareness about health effects, and in helping low-income communities by investing revenues to build health equity in these communities, without causing job losses (in some cases, jobs in the food sector actually increase following SSB taxes).[37] SSB tax revenues in U.S. cities are supporting healthy eating initiatives, including subsidies for purchases of fruits and vegetables; education and early childhood programs; improvements to parks, recreation centers, and libraries; and efforts to improve health equity through health promotion, general wellness programs, and chronic disease prevention.[38] Such investments make SSB taxes an economically progressive policy, transferring revenues collected from people with higher incomes to programs that benefit less-affluent people. The dollar amount of tax revenues funding programs targeted towards people with lower incomes is greater than the amount they pay in taxes.[39] SSB taxes are spreading globally, and as of January 2021, 44 countries and seven localities and the Navajo Nation in the United States have adopted some form of SSB taxes.[40]

Governments have also introduced different forms of front-of-package nutrition labeling (FOPNL), which provide simplified nutrition information on the front of packaged foods and beverages. Nutrient-specific interpretive FOPNL systems, which provide nutrition information for one or more nutrients, all include sugars as a target using traffic light labels (red, yellow, and green), warning labels, or "high in" symbols. These promote nutritional awareness of a product's contents,[41] help consumers make healthier choices, provide incentives for reformulating processed food and drink products,[41] and increase consumption of healthier food and beverage options.[42] Recent studies have shown that FOPNL warning label systems outperform traffic light, Health Star, and nutrition grade (e.g., NutriScore) labels in capturing consumers' attention, improving their ability to identify products high in concerned nutrients, and increasing their intention to buy a relatively healthier option.[43] Countries in Latin America are especially active in adopting warning labels; SSB purchases declined by 23.7% following Chile's implementation of warning labels.[43] Some countries in the region have also begun to restrict marketing of ultra-processed foods, including SSBs, to children (e.g., Mexico).[21,44]

Addressing the health consequences of the SSB industry will require a suite of integrated policies and actions.[45] New strategies that build on the foundation of current activities are emerging. Limiting sales and promotion of SSBs in retail settings, such as restrictions on product promotion and placement targeting the largest source of SSB purchases, is beginning in the United States, United Kingdom, and Australia.[46] There is growing interest in disallowing use of funds from public nutrition programs such as the SNAP program for SSB purchases in the United States. The World Health Organization's Tobacco Control Framework Section 5.3 exclusion of industry from public health policy processes could be applied to the SSB industry. Countermarketing campaigns and further restrictions on SSB marketing could blunt the effects of industry promotional activities.

14.6 CONCLUSION

Recognizing the SSB industry as a vector of disease under the commercial determinants of health framework is important for understanding the industry's impact in driving the growing global NCD epidemic. Current efforts, many of which focus on proximal determinants of health, have been unsuccessful in reversing the rise of NCDs. Future policy, advocacy, and scholarship should focus upstream on the distal determinants of health, including the SSB industry's structural, discursive, and instrumental strategies that undermine efforts to address the NCD epidemic. Current effective strategies such as taxation and labeling policies and limiting SSB marketing should be scaled up and implemented as an integrated set of interventions. Development and evaluation of new strategies such as frameworks to exclude industry from public health policy processes are also needed. Public health advocates will succeed in reducing the health burden of SSBs and reversing the NCD epidemics only if they pursue such a comprehensive approach.

REFERENCES

1. Benziger CP, Roth GA, Moran AE. The Global Burden of Disease Study and the preventable burden of NCD. *Glob Heart*. 2016; 11(4): 393–397. doi:10.1016/j.gheart.2016.10.024
2. World Health Organization. Think piece: Why is 2018 a strategically important year for NCDs? May 2018. Accessed April 10, 2021. https://www.who.int/ncds/governance/high-level-commission/why-2018-important-year-for-NCDs.pdf
3. World Health Organization. Global status report on noncommunicable diseases 2014. 2014. Accessed April 27, 2017. http://apps.who.int/iris/bitstream/10665/148114/1/9789241564854_eng.pdf?ua=1
4. Malik VS, Hu FB. The role of sugar-sweetened beverages in the global epidemics of obesity and chronic diseases. *Nat Rev Endocrinol*. 2022 Apr; 18(4): 205–218. doi:10.1038/s41574-021-00627-6. Epub 2022 Jan 21. PMID: 35064240; PMCID: PMC8778490.
5. Belanger MJ, Hill MA, Angelidi AM, Dalamaga M, Sowers JR, Mantzoros CS. COVID-19 and disparities in nutrition and obesity. *N Engl J Med*. 2020; 383(11): e69. doi:10.1056/NEJMp2021264
6. Clark J. Medicalization of global health 1: Has the global health agenda become too medicalized? *Glob Health Action*. 2014; 7: 23998. doi:10.3402/gha.v7.23998
7. Arah OA, Westert GP, Delnoij DM, Klazinga NS. Health system outcomes and determinants amenable to public health in industrialized countries: A pooled, cross-sectional time series analysis. *BMC Public Health*. 2005; 5: 81. doi:10.1186/1471-2458-5-81
8. Macrotrends. Coca-Cola net worth 2006–2020. April 12, 2021. Accessed April 13, 2021. https://www.macrotrends.net/stocks/charts/KO/cocacola/net-worth
9. Crosbie E, Schillinger D, Schmidt LA. State preemption to prevent local taxation of sugar-sweetened beverages. *JAMA Intern Med*. 2019; 179(3): 291–292. doi:10.1001/jamainternmed.2018.7770
10. Statista. Advertising spending of selected beverage brands in the United States in 2019. January 30, 2021. Accessed April 26, 2021. https://www.statista.com/statistics/264985/ad-spend-of-selected-beverage-brands-in-the-us
11. Pandemic lockdowns fuel 2020 soda sales growth. *Beverage Digest*. November 11, 2020. Accessed April 20, 2021. https://www.beverage-digest.com/articles/372-pandemic-lockdowns-fuel-2020-soda-sales-growth?v=preview
12. Martinez-Belkin N. Nielsen numbers: Big soda volume struggles; Water, energy, sports drinks swell. *Bevnet*. May 26, 2015. Accessed May 10, 2021. https://www.

bevnet.com/news/2015/nielsen-numbers-big-soda-volume-struggles-water-ene
rgy-sports-drinks-swell

13. UCONN Rudd Center for Food Policy & Obesity. Sugary drink advertising to youth: Continued barrier to public health progress. 2020. Accessed April 25, 2021. https://www.sugarydrinkfacts.org/resources/Sugary%20Drink%20FA CTS%202020/Sugary_Drink_FACTS_Full%20Report_final.pdf

14. Barnhill A, Ramírez AS, Ashe M, Berhaupt-Glickstein A, Freudenberg N, Grier SA, Watson KE, Kumanyika S. The racialized marketing of unhealthy foods and beverages: Perspectives and potential remedies. *J Law Med Ethics*. 2022; 50(1): 52–59. doi:10.1017/jme.2022.8. PMID: 35243999; PMCID: PMC9014864.

15. Bragg MA, Miller AN, Roberto CA, et al. Sports sponsorships of food and nonalcoholic beverages. *Pediatrics*. 2018; 141(4): e20172822. doi:10.1542/peds.2017-2822

16. Mialon M, Chantal J, Hercberg S. The policy dystopia model adapted to the food industry: The example of the Nutri-Score saga in France. *World Nutr*. 2018; 9(2): 109–120.

17. Ravuvu A, Friel S, Thow AM, Snowdon W, Wate J. Monitoring the impact of trade agreements on national food environments: Trade imports and population nutrition risks in Fiji. *Global Health*. 2017; 13(1): 33. doi:10.1186/s12992-017-0257-1

18. Blouin C, Chopra M, van der Hoeven R. Trade and social determinants of health. *Lancet*. 2009; 373(9662): 502–507. doi:10.1016/S0140-6736(08)61777-8

19. Labonte R, Crosbie E, Gleeson D, McNamara C. USMCA (NAFTA 2.0): Tightening the constraints on the right to regulate for public health. *Global Health*. 2019; 15(1): 35. doi:10.1186/s12992-019-0476-8

20. Crosbie E, Gonzalez M, Glantz SA. Health preemption behind closed doors: Trade agreements and fast-track authority. *Am J Public Health*. 2014; 104(9): e7–e13. doi:10.2105/AJPH.2014.302014

21. Crosbie E, Carriedo A, Schmidt L. Hollow threats: Transnational food and beverage companies' use of international agreements to fight front-of-pack nutrition labeling in Mexico and beyond. *Int J Health Policy Manage*. 2022; 11(6): 722–725. doi:10.34172/ijhpm.2020.146

22. Thow AM, Jones A, Hawkes C, Ali I, Labonte R. Nutrition labelling is a trade policy issue: Lessons from an analysis of specific trade concerns at the World Trade Organization. *Health Promot Int*. 2018; 33(4): 561–571. doi:10.1093/heapro/daw109

23. Crosbie E, Hatefi A, Schmidt L. Emerging threats of global preemption to nutrition labelling. *Health Policy Plan*. 2019; 34(5): 401–402. doi:10.1093/heapol/czz045

24. Thow AM, Jones A, Huckel Schneider C, Labonte R. Increasing the public health voice in global decision-making on nutrition labelling. *Global Health*. 2020; 16(1): 3. doi:10.1186/s12992-019-0533-3

25. Crosbie E, Pomeranz JL, Hoeper S, Wright K, Schmidt L. State preemption: An emerging threat to local sugar-sweetened beverage taxation. *Am J Public Health*. 2021; 111(4): 677–686.

26. Crosbie E, Schmidt LA. Preemption in tobacco control: A framework for other areas of public health. *Am J Public Health*. 2020; 110(3): 345–350. doi:10.2105/AJPH.2019.305473

27. Barlow P, Serodio P, Ruskin G, McKee M, Stuckler D. Science organisations and Coca-Cola's "war" with the public health community: Insights from an

internal industry document. *J Epidemiol Commun Health*. 2018; 72(9): 761–763. doi:10.1136/jech-2017-210375

28. Niederdeppe J, Gollust SE, Jarlenski MP, Nathanson AM, Barry CL. News coverage of sugar-sweetened beverage taxes: Pro- and antitax arguments in public discourse. *Am J Public Health*. 2013; 103(6): e92–e98. doi:10.2105/AJPH.2012.301023

29. Pedroza-Tobias A, Crosbie E, Mialon M, Carriedo A, Schmidt L. Food and beverage industry interference in the science of soda taxation: Industry's efforts to prevent international diffusion. *BMJ Glob Health*. 2021; 6(8): e00566.

30. Bes-Rastrollo M, Schulze MB, Ruiz-Canela M, Martinez-Gonzalez MA. Financial conflicts of interest and reporting bias regarding the association between sugar-sweetened beverages and weight gain: A systematic review of systematic reviews. *PLoS Med*. 2013; 10(12): e1001578; discussion e1001578. doi:10.1371/journal.pmed.1001578

31. Steele S, Ruskin G, Sarcevic L, McKee M, Stuckler D. Are industry-funded charities promoting "advocacy-led studies" or "evidence-based science"?: A case study of the International Life Sciences Institute. *Global Health*. 2019; 15(1): 36. doi:10.1186/s12992-019-0478-6

32. Nestle M. *Soda Politics: Taking on Big Soda (and Winning)*. University of California Press; 2018.

33. Nguyen KH, Glantz SA, Palmer CN, Schmidt LA. Tobacco industry involvement in children's sugary drinks market. *BMJ*. 2019; 364: l736. doi:10.1136/bmj.l736

34. Nguyen KH, Glantz SA, Palmer CN, Schmidt LA. Transferring racial/ethnic marketing strategies from tobacco to food corporations: Philip Morris and Kraft General Foods. *Am J Public Health*. 2020; 110(3): 329–336. doi:10.2105/AJPH.2019.305482

35. Schmidt L, Mialon M, Kearns C, Crosbie E. Transnational corporations, obesity and planetary health: Coca-Cola in Colombia. *Lancet Planet Health*. 2020; 4(7): E266–E267.

36. Andreyeva T, Marple K, Marinello S, Moore TE, Powell LM. Outcomes following taxation of sugar-sweetened beverages: A systematic review and meta-analysis. *JAMA Netw Open*. 2022 Jun 1; 5(6): e2215276. doi:10.1001/jamanetworkopen.2022.15276. PMID: 35648398; PMCID: PMC9161017.

37. Marinello S, Leider J, Pugach O, Powell LM. The impact of the Philadelphia beverage tax on employment: A synthetic control analysis. *Econ Hum Biol*. 2021 Jan; 40: 100939. doi:10.1016/j.ehb.2020.100939. Epub 2020 Oct 29.

38. Krieger J, Magee K, Hennings T, Schoof J, Madsen KA. How sugar-sweetened beverage tax revenues are being used in the United States. *Prev Med Rep*. 2021; 23: 101388. doi:10.1016/j.pmedr.2021.101388

39. Jones-Smith JC, Knox MA, Coe NB, Walkinshaw LP, Schoof J, Hamilton D, Hurvitz PM, Krieger J. Sweetened beverage taxes: Economic benefits and costs according to household income. *Food Policy*. 2022; 110: 102277. https://doi.org/10.1016/j.foodpol.2022.102277

40. Popkin BM, Ng SW. Sugar-sweetened beverage taxes: Lessons to date and the future of taxation. *PLoS Med*. 2021; 18(1): e1003412. doi:10.1371/journal.pmed.1003412. https://www.globalfoodresearchprogram.org/wp-content/uploads/2022/05/Sugary_Drink_Tax_maps_upload.pdf. Accessed June 17, 2022.

41. Neal B, Crino M, Dunford E, et al. Effects of different types of front-of-pack labelling information on the healthiness of food purchases—A randomised controlled trial. *Nutrients*. 2017; 9(12): 1284. doi:10.3390/nu9121284

42. Pan American Health Organization. Front-of-package labeling as a policy tool for the prevention of noncommunicable diseases in the Americas. November 2020. Accessed May 10, 2021. https://iris.paho.org/bitstream/handle/10665.2/52740/PAHONMHRF200033_eng.pdf?sequence=6&isAllowed=y

43. Global Food Research Program. Front-of-package (FOP) food labelling: Empowering consumers to make healthy choices. September 2020. Accessed April 22, 2021. https://globalfoodresearchprogram.web.unc.edu/wp-content/uploads/sites/10803/2020/08/FOP_Factsheet_UNCGFRP_2020_September_Final.pdf

44. Taillie LS, Reyes M, Colchero MA, Popkin B, Corvalan C. An evaluation of Chile's Law of Food Labeling and Advertising on sugar-sweetened beverage purchases from 2015 to 2017: A before-and-after study. *PLoS Med*. 2020; 17(2): e1003015. doi:10.1371/journal.pmed.1003015

45. Krieger J, Bleich SN, Scarmo S, Ng SW. Sugar-sweetened beverage reduction policies: Progress and promise. *Annu Rev Public Health*. 2021; 42: 439–461. doi:10.1146/annurev-publhealth-090419-103005

46. Brimblecombe J, McMahon E, Ferguson M, et al. Effect of restricted retail merchandising of discretionary food and beverages on population diet: A pragmatic randomised controlled trial. *Lancet Planet Health*. 2020; 4(10): e463–e473. doi:10.1016/S2542-5196(20)30202-3

SECTION 4

Cross-Industry Mechanisms

CHAPTER 15

Marketing

SIMONE PETTIGREW AND ALEXANDRA JONES

15.1 INTRODUCTION

The American Marketing Association's definition of marketing is "creating, communicating, delivering, and exchanging offerings that have value for customers, clients, partners, and society at large."[1] This apparently benevolent definition fails to acknowledge the inevitable tension between profit maximization on the one hand and human health and planetary welfare on the other. This tension is manifest in the many health, social, and environmental problems resulting from the large-scale consumption of heavily marketed products that can be classified as commercial determinants of health.

The World Health Organization's (WHO) "best buys" policies for creating healthy environments relate to four primary intervention areas: tobacco, alcohol, poor diet, and physical inactivity.[2] Three of these—tobacco, alcohol, and poor diet—are recognized as powerful commercial determinants of health that individually and in combination account for substantial burdens of disease globally.[3] The marketing budgets of these industries are astronomical, greatly dwarfing the public resources available to counteract their efforts. This state of affairs is reflected in a particular focus in the WHO's best buys recommendations on strategies for constraining the marketing activities of these industries. Recommendations include advertising bans, mandating the use of warnings on product packages, restrictions on availability, product reformulation, and taxes.

Marketing is often operationalized as the "4 Ps" of product, promotion, place, and price. Addressing these 4 Ps is key to addressing the negative health burden imposed by corporate activity. This chapter outlines each of the 4 Ps in the context of current industry practices and the implications for

Simone Pettigrew and Alexandra Jones, *Marketing* In: *The Commercial Determinants of Health*.
Edited by: Nason Maani, Mark Petticrew, and Sandro Galea, Oxford University Press. © Oxford University Press 2023.
DOI: 10.1093/oso/9780197578742.003.0015

governments and other agencies tasked with reducing the harms associated with these activities. Consideration is also given to research gaps that need to be addressed to develop and implement more effective countermeasures to current strategies being used to market unhealthy products.

15.2 PRODUCT

Marketing strategies relating to the product "P" are those encompassing the development and modification of products sold in the marketplace. They also involve branding and packaging elements that coalesce in consumers' minds to represent the totality of the product. Constant innovation is the lifeblood of commercial success, including in mature product markets in which overall consumer demand is stable. For example, although per capita alcohol consumption has plateaued in many countries, new products are continually brought to market as competitors seek to optimize their share of the available profits.

New product development and product modification represent opportunities for producers to circumvent existing and proposed actions that seek to constrain the marketing of harmful products. Two examples are outlined here.

15.2.1 E-Cigarettes

In many areas of the world, tobacco use has been declining in response to the implementation of a suite of public health interventions that in many cases are supported by laws and regulations. The emergence of e-cigarettes has provided the opportunity for the tobacco industry to invest in nicotine-dispensing products that are exempt from the restrictions placed on tobacco products. The evidence relating to the ability of e-cigarettes to facilitate smoking cessation remains contested, while there is increasing evidence that these products provide a "gateway" via which youth who would not otherwise have smoked traditional cigarettes are introduced to the behavior.[4] This is achieved in part through the availability of e-cigarettes in a wide range of flavors that are attractive to youth, such as candy apple and fairy floss. At least some of these young e-cigarette users graduate to traditional tobacco products once they have become addicted to nicotine.[5]

15.2.2 Zero-Alcohol Products

Recent years have seen the rapid growth of a wide range of zero-alcohol products that achieve a similar taste experience to their alcohol-containing counterparts. These products provide the alcohol industry with a method of maintaining sales in the face of growing evidence of the harms associated with alcohol consumption, even at low doses. For example, the International Agency for Research on Cancer reports causal association between alcohol consumption and seven different types of cancer.[6] At first glance, the growing availability of palatable zero-alcohol products would appear to be a positive outcome due to a presumed associated decrease in alcohol ingestion at the population level. However, there are several possible negative outcomes that have yet to be adequately assessed. For example, these products can be sold and promoted in ways that are not permitted for their alcohol product equivalent. Alcohol companies can brand and package their zero-alcohol products in ways that make them virtually indistinguishable from their alcohol-containing counterparts, allowing them to build brand awareness and preference relating to new usage contexts (e.g., while driving and operating machinery) and among new market segments (e.g., pregnant women and children).[7]

15.3 PROMOTION

The available options for marketers to promote their products have grown rapidly. Traditional "above the line" promotion methods such as television, radio, and outdoor advertising are complemented by a wide range of "below the line" methods, notably digital advertising. Examples of the latter include targeted campaigns disseminated via social media and email. Efforts to prevent the promotion of harmful products via traditional media are typically weak and poorly monitored. Advertising via digital platforms compounds these regulatory weaknesses due to the ability of marketers to segment potential customers down to the individual level to deliver tailored messages at places and times when they are most likely to be effective.[8] This individualized promotion is all but invisible to regulators and researchers, preventing appropriate levels of scrutiny and oversight.

In some instances, traditional and new forms of advertising are intersecting to produce highly effective methods of engaging with target market segments. An example is sports sponsorship as a form of promotion that can circumvent advertising bans and reach consumers in a manner that can reduce their likelihood of activating the cognitive defenses they would apply to more explicit forms of advertising.[9] Consider an alcohol company that sponsors a football team. Its brand logo is visible each time players' jerseys are on-screen and when the camera pans to the on-field advertising signage that is part of the sponsorship package. This footage can be available when the game is screened live and from digital versions available via a range of platforms. In this way, high levels of brand exposure can be obtained despite the existence of any regulations preventing alcohol advertising in the ad breaks within the broadcast. In addition, the alcohol company will capitalize on the sponsorship investment by promoting it across its media activities, including engagement with fans on its website and social media networks.[10-12] This engagement has been found to feature attributes that are especially attractive to youth, including interactivity, shareability, and the adulation of sporting heroes.[13]

Consumers' immersion in both real-world and online environments that are characterized by high levels of promotion for unhealthy products has substantial potential negative consequences. Much decision-making occurs at a subconscious level, making individuals susceptible to influence from repeated exposure to well-resourced promotional campaigns for harmful products.[14] The "mere exposure" effect is the process by which this repeated exposure results in an automatic assumption of the acceptability and desirability of the promoted products.[15] A further mechanism to influence consumers is the use of messages that are ostensibly seeking to reduce harm but in effect promote the use of the product. Examples include "warnings" such as "DrinkWise" on alcohol containers and "TreatWise" on confectionary packets. Such messages can be interpreted by consumers as normalizing consumption while simultaneously preventing more effective regulatory measures from being implemented by persuading policymakers that the industries in question are taking responsibility for communicating potential harm to users.[16]

15.4 PLACE

This "P" covers marketing activities relating to the places in which products are sold and how they are distributed. Technological advancements have resulted in substantial changes to the ways products move through the supply chain from the point of production to the point of consumption. There is now unparalleled access to harmful products on a mass scale. In the case of unhealthy foods, this is apparent in the rapid growth of online food ordering platforms such as Uber Eats, Grubhub, DoorDash, and Deliveroo. Currently valued at approximately $100 billion, this market is forecast to continue to expand quickly as high-speed internet access and smartphone ownership increase in coverage and consumers become accustomed to the convenience of home delivery.[17] This trend is problematic given that foods ordered online are predominantly unhealthy.[18] Also of concern is the increased availability of alcohol products via online ordering, especially where this enables inebriated individuals to order more alcohol when they are too intoxicated to go out to purchase it themselves. The relaxation of alcohol delivery regulations in some jurisdictions during COVID-19 has opened a gate that may be very difficult to close.[19]

The increased availability of unhealthy foods and beverages, including via online ordering platforms, has implications for the effectiveness of place-based food availability policies that seek to create healthy environments for specific population subgroups. Examples include healthy food policies being implemented in schools, hospitals, and workplaces. In Australia, for instance, nutrition policies have been introduced in many schools and hospitals to preclude the sale of sugar-sweetened beverages and other unhealthy products.[20] This hard-won progress is now under threat from the availability of cheap, unhealthy food delivered anytime, anywhere. The consequences are particularly challenging for schools seeking to prevent unhealthy foods being delivered to campus due to the implications for students' diets and safety issues around delivery vehicles.[21] The difficulties of containing the online delivery explosion across all contexts will be exacerbated once foods and beverages are also available via drone delivery. Domino's drone pizza delivery trial has already established the feasibility of this distribution method.[22]

15.5 PRICE

A key element in the armory of unhealthy product marketers is ensuring affordability for target segments. For mass-disseminated harmful products (e.g., many forms of tobacco, alcohol, and unhealthy food), affordability is assured in two primary ways: keeping unit costs low through large-scale distribution (e.g., mass-produced, highly processed foods with a long shelf-life) and producing pack sizes that enable lower income consumers to participate in the market (e.g., selling cigarettes in small packs or by the stick). Of particular concern is that making harmful products available at "pocket money" prices allows marketers to introduce children to their brands and groom them to become loyal future consumers. Similarly, entering developing countries with affordable products provides access to enormous markets that are typically characterized by less regulation and huge profit potential as incomes increase over time.[23]

Pricing strategies can intersect with the other three Ps discussed above. For instance, bulk alcohol products (e.g., 3-liter wine cartons) are heavily promoted, often available at lower per standard drink prices than bottled water, and widely distributed via brick-and-mortar stores and online ordering platforms.[24] This makes these products highly visible, affordable, and available. Similarly, the increased distribution of unhealthy foods via digital ordering platforms and automated delivery mechanisms increases demand and reduces per-order costs, allowing marketers to provide their offerings at low prices that fuel further demand. Customer targeting via digital profiling enables companies to tailor price discounts to individuals at the times of the day, week, and year when they are most susceptible to temptation.[8]

15.6 POLICY AND RESEARCH IMPLICATIONS

15.6.1 Policy

The previously mentioned WHO best buys recommend a comprehensive suite of policy interventions for governments to address the 4 Ps in the context of tobacco, alcohol, and unhealthy diets. These recommendations recognize that the current economic environment increases exposure to harmful products and services, and if left unchecked, the industry imperative to maximize profits presents risks to public health that require government intervention.

In the context of tobacco, policy guidance is provided by the Framework Convention on Tobacco Control, an international treaty negotiated under the auspices of WHO.[25] The Convention entered into force in 2005, and by 2021 it covered 182 countries and more than 90% of the world's population. Countries that are party to the Convention are obliged to implement national laws to reduce both the demand and the supply of tobacco. To address the price P, for example, nearly all parties have implemented some form of tobacco taxation to discourage consumption.[26] To address the promotion P, most countries have now implemented comprehensive bans on tobacco advertising, promotion, and sponsorship. For the product P, rapid progress has been made by countries implementing requirements for packaging and labeling, such as pictorial warnings to advise consumers of the harms of tobacco smoking. For the place P, most countries have prohibited tobacco sales to minors. Although significant progress has been made in addressing tobacco marketing in all its forms, continued innovation by the tobacco industry to maintain sales and profits, such as through e-cigarettes and digital marketing, means that governments must also continue to innovate their policy responses to preserve public health gains.

Countries do not yet have the equivalent benefit of policy guidance from a binding international treaty for reducing the harmful use of alcohol and addressing unhealthy diets. However, the WHO best buys are similar in their recommendation of evidence-based policies such as taxes and labeling regulations.[2] For example, at least 40 countries worldwide now have health-related taxes on sugar-sweetened beverages, and most require packaged foods to carry mandatory nutrient declarations on the back of the pack.[27,28]

Although the WHO also recommends restrictions on the promotion of alcohol and unhealthy foods, in many countries these have been implemented in partnership with industry through voluntary agreements that have been shown to be ineffective.[9,29,30] An exception has been the French Loi Évin model that stipulates what alcohol marketers can do rather than what they cannot. This law requires alcohol marketers to limit their promotional efforts to the provision of factual information using prespecified media platforms. In the area of product content, the food industry continues to push for voluntary targets for food reformulation (e.g., to reduce salt and sugar) as part of efforts to stave off stricter mandatory limits on food composition.[29] In contrast to tobacco control, the limited progress made in promoting healthier diets and reducing alcohol harm suggests the need for stronger policy responses, including mandatory legislation, to address the commercial determinants of health in these areas.

As the markets for tobacco, alcohol, and unhealthy food continue to evolve, challenges for governments include the inherent difficulties associated with restricting the introduction of new products that are likely to be harmful but for which data are lacking to provide tangible evidence of the nature and scale of potential harm, particularly in the longer term. The globalized nature of markets also brings continued challenges in regulating the cross-border flow of harmful products and their marketing. Countries implementing progressive policies may face threatened or real litigation from affected industries and their representatives as an intentional strategy to deter policy innovation.

15.6.2 Research

As per the evidentiary justification for the WHO's best buys policy recommendations, there is now ample evidence of the types of regulatory reforms and other public health initiatives that are likely to be effective in addressing the commercial determinants of health. This suggests that one of the most important research tasks is to explicate the factors preventing the introduction of such policies.[31] These factors are likely to fall into two main categories: political and technical.[7] Political barriers relate primarily to the effects of industry influence on governments' will to implement effective policies. Technical issues include the complexities associated with anticipating, monitoring, and addressing the constantly changing digital environments that flout international barriers and often reside beyond regulators' line of sight.

A potential means of strengthening political will is to demonstrate public support for effective policies.[32] Researchers have an important role to play in assessing current community sentiment and identifying methods of increasing community understanding of and support for evidence-based approaches to addressing the commercial determinants of health. Such work is an important complement to a broad range of other research foci, including (a) documenting industry preemptive and post-introduction reactions to varying policy changes; (b) modeling the impacts of proposed policy changes on short-, mid-, and long-term health outcomes; and (c) developing new tools to monitor digital marketing activities. Across this research, of particular importance will be a focus on the needs of vulnerable consumers such as children and those with lower levels of health literacy.

15.7 CONCLUSION

Producers of unhealthy products will always seek opportunities to maximize their profits through innovative marketing approaches. Effectively preventing harms associated with the commercial determinants of health is likely to involve applying controls that specify what marketers can do, rather than what they cannot. A potential approach to this task could be to develop a theory of change[33] that conceptualizes an acceptable level of availability of harmful products and working backwards to determine policy interventions that would produce this scenario. This approach would require a level of political bravery well beyond that demonstrated to date.

REFERENCES

1. The American Marketing Association. What is marketing? 2017. Accessed April 14, 2021. https://www.ama.org/the-definition-of-marketing-what-is-marketing
2. World Health Organization. *Tackling NCDs: "Best Buys" and Other Recommended Interventions for the Prevention and Control of Noncommunicable Diseases*. World Health Organization; 2017.
3. Murray CJL, Aravkin AY, Zheng P, et al. Global burden of 87 risk factors in 204 countries and territories, 1990–2019: A systematic analysis for the Global Burden of Disease Study 2019. *Lancet*. 2020; 396(10258): 1223–1249. doi:10.1016/S0140-6736(20)30752-2
4. Pierce JP, Chen R, Leas EC, et al. Use of e-cigarettes and other tobacco products and progression to daily cigarette smoking. *Pediatrics*. 2021; 147(2): e2020025122. doi:10.1542/peds.2020-025122
5. Chan GCK, Stjepanovic D, Lim C, et al. Gateway or common liability? A systematic review and meta-analysis of studies of adolescent e-cigarette use and future smoking initiation. *Addiction*. 2021: 116(4): 743–756.
6. International Agency for Research on Cancer. *Alcohol and Cancer in the WHO European Region*. World Health Organization; 2020.
7. Miller M, Pettigrew S, Wright C. Zero-alcohol beverages—Harm-minimisation tool or gateway drink? Drug Alcohol Rev. 2022: 41(3): 546–749.
8. Villanova D, Bodapati A, Puccinelli N, et al. Retailer marketing communications in the digital age: Getting the right message to the right shopper at the right time. *J Retailing*. 2021: 9741(1): 116–132. doi:10.1016/j.jretai.2021.02.001
9. Pettigrew S, Grant H. Policy implications of the extent, nature and effects of young people's exposure to alcohol promotion in sports-related contexts. *Evidence Base*. 2020; 2020(2): 62–78. doi:10.21307/eb-2020-003
10. Gupta H, Lam T, Pettigrew S, Tait RJ. A cross-national comparison of the Twitter feeds of popular alcohol brands in India and Australia. *Drugs Educ Prev Policy*. 2019; 26(2): 148–156.
11. Gupta H, Pettigrew S, Lam T, Tait RJ. How alcohol marketing engages users with alcohol brand content on Facebook: An Indian and Australian perspective. *Crit Public Health*. 2018; 28(4): 402–411.

12. Gupta H, Lam T, Pettigrew S, Tait RJ. Alcohol marketing on YouTube: Exploratory analysis of content adaptation to enhance user engagement in different national contexts. *BMC Public Health*. 2018; 18(1): Article 141.

13. Westberg K, Stavros C, Smith ACT, Munro G, Argus K. An examination of how alcohol brands use sport to engage consumers on social media. *Drug Alcohol Rev*. 2018; 37(1): 28–35. https://doi.org/10.1111/dar.12493

14. Chartrand TL, Fitzsimons GJ. Editorial note: Nonconscious consumer psychology. *J Consumer Psychol*. 2011; 21(1): 1–3.

15. Fang X, Singh S, Ahluwalia R. An examination of different explanations for the mere exposure effect. *J Consumer Res*. 2007; 34(1): 97–103. doi:10.1086/513050

16. Pettigrew S. Reverse engineering a "responsible drinking" campaign to assess strategic intent. *Addiction*. 2016; 111(6): 1107–1113.

17. Belanche D, Flavián M, Pérez-Rueda A. Mobile apps use and WOM in the food delivery sector: The role of planned behavior, perceived security and customer lifestyle compatibility. *Sustainability*. 2020; 12(10): 4275. doi:10.3390/su12104275

18. Poelman MP, Thornton L, Zenk SN. A cross-sectional comparison of meal delivery options in three international cities. *Eur J Clin Nutr*. 2020; 74(10): 1465–1473. doi:10.1038/s41430-020-0630-7

19. Reynolds J, Wilkinson C. Accessibility of "essential" alcohol in the time of COVID-19: Casting light on the blind spots of licensing? *Drug Alcohol Rev*. 2020; 39(4): 305–308. https://doi.org/10.1111/dar.13076

20. Rosewarne E, Hoek AC, Sacks G, et al. A comprehensive overview and qualitative analysis of government-led nutrition policies in Australian institutions. *BMC Public Health*. 2020; 20(1): 1038. doi:10.1186/s12889-020-09160-z

21. Stephens J, Miller H, Militello L. Food delivery apps and the negative health impacts for Americans. *Front Nutr*. 2020; 7: 14. doi:10.3389/fnut.2020.00014

22. Park J, Kim S, Suh K. A comparative analysis of the environmental benefits of drone-based delivery services in urban and rural areas. *Sustainability*. 2018; 10(3): 888. doi:10.3390/su10030888

23. Baker P, Friel S. Food systems transformations, ultra-processed food markets and the nutrition transition in Asia. *Global Health*. 2016; 12(1): 80. doi:10.1186/s12992-016-0223-3

24. Johnston R, Stafford J, Pierce H, Daube M. Alcohol promotions in Australian supermarket catalogues. *Drug Alcohol Rev*. 2017; 36(4): 456–463. https://doi.org/10.1111/dar.12478

25. World Health Organization. *WHO Framework Convention on Tobacco Control*. World Health Organization; 2003.

26. World Health Organization. *Global Progress Report on Implementation of the WHO Framework Convention on Tobacco Control*. World Health Organization; 2018.

27. World Bank. *Taxes on Sugar-Sweetened Beverages: International Evidence and Experiences*. World Bank; 2020.

28. World Health Organization. *Global Nutrition Policy Review 2016–2017*. World Health Organization; 2018.

29. Seferidi P, Millett C, Laverty AA. Industry self-regulation fails to deliver healthier diets, again. *BMJ*. 2021; 372: m4762. doi:10.1136/bmj.m4762

30. Pierce H, Stafford J, Pettigrew S, Kameron C, Keric D, Pratt IS. Regulation of alcohol marketing in Australia: A critical review of the Alcohol Beverages Advertising Code Scheme's new Placement Rules. *Drug Alcohol Rev*. 2018; 38(1): 16–24. doi:10.1111/dar.12872

31. O'Brien KS, Carr SM. Commentary on de Bruijn et al. (2016): Effective alcohol marketing policymaking requires more than evidence on alcohol marketing effects—Research on vested interest effects is needed. *Addiction*. 2016; 111(10): 1784–1785. https://doi.org/10.1111/add.13489

32. Diepeveen S, Ling T, Suhrcke M, Roland M, Marteau TM. Public acceptability of government intervention to change health-related behaviours: A systematic review and narrative synthesis. *BMC Public Health*. 2013; 13(1): 756. doi:10.1186/1471-2458-13-756

33. Breuer E, Lee L, De Silva M, Lund C. Using theory of change to design and evaluate public health interventions: A systematic review. *Implement Sci*. 2016; 11(1): 63. doi:10.1186/s13012-016-0422-6

CHAPTER 16

Corporate Social Responsibility

Past, Present, and Future

NINO PAICHADZE, VINU ILAKKUVAN, MULUKEN GIZAW,
AND ADNAN A. HYDER

16.1 INTRODUCTION

In recent decades, the public health community has begun acknowledging
threats stemming from industries such as alcohol, tobacco, firearms, foods,
beverages, and pharmaceuticals. This recognition has created a shift in the
focus of research and practice from individual- or community-level factors
toward the role played by corporations whose products and practices impact
health, lifestyle, economy, international trade and political systems globally.[1]
Corporations use a myriad of tactics and practices, either singularly or in
combination, to influence health policy and practice.[2] One frequently utilized
approach is corporate citizenship, often referred to as corporate social responsibility (CSR). CSR includes policies and practices that industries use to—in
theory—have a positive influence on society.[3] Although these activities may
appear to have societal benefit, there is substantial evidence of industries
adopting CSR in order to increase their growth and profitability by influencing consumption of their products as well as broader public and policy perceptions. This includes companies using CSR to self-regulate (and thus discourage
stronger policy regulations) and to distract from negative public health consequences related to their products and operations.

This chapter provides an overview of the concept of CSR and how it has
been operationalized with a special focus on the public health implications.
The chapter explores how CSR has been defined and the impact of CSR on

Nino Paichadze, Vinu Ilakkuvan, Muluken Gizaw, and Adnan A. Hyder, *Corporate Social Responsibility* In: *The Commercial
Determinants of Health*. Edited by: Nason Maani, Mark Petticrew, and Sandro Galea, Oxford University Press.
© Oxford University Press 2023. DOI: 10.1093/oso/9780197578742.003.0016

industries and consumers, and it reviews existing policies to regulate CSR. It then proposes recommendations to try to address the consequences of unregulated CSR efforts globally.

16.2 DEFINING CORPORATE SOCIAL RESPONSIBILITY

Several definitions of CSR have been proposed by authors, academics, industry members, and public health practitioners. Over time, the definitions of CSR have varied, particularly when they are discussed by industry members versus public health practitioners. Therefore, in order to understand CSR, it is important to review a diverse set of CSR definitions and frameworks. These can be grouped into three categories: (a) business and industry definitions, which focus solely on the obligation of companies to give back to society; (b) transformative definitions, which recognize the transformative power of CSR to influence consumer perceptions and choices; and (c) public health definitions, which recognize the potential health consequences of CSR and aim to combat them.

The first category includes definitions such as that by Howard Bowen,[4,5] which suggested that businesses were responsible for their impacts on communities and the environment as well as to their stakeholders, and as such, had to engage in socially responsible activities. We propose to rely less on industry-generated definitions.

In the second category, Dorfman et al. recognized how the unhealthy commodity industries could use these tactics, and they reflected on the ethical principles related to such strategies.[6] They proposed two separate ways to conceptualize CSR. The first was from the perspective of proponents of CSR, noting that it can help companies meet their essential needs while addressing their "higher" social responsibilities.[7] In an attempt to be accountable to groups beyond their shareholders, companies accept ethical obligations to society at large.[8] The second was from the perspective of critics of CSR, who describe CSR as primarily a public relations strategy that is designed to achieve "innocence by association" as corporations align themselves with good causes to burnish their public image and protect their core business.[9,10] When corporations fear a threat to their profitability, they often introduce CSR initiatives because these can boost a firm's bottom line both directly through sales and indirectly by moderating the risk for regulation and improving the overall business climate.[6,11] These two competing perspectives emphasized the shift in CSR from just encompassing socially responsible actions to using such actions to benefit the company itself.

Burke and Logsdon even identified the "payoff" of CSR as a subject worth studying, providing a framework that businesses can use to identify the value of their CSR initiatives not in contributions to society but, rather, in the economic benefits a firm should expect to receive from such initiatives (Figure 16.1).[12] These definitions begin to recognize and reflect on the power of CSR initiatives to transform consumer perceptions of a company, and therefore their purchase of products and services to drive economic growth among industries.

A third category of definitions emerges from scholars who aim to draw attention to the need for health research, interventions, and policies for CSR among unhealthy commodity industries. Kickbusch et al. described CSR as a tool to "deflect attention and whitewash tarnished reputations."[13] Similarly, Babor and Robaina defined CSR as business practices that help companies manage their economic, social, and environmental impacts and their relationships in key areas of influence, such as the marketplace, the supply chain, the community, and the public policy arena.[14] They went further to specify four different types of CSR efforts, citing the alcohol industry as an example, including (a) the sponsorship of scientific research, (b) industry efforts to influence public perceptions of research findings, (c) the dissemination of scientific information, and (d) industry-funded public policy initiatives.[14] Such

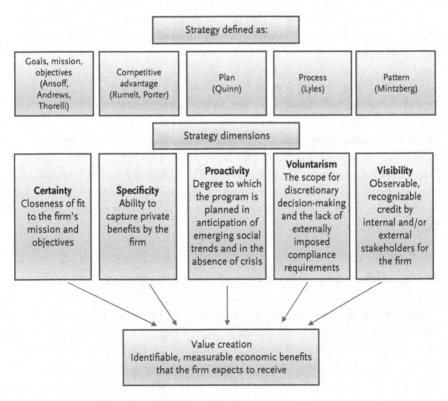

Figure 16.1 A conceptual framework for CSR.
Adapted from Burke and Logsdon.[12]

industries create social aspects and public relations organizations (SAPROs) in order to help further these agendas and manage industry issues that overlap with public health, such as policymaking or medical research findings.[14] By creating SAPROs, which are framed as socially responsible, industries are able to divert attention away from the public health ramifications of the consumption of their products.

CSR has also been described as a source of structural power; for example, supermarkets are able to use CSR to set limits on the range of choices available to other food system actors (e.g., growers, manufacturers, and consumers) by agenda-setting and rule-setting.[15] Similarly, the use of CSR among tobacco companies has been defined simply as a "tax-deductible form of lobbying," such as Philip Morris strategically using philanthropy to "improve company image, influence policymakers, and influence public health policies."[16] Researchers have also noted the use of CSR as a tax avoidance strategy, which has significant downstream public health implications. One study of listed firms in China found more aggressive tax avoidance among companies employing CSR, implying that these companies are using CSR as a risk management strategy.[17] Another study of listed companies from 35 countries also found CSR is positively related to tax avoidance, further noting that "in countries with weak country-level governance, firms with higher CSR scores engage in less tax avoidance, implying that CSR and country-level governance are substitutes."[18]

16.3 EXAMPLES OF CSR ACTIVITIES ACROSS INDUSTRY SECTORS

There are several types of CSR activities common across industries; a non-exhaustive list with selected examples is provided in Table 16.1. At first glance, these activities may seem beneficial to society, but a closer look at how companies engage in these efforts illustrates how they can ultimately be harmful to public health. They demonstrate the diversity of approaches used by industry under the general rubric of CSR.

16.4 EXAMPLES OF CURRENT INTERVENTIONS FOR CSR

Given the strategic use of CSR by companies to influence consumption of their products, strengthen consumer perception, and moderate the risk of regulation and increased taxation—all of which have significant health consequences—it is important to consider how CSR should be regulated. As Lin notes, CSR is typically assumed to be a voluntary initiative, but in recent years, a number of countries, particularly low- and middle-income countries (LMICs), have proposed or adopted laws that encourage and reward—or even

Table 16.1 ILLUSTRATIVE EXAMPLES OF CSR ACTIVITIES

Type of CSR Activity	Illustrative Example
Cause marketing	Corporations engage in "pinkwashing" of products to show support for breast cancer awareness, putting the focus on relatively ineffective approaches (i.e., individual awareness and routine screening) instead of the structural health and environmental root causes of the disease (e.g., toxic chemicals, exposure to carcinogens, and lack of chemical regulation policies), which many of these corporations are contributing to, sometimes via the pinkwashed products themselves.[19-21]
Charitable and in-kind giving	Philip Morris' "PM21" campaign in 1999 included heavily advertised charitable contributions related to homelessness, domestic abuse, and the arts, as well as attempts to co-opt groups that opposed the tobacco industry. The company described the campaign as "a multifaceted, cross functional effort to change the public's perception of Philip Morris and to improve the public's attitude towards the company and the people who work for it."[6]
Community grants and sponsorships	Coca-Cola, PepsiCo, and other beverage companies use community grants and sponsorships related to physical activity and other initiatives to "link their brands to health and wellness rather than illness and obesity; create partnerships with respected health and minority groups to win allies, silence potential critics, and influence public health policy decisions; garner public trust and goodwill to increase brand awareness and brand loyalty; [and] court growing minority populations to increase sales and profits."[22]
Environmental sustainability initiatives	Companies often make sustainability claims to distract from a problematic environmental track record, a practice termed "greenwashing." They may also disingenuously promote practices such as recycling to assuage consumer concerns about their products. For instance, oil and gas companies, the makers of plastic, have spent millions promoting recycling well aware that recycling plastic is not viable, with less than 10% of plastic recycled in the past 40 years.[19,23,24]
Voluntary self-regulation	The Winchester Repeating Arms Company has directed their CSR campaigns toward programs intended to help prevent "straw purchases" (i.e., illegal purchase of a firearm by one person for another) and thefts from firearm retailers.[25] Such self-regulatory attempts are often ineffective and can help companies undercut stronger regulatory proposals at the state and national level.

explicitly require—the inclusion of CSR activities in company operations.[19] On the other hand, recognizing the aforementioned strategic use of CSR to bolster company reputation and profits—often at the expense of public health and well-being—some regulatory bodies and governments have banned CSR activities or the publicizing of such activities by certain industries, most commonly the tobacco industry. Lin also categorized several types of CSR interventions, including (a) mandatory CSR disclosure, (b) mandatory CSR philanthropy, and (c) mandatory CSR due diligence.[19] These are discussed in further detail next, along with an exploration of CSR bans and lessons from the tobacco industry.

16.4.1 Mandatory CSR Disclosure

Mandatory disclosure or reporting related to a company's environmental, social, and governance performance is perhaps the most common form of CSR regulation. According to a 2020 analysis of the latest trends in CSR reporting provisions, covering 614 reporting requirements and resources across more than 80 countries, most of these provisions are issued by governmental bodies and financial regulators and approximately 90% target the private sector, particularly large and listed companies.[20] Key topic areas covered by disclosure requirements include climate change, human rights, labor, and anti-corruption. Although the volume of mandatory CSR disclosure provisions continues to trend upward globally, disclosure types and reporting formats are not standardized, and there are significant gaps in ensuring disclosures are high quality or useful in informing decisions.[20]

16.4.2 Mandatory CSR Philanthropy

Although current conceptions of CSR have expanded far beyond only corporate philanthropy, it persists as both a key component of CSR and a target of regulation, particularly in LMICs.[19] For example, India adopted a law in 2013 that requires companies meeting certain financial thresholds to spend at least 2% of their profits on CSR activities.[21] This now includes fines for noncompliance as well as requirements for independent impact assessments of large projects.[21,22]

Other countries have stopped short of mandating such contributions but have taken steps to encourage or reward them. A bill approved by the House of representatives in 2020 and currently under consideration by the Senate in the Philippines, for example, would allow companies to retain additional profits to use for expanding CSR activities and would mandate the country's Department of Trade and Industry to "recognize and reward" businesses for "outstanding, innovative, and world-class" CSR initiatives. It would also require local governments to provide necessary assistance to businesses in executing their CSR projects.[23]

16.4.3 Mandatory CSR Due Diligence

The conceptualization of CSR as a management process has prompted process-oriented legislation that mandates CSR due diligence—the identification, prevention, mitigation, and accounting of the social, environmental, and human rights risks associated with a company's supply chain and business operations more broadly.[19,24] Unlike laws that only mandate disclosure of voluntary due diligence (or lack thereof), laws that mandate CSR due diligence—such as France's 2017 law—require it and, in theory, allow civil action from those harmed by the failure of a company to do so.[19,25] However, the French law only requires that corporations establish and implement a plan, not guarantee the results of it. This, in combination with the challenge of proving causation, likely explains why no such actions have been reported to date in France.[19,26]

16.4.4 CSR Bans: The Case of Tobacco

Although some countries are using legislation to encourage or mandate CSR within companies across all industries, there has also been a push to ban companies from engaging in, or at least publicizing, their CSR activities, especially by industries widely understood to harm public health, such as the tobacco industry. Notably, the World Health Organization (WHO) considers CSR activities by the tobacco industry "an inherent contradiction."[27] According to implementation guidance for Article 13 of the WHO Framework Convention on Tobacco Control (FCTC), tobacco industry CSR philanthropy is a form of sponsorship, and publicizing their CSR activities is a form of advertising.[28] Article 13 recommends a comprehensive ban of all forms of tobacco advertising, promotion, and sponsorship or, where that is not possible for constitutional reasons, substantial restrictions.[29] A number of countries have specifically banned tobacco CSR activities or publicizing of such activities.[30]

The tobacco industry has also been singled out as an exception to legislation that otherwise requires CSR activities. For example, advocates in India took to the courts their concerns that the nation's aforementioned mandatory CSR philanthropy law conflicted with both India's 2003 Cigarettes and Other Tobacco Products Act (which prohibits tobacco advertising) and the FCTC's recommendations to ban tobacco industry CSR activities.[31,32] Ultimately, the Ministry of Corporate Affairs issued a circular which clarified that companies engaging in CSR activities cannot violate existing laws.[31,33] Yadav et al. noted that this meant that while doing CSR, all companies must conform to the ban on direct and indirect advertising, promotion, and sponsorship of tobacco products.[31]

Similarly, with respect to the proposed Philippines corporate philanthropy law, advocates are working to exclude tobacco from this bill, disallowing future opportunities for tobacco companies to promote their donations and get access to policymakers.[34]

16.5 CONSIDERATIONS FOR CSR REGULATION

The most prevalent form of CSR regulation (mandatory CSR disclosure) appears to be inadequate in informing decisions or leading to organizational change. The stated goal of such legislation is to increase the contribution of companies to social and environmental causes (e.g., eradicating hunger and poverty, promoting education and health care, and mitigating climate change). However, a question has been raised: Why would governments employ this approach when they have the ability to directly regulate and tax companies in ways that serve these social and environmental causes? In fact, these would be more effective and would avoid the indirect consequence of "mandat[ing] public relations management" that unfortunately serves to improve corporate reputations.[19]

Lin discusses the concept of "implicit CSR legislation," which captures a wide range of legislative efforts to raise social, labor, environmental, or human rights standards, including via labor and environmental regulations.[19] Others have argued for "taxation as CSR,"[35,36] whereas Fisher states that the doctrine of corporate social responsibility provides a logical rationale for multinational corporations to adopt anti-avoidance practices, and that the harm caused by tax avoidance outweighs any financial benefit that results from these practices.[37]

Yadav et al. recommend that mandatory CSR activities under India's aforementioned law be banned for tobacco companies and replaced with an equivalent 2% tax on these companies' net profits.[31] Although some countries have banned CSR activities by the tobacco industry, it may not make sense to ban CSR activities by industries across the board given that it is in the interest of public health and well-being to have companies act in ways that are socially responsible. Thus, robust due diligence requirements that go beyond merely reporting are vital; companies should be held responsible for the identification, prevention, mitigation, and accounting of the social, environmental, and human rights risks associated with their business practices.[19,24]

For example, a recent study of the implementation of CSR, particularly due diligence requirements for companies in the European Union, recommended a region-wide legislative initiative regarding "substantive" social and environmental due diligence that goes beyond reporting to require companies to "engage actively in analyzing, mitigating, as well as remedying any adverse impacts on human rights" related to their business activities.[24] And Lin recommends CSR due diligence laws be improved "with government monitoring, legal punishment for non-compliance, and stakeholder recourse against companies that do not comply."[19] In the spirit of due diligence, some scholars have also suggested that CSR activities be independently audited or assessed specifically for impact on population health and well-being.[38,39]

The previously discussed considerations and recommendations provide a starting point for how countries and other regulatory bodies might approach efforts to strengthen CSR laws in a way that reshapes business practices to prioritize social and environmental concerns and improve public health and well-being. However, this chapter recommends a framework akin to the "precautionary" principle used in environmental health[40-48] because everything about the industry practices and products cannot be known contemporaneously. This means that it ought not to be the purview of society to show the negative health and associated impacts of industry activities; rather, it ought to be incumbent on the industry to *prove* that its products, services, and activities are not harmful to health. This shift in perspectives will reframe the goal of CSR and make it dual purpose: (a) to showcase the evidence of lack of health impact (or positive health impact) and to keep it current and (b) to demonstrate societal engagement and welfare by the industry. We believe that such a goal will fundamentally change the discourse on commercial determinants of health.

REFERENCES

1. Freudenberg N. *Lethal But Legal: Corporations, Consumption, and Protecting Public Health*. Oxford University Press; 2014.
2. Wiist WH. The corporation: An overview of what it is, its tactics, and what public health can do. In: Wiist WH, ed. *The Bottom Line or Public Health*. Oxford University Press; 2010: 3–71.
3. Torugsa NA, O'Donohue W, Heckler R. Capabilities, proactive CSR and financial performance in SMEs: Empirical evidence from an Australian manufacturing indurstry sector. *J Bus Ethics*. 2012; 109: 483–500.
4. Agudelo MAL, Jóhannsdóttir L, Davídsdóttir B. A literature review of the history and evolution of corporate social responsibility. *Int J Corporate Social Responsibility*. 2019; 4(1): 1–23.
5. Bowen HR. *Social Responsibilities of the Businessman*. University of Iowa Press; 1953.
6. Dorfman L, Cheyne A, Friedman LC, Wadud A, Gottlieb M. Soda and tobacco industry corporate social responsibility campaigns: How do they compare? *PLoS Med*. 2012; **9**(6): e1001241.

7. Lee SY, Carroll CE. The emergence, variation, and evolution of corporate social responsibility in the public sphere, 1980–2004: The exposure of firms to public debate. *J Bus Ethics*. 2011; 104: 115–131.

8. Garriga E, Melé D. Corporate social responsibility theories: Mapping the territory. *J Bus Ethics*. 2004; 53: 51–71.

9. Johns G. Deconstructing corporate social responsibility. *Agenda*. 2005; 12(4): 369–384.

10. Doane D. The myth of CSR2005. *Stanford Soc Innovation Rev*. Fall 2005. https://ssir.org/articles/entry/the_myth_of_csr#

11. Siegel DS, Vitaliano DF. An empirical analysis of the strategic use of corporate social responsibility. *J Econ Manage Strategy*. 2007; 16(3): 773–792.

12. Burke L, Logsdon JM. How corporate social responsibility pays off. *Long Range Planning*. 1996; 29(4): 495–502.

13. Kickbusch I, Allen L, Franz C. The commercial determinants of health. *Lancet*. 2016; 4(12): 895–896.

14. Babor TF, Robaina K. Public health, academic medicine, and the alcohol industry's corporate social responsibility activities. *Am J Public Health*. 2013; 103(2): 206–214.

15. Clapp J, Fichs D. Agrifood corporations, global governance, and sustainability: A framework for analysis. In: Clapp J, Fuchs D, eds. *Corporate Power in Global Agrifood Governance* [Online]. MIT Press; 2009.

16. Tesler LE, Malone RE. Corporate philanthropy, lobbying, and public health policy. *Am J Public Health*. 2008; 98: 2123–2133.

17. Mao C-W. Effect of corporate social responsibility on corporate tax avoidance: Evidence from a matching approach. *Qual Quant*. 2019; 53: 49–67.

18. Zeng T. Relationship between corporate social responsibility and tax avoidance: International evidence. *Social Responsibility J*. 2018; 15(2): 244–257.

19. Lin L-W. Mandatory corporate social responsibility legislation around the world: Emergent varieties and national experiences. *University Pennsylvania J Bus Law*. 2020. https://ssrn.com/abstract=3678786

20. Wijs PPvd, Lugt Cvd. *Sustainability Reporting Policy: Global Trends in Disclosure as the ESG Agenda Goes Mainstream* [Online]. Carrots & Sticks; 2020.

21. Beliveau A-ML, Binder NV, Littenberg MR. Corporate social responsibility in India: New requirements for U.S.-based multinationals on the horizon. 2020. Accessed May 10, 2021. https://www.lexology.com/library/detail.aspx?g=b5c2a053-eee0-4aae-884c-bf7a785bd04e

22. Rishi R, Antani M. India-amendments to CSRR rules: A game changer. 2021. Accessed May 10, 2021. https://www.natlawreview.com/print/article/india-amendments-to-csr-rules-game-changer

23. Rosario B. House approves "CSR Act" on third and final reading. *Manila Bulletin*. 2020. Accessed May 10, 2021. https://mb.com.ph/2020/05/22/house-approves-csr-act-on-third-and-final-reading

24. Noti K, Mucciarelli FM, Angelici C, Pozza Vd, Pillinini M. *Corporate social responsibility (CSR) and its implementation into EU Company Law* [Online]. Policy Department for Citizen's Rights and Constitutional Affairs; 2020.

25. Cossart S, Chaplier J, Lomenie TBD. The French law on duty of care: A historic step towards making globalization work for all. *Bus Hum Rights J*. 2017; 2: 317–323.

26. Brabant S, Savourey E. A closer look at the penalties faced by companies. *Int J Compliance Bus Ethics*. 2017; supplement to *Business and Business Legal Week* No. 50.

27. World Health Organization. *Tobacco Industry and Corporate Social Responsibility . . . An Inherent Contradiction*. World Health Organization; 2004.

28. World Health Organization. *Elaboration of Guidelines for Implementation of Article 13 of the Convention* [Online]. World Health Organization; 2008.

29. World Health Organization. *WHO Framework Convention on Tobacco Control*. Geneva, World Health Organization; 2003.

30. World Health Organization. *Ban on Tobacco Companies/the Tobacco Industry Publicizing Their CSR Activities (Tobacco control: Enforce bans): The Global Health Observatory* [Online]. World Health Organization; 2020.

31. Yadav A, Lal P, Sharma R, Pandey A, Singh RJ. Tobacco industry corporate social responsibility activities amid COVID-19 pandemic in India. *Tob Control*. 2021. doi:10.1136/tobaccocontrol-2020-056419

32. Madras High Court. Cyril Alexander versus Union of India. High Court of Judicature; 2016.

33. Ministry of Corporate Affairs. New Delhi clarification with regard to provisions of corporate social responsibility under section 135 of the Companies Act, 2013. Government of India; 2016.

34. STOP. Trading "philanthropy" for favors: Tobacco industry CSR during COVID-19. August 17, 2020. https://exposetobacco.org/news/ban-ti-csr

35. Rangan S. Tax as CSR—Not CSR as tax! 2019. Accessed May 10, 2021. http://www.lawstreetindia.com/experts/column?sid=319

36. Israel E. Corporate responsibility: It's the tax disclosure, stupid! 2021. Accessed May 10, 2021. https://skytopstrategies.com/corporate-responsibility-its-the-tax-disclosure-stupid

37. Fisher J. Fairer shores: Tax heavens, tax avoidance, and corporate social responsibility. *Boston Univ Law Rev*. 2014; 94: 337–365.

38. Galea G, McKee M. Public–private partnerships with large corporations: Setting the ground rules for better health. *Health Policy*. 2014; 115(2–3): 138–140.

39. Maani N, Schalkwyk MCV, Petticrew M, Galea S. The commercial determinants of three contemporary national crises: How corporate practices intersect with the COVID-19 pandemic, economic downturn, and racial inequity. *Milbank Q*. 2021; 99(2): 503–518.

40. Kriebel D, Tickner J, Epstein P, et al. The precautionary principle in environmental science. *Environ Health Perspect*. 2001; 109: 871–876.

41. Ansoff HI. *Corporate Strategy: An Analytic Approach to Business Policy for Growth and Expansion*. McGraw-Hill, New York; 1965.

42. Thorelli HB, ed. *Strategy Plus Structure Equals Performance*. Indiana University Press: Bloomington, IN; 1977.

43. Andrews KR. *The Concept of Corporate Strategy*. Richard D. Irwin: Homewood, IL; 1980.

44. Porter ME. *Competitive Advantage*. Free Press: New York; 1985.

45. Rumelt R. The evaluation of business strategy. In: Glueck WF, ed. *Business Policy and Strategic Management*, 3rd edn, McGraw-Hill: New York; 1980.

46. Quinn JB. *Strategies for Change: Logical Incrementalism*. Richard D. Irwin: Homewood, IL; 1980.

47. Lyles MA. Strategic problems: How to identify them. In: Fahey L, ed. *The Strategic Planning Management Reader*. Prentice Hall: Englewood Cliffs, NJ; 1985.

48. Mintzberg H. Opening up the definition of strategy. In: Quinn JB, Mintzberg H, James RM, eds. *The Strategy Process*. Prentice Hall: Englewood Cliffs, NJ; 1988.

CHAPTER 17

The Institutionalization of Corporate Power Within Policy

GARY FOOKS

17.1 INTRODUCTION

Addressing corporations' effects on health requires fundamental changes in markets. Among other things, these changes relate to what products and services are sold, at what price, how and to whom, the conditions under which people live and work, and maximum thresholds of industrial pollution. States' capacity to regulate corporations is central to this process. As the area of law and public policy that mediates between public and private interests, regulation goes to the heart of effective democratic control of corporations. Specifically, regulation works to prevent corporations from shifting the costs associated with their activities onto the general population and, in this sense, provides a system of rules to protect the planet and its people from profit-driven externalities.

In practice, states do not have complete freedom over how they regulate. In fact, governments' policy space—the freedom, scope, and mechanisms that they have to choose, design, and implement public policy and regulation[1]— has steadily contracted during the past 40 years as a result of a combination of processes, which have worked to strengthen corporate power within policy-making. This chapter is concerned with one of these processes—the emergence of cost–benefit analysis and new regulatory oversight mechanisms, which increasingly govern how policies and regulations (hereafter referred to as policy) are developed. The chapter is based on the premise that understanding health policy in the context of the commercial determinants of health requires us to

Gary Fooks, *The Institutionalization of Corporate Power Within Policy* In: *The Commercial Determinants of Health.* Edited by: Nason Maani, Mark Petticrew, and Sandro Galea, Oxford University Press. © Oxford University Press 2023. DOI: 10.1093/oso/9780197578742.003.0017 look behind discrete forms of business political activity, such as lobbying, and focus on how corporations *institutionalize* their advantage in policymaking.

17.2 COST–BENEFIT ANALYSIS

17.2.1 Theoretical Benefits

Since the 1980s, many countries have transformed their approach to developing new policies that affect business. In practice, these changes have worked to increase the business voice within policymaking through a combination of horizontal policy instruments that apply to all policymaking, such as cost–benefit analysis and mandatory stakeholder consultation, and regulatory oversight bodies, such as the U.S. Office of Information and Regulatory Affairs (OIRA). Although the precise combination and effect of these changes vary from jurisdiction to jurisdiction, in the main they have reduced policymaker discretion and steadily "economized" policymaking by integrating the working assumptions and professional tools of microeconomics into what is, in effect, a new governing framework of policymaking. The justification for reducing policymaker discretion rests on a combination of arguments that draw on questions of social equity and efficiency.[2,3] Policy instruments associated with economic analysis have been said to reduce "the mental heuristics, blind spots, personal agendas, institutional inertias, and political pressures" that can cause policy actors to overlook or discount important policy-related effects[2] and help ensure that policy impacts on both the powerful and politically marginalized are comprehensively assessed.[2] The net effect, according to these and other commentators, is that cost–benefit analysis shapes policymaking and policies in ways that that ultimately "increase the net welfare of the community."[4]

Importantly, however, but perhaps not surprisingly, in many jurisdictions these changes have come about in response to persistent lobbying by large corporations with significant negative impacts on health and the environment, such as British American Tobacco (BAT), Shell, Coca-Cola, Mars, Dow, Unilever, and Bayer.[5,6] To understand the interest of these companies in policymaking governance and, more generally, how the new policymaking architecture works, on balance, to institutionalize their influence and interests within policymaking, it is important to understand three overlapping issues: how information is collated and integrated into cost–benefit policy instruments; the risk of "regulatory budget" rules in ossifying policymaking; and the role that regulatory oversight bodies play in both managing how information is organized and remodeled within cost–benefit instruments and creating veto points, which weaken the operation of the precautionary principle within policymaking.

17.2.2 Information and Corporate Influence Within Cost–Benefit Instruments

In most countries, cost–benefit analysis is realized through ex ante impact assessments. In theory, these are meant to assess the risks to public and environmental welfare of the problem under consideration; pool together all the relevant evidence concerning the economic, social, and environmental impacts of different policy options; and calculate their relative costs and benefits. A key method for obtaining this information is mandatory stakeholder consultations, which involve government departments and regulatory agencies calling upon interested parties to volunteer relevant data, research, and arguments, which, where relevant, are then integrated into impact assessments. In this way, impact assessments, aligned closely with mandatory stakeholder consultation, are said to optimize the net benefits of new policies and ensure that decisions are based on strong evidence and a thorough analysis of options, each with its corresponding benefits and costs.

In practice, however, this highly idealized account of impact assessments and stakeholder consultations overlooks several interlocking factors that shape how evidence is created, selected, and processed, which are key to understanding the political and organizational ecology of business advantage within contemporary policymaking. There is, for example, good evidence to suggest that business interests are overrepresented in stakeholder consultations[7-12] and, importantly, that, in the United States at least, corporations' influence over policy outcomes rises in proportion to their involvement in consultations.[12,13] Although the evidence is mixed,[12,14] this influence on policy outcomes is unlikely to be reducible simply to corporations' outsized presence in consultations. Just as important are business's superior resources and governments' structural dependence on business for policy-relevant information. In relation to the former, corporations are more likely to have the capacity to understand the complex, technical data and studies that are often relevant to policy deliberations. In relation to the latter, consideration needs to be given to deep-seated information asymmetries between regulated businesses and policy actors.[15]

17.2.3 Information Asymmetries

In assessing the impact of policy decisions, policymakers are often imperfectly informed about the potential economic impacts of policy decisions[16] and are dependent on information from affected businesses, which typically appear to know more about the costs of policy alternatives and their expected consequences and represent an inexpensive way of obtaining these data.[14] This apparent information advantage partly reflects their control over different types of information essential to working out policy impacts, such as the number of workers they employ, sales volumes, and the costs of production.[16,17] Equally, in many cases, corporations generate policy-relevant information as a simple byproduct of doing business—so they automatically possess data about costs and demand and technological expertise. Even with respect to product risks, corporations are likely to hold better information about the underlying problem through the normal course of business or to be able to obtain such information more easily than governments.[14,18,19] Chemical firms, for instance, knew about the health risks from vinyl chloride emissions long before governments became aware of them.[18] More generally, many large companies have internal tracking systems through which they can identify risks from their products and manufacturing processes.[14] Another important component of corporations' information advantage concerns policymakers' capacity constraints, which are particularly acute in lower income countries. This is compounded by the fact that policy actors must spread their resources across a range of policy areas, whereas corporations only need to focus on producing evidence with respect to specific policy issues that affect them. Furthermore, because political decisions are often important for specific industrial sectors, they have strong incentives to pool resources to produce research relevant to policy issues, which strengthens their hand in shaping the evidence base of policy-related cost.

17.2.4 Business Overestimation of Costs

Information asymmetries have played an important role in driving the adoption of impact assessments and mandatory stakeholder consultations. BAT, which played a decisive role in integrating impact assessment into European Union (EU) policymaking, had been advised that impact assessments—tied to mandatory consultation—would strengthen their capacity to direct policymakers to their preferred sources of data and analysis,[6] "unavailable to government officials," including "industry developed statistical series" and industry-sponsored "economic assessment studies."[6] This asks us to consider how information generated by business may differ from other sources of information. Here, the important point to recognize is that affected businesses typically have an incentive to overestimate policy-related costs, and the evidence suggests this is a relatively routine practice across industrial sectors.[17,20-22] For instance, a recent study examining the soft drink industry's use of economic data in South Africa's 2016 consultation on a proposed sugar tax found that the industry used several interdependent techniques, which worked cumulatively to exaggerate the impact of the tax on jobs, public revenue generation, and gross domestic product.[17] Equally, when the EU's chemical regulation, REACH, was first proposed, the peak business association for the European chemical industry—the European Chemical Industry Council—estimated that REACH would cost the industry between €20 and €30 billion.[23] Other industry-funded reports predicted huge job losses in EU member states.[22] The actual costs have proved to be far lower. Among the REACH processes, registration is the main cost driver for the chemicals industry. An interim evaluation by the European Commission calculated that the regulation had cost the industry €3 billion over 11 years.[24]

This pattern of overestimation runs up against a common assumption that businesses have an interest in maintaining their reputation as suppliers of reliable information. In practice, however, the assumption neglects the fact that overestimates are typically achieved using relatively opaque methods.[16,17] In the South African sugar tax case, even relatively simple methods—such as double-counting projected job losses—were deeply buried in industry-funded analyses.[17] More sophisticated methods, which involved unverifiable steps in economic modeling, the failure to undertake sensitivity analyses in response to highly uncertain and effectively unknowable input variables, and questionable assumptions about how the public would respond to the introduction of the tax, were even more difficult to detect.[17] One problem for policymakers is that outwardly innocuous, indiscernible choices regarding what eventualities get modeled can have major effects on economic estimates of policy-related impacts, which are compounded by the fact that key data underpinning industry economic estimates are privately held and not automatically made available to public officials.[17]

17.2.5 Government Overestimation of Costs

In practice, governments are not formally compelled to accept industry estimates and are able to reject them or adjust them downwards. However, the evidence—albeit limited to the United Kingdom—suggests that projected costs in impact assessments rely heavily on business estimates,[16] that public officials accept business information at face value (which affords little disincentive for overestimation and provides an enabling context for inflated cost estimates in final impact assessments),[16] and that information originating from businesses serves to increase estimated costs between pre- and-post-consultation impact assessments.[16] In practice, these factors may help explain why cost–benefit analyses across jurisdictions routinely overestimate business costs, sometimes by quite large margins.[16]

17.3 REGULATORY BUDGETS AND POLICY OFFSETTING

Increasingly, governments have become concerned with "regulatory budgets,"[25-27] which although not strictly institutionalizing corporate *power* within policy development, nonetheless can institutionalize their *interests* at the expense of public health. In essence, regulatory budget rules require deregulatory action as a mandatory condition for introducing new policy. This can take various forms. In the United States, for instance, Executive Order 13771 requires administrative agencies to offset each new regulation by removing two existing regulations and sets a cap on total incremental regulatory costs.[25] The United Kingdom, by contrast, observes a "one-in-three-out" rule, where government departments and agencies are required to find three pounds of net savings from deregulatory measures for every pound of additional net cost imposed on business by new policies.[26]

Policy offsetting creates three overlapping risks to the formation of public health policies. First, it potentially creates a chilling effect on new policies, particularly where the only available policies for removal produce socially beneficial effects. Second, it can lower health protection where selected policies for removal provide genuine social protection. Third, government departments and agencies face the possibility of having new policies blocked if they are unable to adequately offset.

In practice, these risks are exacerbated by the fact that both non-business (e.g., health, environmental welfare, and social equality) and indirect business benefits of regulation are typically disregarded for the purposes of policy offsetting.[25] In the United Kingdom, regulatory "ins" and "outs" are calculated exclusively with reference to monetized direct costs on and savings to business, expressed as the equivalent annual net cost to business (EANCB).[28] This means that even where a proposed policy yields significant social benefits, it is nonetheless considered to be an "in" if the direct costs to business are larger than the direct savings. This is particularly relevant in the context of the commercial determinants of health, where there is a relatively strong correlation between costs to business and health benefits.

17.4 REGULATORY OVERSIGHT BODIES

In some cases, the problems outlined above have little effect on policy outcomes because ministry and agency officials in many jurisdictions still exercise considerable autonomy over how they engage with the results of impact assessments.[29] However, efforts to strengthen policymaking oversight through the introduction of regulatory oversight bodies (ROB), such as OIRA, the Regulatory Policy Committee (RPC) in the United Kingdom, and Regulatory Scrutiny Board (RSB) in the EU, have worked to narrow this autonomy.

ROBs' mandates and powers differ significantly and include reviewing impact assessments and recommending or requiring changes to them to, rejecting proposed regulations (where "costs" exceed "benefits" or where they are not supported by adequate analysis), and setting or enforcing regulatory budgets. Despite this variation, the direction of policy travel involves ROBs assuming greater power over ministries and regulatory agencies.[29] The implications of enhanced ROB for the institutionalization of corporate power in health policy are fourfold.

17.4.1 A Presumption Against Regulation

Because ROBs' powers are effectively limited to action by government departments and regulatory agencies, not inaction, regulatory review is effectively organized against regulation.[30] In the United States, for example, OIRA is far more likely to seek changes that make regulations less protective of human health and the environment and less costly for business.[31] Furthermore, changes triggered by OIRA review to rules proposed by government agencies whose rule-making is highly relevant to health—such as the U.S. Department of Health and Human Services and the U.S. Environmental Protection Agency—are typically more significant than rules proposed by other government agencies.[32]

17.4.2 Low-Visibility Access Points and Corporate Lobbying

Regulatory review also changes the opportunity structures within which corporations can influence policy by providing an additional access point for corporate lobbyists. Several studies, for instance, have found that OIRA meets far more regularly with business actors.[30,33-35] Importantly, lobbying OIRA is strongly and positively associated with policy change, particularly for well-resourced industry groups,[35] and facilitated by the opacity of the process.[30,33,36]

17.4.3 The Precautionary Principle

Review by ROBs with a de facto veto power on policy sign-off—such as OIRA,[37] RPC,[28,38] and RSB[29,39]—can work to shape how the precautionary principle is operationalized in policymaking.[37] In the United Kingdom, this is an indirect effect of the standard of evidence the RPC requires agencies and departments to meet in specifying the policy problem within impact assessments. A case in point is the Medicine and Healthcare Products Regulatory Agency's (MHRA) consultation on introducing new regulations on nicotine-containing products.[40] In its opinion on MHRA's efforts to extend its regulation of nicotine-containing products,[41] RPC reported that the agency had failed to provide "sufficient evidence" to suggest that there was a significant risk to public health from unlicensed nicotine-containing products that would "justify the future regulation of these products," noting that the MHRA had itself acknowledged that the risk to public health from such products was "unknown."[40] MHRA regulation of e-cigarettes eventually took effect in 2016, 6 years after its initial impact assessment.[42]

17.4.4 Cost–Benefit Methodologies

ROBs also play an instrumental role in shaping cost–benefit methodologies, which by ossifying policy development work to institutionalize corporate advantage within policymaking. An instructive illustration relates to RPC's responsibility of validating departmental calculations for EANCB. Formally, only business costs and benefits *directly* attributable to a policy are considered within the scope for calculating EANCB.[38] Subsequent effects that occur as a result of direct impacts, including behavior change, are considered to be indirect and out of scope.[38] In principle, this means that the impact of new policies that reduce the demand for healthful commodities—and, therefore, company earnings—should be treated as a second-order effect.

Historically, this approach had been applied successfully by the Department of Health (DoH) in tobacco control-related impact assessments with the approval of RPC.[43-46] However, when the DoH sought to characterize loss of profits to tobacco companies due to reduced consumption of cigarettes and down trading as indirect effects in its interim impact assessments for the standardized packaging for tobacco products, RPC demurred.[47-49] The DoH was forced to accept RPC's position. The practical effect was to increase EANCB from zero to £36.78 million, which required the DoH to remove existing policies imposing £73 million in costs to business.[1] But it is within RPC's reasoning that we find the true significance of the decision.

RPC's position was based on the simple assertion that

> policies which ban or severely restrict a particular activity, that explicitly prohibits a form of promotional activity, and have a primary objective to reduce sales (even if by promoting behaviour change) should be considered as having a direct impact on businesses.[50]

Considering loss of profits as an indirect cost, it later claimed, would produce a "counter-intuitive outcome"[51] by scoring standardized packaging as net beneficial to tobacco companies. The justification illustrates the *self-authenticating* nature of cost–benefit analysis as a style of reasoning—that is, it defines its own criteria of validity and objectivity in response to preferred outcomes. EANCB and similar offsetting concepts are little more than artifacts, which are not concerned with costs to business overall. These would have been neutral because money not spent on cigarettes is simply spent elsewhere in the economy. Instead, where health and environmental protection are at issue, offsetting calculi are solely concerned with ensuring that efforts to extinguish the externalizing costs of regulated industries are converted into deregulatory measures elsewhere: In most cases, the larger the externality addressed, the greater the deregulation. Viewed in this way, the RPC was, in effect, seeking an ostensibly logical outcome from an illogical, arbitrary calculus.

17.5 LITIGATION RISK

By providing a more bureaucratic, rule-bound system of decision-making, formal integration of cost–benefit analysis into policymaking also opens the door to judicial review of policy development. Deliberations by the European Court of Justice, for example, suggest appellate courts may consider alleged deviations from "Better Regulation" rules in determining breaches of binding legal principles (e.g., the principle of proportionality) outlined in legislation.[52]

17.6 CONCLUSION

There are fundamental inconsistencies between public health goals and the new policymaking architecture.[53] Population-level policy instruments that manage the market environment for unhealthful products represent some of the most cost-effective means of promoting health,[54] but because of their effects on business earnings, they run up against the new architecture's primary objective of reducing business costs.[26,55]

Just as important, the new architecture reduces political conflicts to complex assessments of costs and benefits, which are largely processed out of public view. In this respect, it represents another form of "quiet politics" in which business advantages are institutionalized and illustrates how political choices about the balance between public and private interests can become rationalized over time, hidden from view, and incorporated into administrative arrangements, knowledge tools, and professional specialisms.

Finally, the enhanced administrative status attached to regulatory review not only locks in governments' information dependence on business but also embeds a specific style of economic reasoning into policymaking, orienting concepts, ways of thinking about problems, causal assumptions, and approaches to methodology—which represent major challenges to addressing the commercial determinants of health through public policy.

NOTE

1. In 2013, the United Kingdom switched from a "one-in, one-out" system to a "one-in, two-out" system.

REFERENCES

1. Koivusalo M, Schrecker T, Labonté R. Globalization and policy space for health and social determinants of health. In: Labonte R, Schrecker T, Packer C, Runnels V, eds. *Globalization and Health: Pathways, Evidence and Policy*. Routledge; 2009: 105–130.
2. Schwartz J. Approaches to cost–benefit analysis. In: Dunlop CA, Radaelli CM, eds. *Handbook of Regulatory Impact Assessment*. Elgar; 2016: 33–51.
3. Kirkpatrick C, Parker D. Regulatory impact assessment: An overview. In: Kirkpatrick C, Parker D, eds. *Regulatory Impact Assessment: Towards Better Regulation?* Elgar; 2007: 1–15.
4. Radaelli CM, De Francesco F. Regulatory impact assessment. In: Cave M, Baldwin R, Lodge M, eds. *The Oxford Handbook of Regulation*. Oxford University Press; 2010: 279–301.
5. Waterhouse BC. Uncertain victory: Big business and the politics of regulatory reform. In: *Lobbying America*. Princeton University Press; 2014: 174–200.
6. Smith KE, Fooks G, Gilmore AB, Collin J, Weishaar H. Corporate coalitions and policy making in the European Union: How and why British American Tobacco promoted "Better Regulation." *J Health Polit Policy L*. 2015; 2: 2882231.
7. Beyers J, Arras S. Who feeds information to regulators? Stakeholder diversity in European Union regulatory agency consultations. *J Public Policy*. 2020; 40(4): 573–598.
8. Rasmussen A, Carroll BJ. Determinants of upper-class dominance in the Heavenly Chorus: Lessons from European Union online consultations. *Br J Polit Sci*. 2014; 44(2): 445–459.
9. Berkhout J, Hanegraaff M, Braun C. Is the EU different? Comparing the diversity of national and EU-level systems of interest organisations. *West Eur Politics*. 2017; 40(5): 1109–1131.
10. Røed M, Wøien Hansen V. Explaining participation bias in the European Commission's online consultations: The struggle for policy gain without too much pain. *J Common Market Stud*. 2018; 56(6): 1446–1461.
11. Rasmussen A. Participation in written government consultations in Denmark and the UK: System and actor-level effects. *Govern Opposition*. 2015; 50(2): 271–299.
12. Yackee JW, Yackee SW. A bias towards business? Assessing interest group influence on the U.S. bureaucracy. *J Politics*. 2006; 68(1): 128–139.
13. McKay A, Yackee SW. Interest group competition on federal agency rules. *Am Polit Res*. 2007; 35(3): 336–357.
14. Coglianese C, Zeckhauser R, Parson E. Seeking truth for power: Informational strategy and regulatory policymaking. *Minnesota L Rev*. 2004; 89(2): 277–341.
15. Harrington W, Morgenstern RD, Nelson P. On the accuracy of regulatory cost estimates. *J Policy Analysis Manage*. 2000; 19(2): 297–322.

16. Fooks G, Mills T. The tolerable cost of European Union regulation: Leaving the EU and the market for politically convenient facts. *J Social Policy*. 2017; 46(4): 719–743.
17. Fooks GJ, Williams S, Box G, Sacks G. Corporations' use and misuse of evidence to influence health policy: A case study of sugar-sweetened beverage taxation. *Global Health*. 2019; 15(1): 56.
18. Markowitz G, Rosner D. *Deceit and Denial: The Deadly Politics of Industrial Pollution*. University of California Press; 2013.
19. Rosner D, Markowitz G. *Deadly Dust: Silicosis and the Ongoing Struggle to Protect Worker's Health*. University of Michigan Press; 2006.
20. Bailey PD, Haq G, Gouldson A. Mind the gap! Comparing ex ante and ex post assessments of the costs of complying with environmental regulation. *Eur Environ*. 2002; 12(5): 245–256.
21. McGarity T, Ruttenberg R. Counting the cost of health, safety and environmental regulation. *Texas L Rev*. 2002; 80(7): 1997–2058.
22. International Chemical Secretariat. *Cry Wolf—Predicted Costs by Industry in the Face of New Regulations*. International Chemical Secretariat; 2015.
23. Schörling I. *REACH—The Only Planet Guide to the Secrets of Chemicals Policy in the EU: What Happened and Why?* Greens/European Free Alliance in the European Parliament; 2004.
24. European Commission. *Commission Staff Working Document Accompanying the Document, Communication from the Commission to the European Parliament, the Council, and the European Economic and Social Committee, Commission General Report on the Operation of REACH and Review of Certain Elements: Conclusions and Actions*. European Commission; 2018.
25. Weaver HL. One for the price of two: The hidden costs of regulatory reform under Executive Order 13771 comments. *Admin L Rev*. 2018; **70**: i.
26. National Audit Office. *The Business Impact Target: Cutting the Cost of Regulation*. National Audit Office; 2016.
27. Abeele ÉVd. *"One-in, One-out" in the European Union Legal System: A Deceptive Reform?*. European Trade Union Institute for Research; 2020.
28. HM Government. *One-in, One-out (OIOO) Methodology*. Department for Business, Innovation and Skills; 2011.
29. Organisation for Economic Co-operation and Development. Studies of RegWatchEurope Regulatory Oversight Bodies and the European Union Regulatory Scrutiny Board. Organisation for Economic Co-operation and Development; 2018.
30. Livermore MA, Revesz RL. Regulatory review, capture, and agency inaction. *Georgetown L J*. 2012; 101(5): 1337–1398.
31. Bressman LS, Vandenbergh MP. Inside the administrative state: A critical look at the practice of presidential control. *Michigan L Rev*. 2006; 105(1): 47–99.
32. Haeder SF, Yackee SW. Presidentially directed policy change: The Office of Information and Regulatory Affairs as partisan or moderator? *J Public Admin Res Theor*. 2018; 28: 475–488.
33. Steinzor RI, Patoka M, Goodwin J. *Behind Closed Doors at the White House: How Politics Trumps Protection of Public Health, Worker Safety, and the Environment*. Center for Progressive Reform; 2011.
34. Haeder SF, Yackee SW. Out of the public's eye? Lobbying the President's Office of Information and Regulatory Affairs. *Interest Groups Advocacy*. 2020; 9(3): 410–424.

35. Haeder SF, Yackee SW. Influence and the administrative process: Lobbying the U.S. President's Office of Management and Budget. *Am Polit Sci Rev.* 2015; 109(3): 507–522.

36. Wagner W. Participation in the US administrative process. In: Bignami F, Zaring D, eds. *Comparative Law and Regulation.* Elgar; 2016.

37. Driesen DM. Cost–benefit analysis and the precautionary principle: Can they be reconciled. *Michigan State L Rev.* 2013: 771–826.

38. Department for Business Innovation and Skills. *Better Regulation Framework Manual.* Department for Business, Innovation and Skills; 2013.

39. Senninger R, Blom-Hansen J. Meet the critics: Analyzing the EU Commission's Regulatory Scrutiny Board through quantitative text analysis. *Regul Governance.* 2021; 15(4): 1436–1453.

40. Regulatory Policy Committee. *Opinion: Consultation on Regulation of Nicotine Containing Products.* Regulatory Policy Committee; 2010.

41. Medicines and Healthcare Products Regulatory Agency. *Impact Assessment of the Regulation of Nicotine Containing Product.* Medicines and Healthcare Products Regulatory Agency; 2010.

42. Britton J, Bogdanovica I. *Electronic cigarettes: A report commissioned by Public Health England.* Public Health England; 2014.

43. Regulatory Policy Committee. *Opinion: Impact Assessment for the Prohibition on the Sale of Tobacco from Vending Machines* [Final/Enactment]. Regulatory Policy Committee; 2012.

44. Regulatory Policy Committee. *Opinion: The Protection from Tobacco (Sales from Vending Machines) (England) Regulations 2010.* Regulatory Policy Committee; 2010.

45. Department of Health. *Impact Assessment on the Prohibition of Display of Tobacco Products at the Point of Sale in England.* Department of Health; 2011.

46. Department of Health. *Impact Assessment for the Prohibition on the Sale of Tobacco from Vending Machines* [Final]. Department of Health, 2012.

47. Department of Health. Impact Assessment on standardised packaging for tobacco products (consultation). London: Department of Health, 2012.

48. Regulatory Policy Committee. *Opinion: Standardised Packaging for Tobacco Products* [Consultation]. Regulatory Policy Committee; 2014.

49. Department of Health. *Impact Assessment: Standardised Packaging of Tobacco Products* [Consultation]. Department of Health; 2014.

50. Department of Health. *Impact Assessment. Standardised Packaging of Tobacco Products* [Final]. Department of Health; 2015.

51. Regulatory Policy Committee. *Impact Assessment Case Histories. A Practical Guide on How to Interpret Better Regulation Framework Principles and Rules.* Regulatory Policy Committee; 2016.

52. Alemano A. A meeting of minds of impact assessment: When ex ante evaluation meeting ex post judicial control. *Eur Public L.* 2011; 17(3).

53. Smith K, Fooks G, Collin J, Weishaar H, Gilmore A. Is the increasing policy use of impact assessment in Europe likely to undermine efforts to achieve healthy public policy? *J Epidemiol Commun Health.* 2010; 64(6): 478–487.

54. Bloom DE, Chisholm D, Jané-Llopis E. *From Burden to "Best Buys": Reducing the Economic Impact of Non-Communicable Diseases in Low- and Middle-Income Countries.* World Economic Forum; 2011.

55. European Commission. Better Regulation: Why and who. n.d. Accessed March 7, 2017. https://ec.europa.eu/info/law/law-making-process/better-regulation-why-and-how_en

CHAPTER 18

Corporations as Irresponsible Artificial People

Human Rights, Profits, and Public Health

GEORGE J. ANNAS

Few subjects of solemn inquiry have been more unproductive than the study of the modern large corporation. The reasons are clear. A vivid image of what should exist acts as a surrogate for reality. Pursuit of the image then prevents pursuit of the reality.
—John Kenneth Galbraith[1(p85)]

18.1 INTRODUCTION

In Kazuo Ishiguro's deeply disturbing novel, *Klara and the Sun*, Klara recounts her life as an artificial person, designed and sold as an "artificial friend."[2] The human-like robots are wonders of technology that are able to act as a "friend" and companion to a "real" person, and they are even willing to sacrifice their lives for the life of their owner. As robots become increasingly more "life-like," we are invited to better define what we mean by a "person" and what distinguishes a real person from an artificial one. This question has, of course, particular relevance to our ever-evolving notions of a corporation, which is an artificial person created by law.

Corporations have been a staple of the global economy at least since the 1800s. And since the 20th century, they have grown in size, complexity, and even personality to be the most consequential life form on the planet. This includes shaping the health of the planet and its inhabitants. Corporations

George J. Annas, *Corporations as Irresponsible Artificial People* In: *The Commercial Determinants of Health*.
Edited by: Nason Maani, Mark Petticrew, and Sandro Galea, Oxford University Press. © Oxford University Press 2023.
DOI: 10.1093/oso/9780197578742.003.0018

were initially created to consolidate large sums of money (capital) for a specific purpose (often to manufacture a particular product, such as an automobile or a pharmaceutical), whose stockholders were promised limited personal liability—limited to the value of their stock in the corporation.[3] Corporations also have the ability to sue and to be sued by governments, other corporations, and natural persons, and litigation plays a prominent role in the life, growth, and even death (e.g., in bankruptcy) of the corporation. Although technically not "alive," corporations nonetheless have the possibility of immortality because there is no formal limit on their life span, and corporations may soon be endowed with ever more powerful artificial intelligence that will potentially add to their longevity.

In the past three decades, we have witnessed corporations negotiating massive settlements of lawsuits brought against them for the health damage caused by their tobacco products and the death and destruction of lives caused by their false advertising of opioids. In addition to being sued for damages caused to private citizens, corporations can commit crimes and be penalized by governments. It is, however, very rare for those who control the corporation, the chief executive officer and the board of directors, to actually go to jail, even if their malfeasance has caused deaths, as in the case of Perdue Pharma and its bestselling product, OxyCotin. In criminal cases especially, the penalties are paid by the corporation's artificial friend (who may even die for the corporation or be created just to die for the corporation), and the corporation may continue in business or transfer its business to another corporation, giving it a new lease on "life." For example, Pfizer was fined $1.2 billion for fraudulently marketing valdecoxib (Bextra). Federal law required that any company found guilty of such a crime be automatically excluded from the Medicare and Medicaid programs. But government prosecutors thought that this would lead to the collapse of Pfizer, which they considered too big to fail. Accordingly, the prosecutors approved a plan in which a Pfizer subsidiary corporation, Pharmacia & Upjohn, would plead guilty to this crime, pay the fine, and be excluded from Medicare and Medicaid. The parent company, Pfizer, would continue doing its business as usual.

This chapter highlights the contemporary movement to change the formal corporate purpose from maximizing shareholder value to maximizing *stakeholder* value and also the movement to grant corporations new constitutional rights of free speech and freedom of religion. It then discusses how this empowered and powerful artificial person might be tamed in a way that permits governments to channel the activities of corporations, including their adoption of artificial intelligence and gene editing techniques, toward improving the health of the world's people and lessening the impact of climate change on the planet.

18.2 STAKEHOLDER VALUES

At least since Milton Friedman's destructively influential 1970 libertarian essay, "The Social Responsibility of Business Is to Increase its Profits," the corporation has been widely viewed as owing primary, if not exclusive, loyalty to enhancing the value of its stock, and therefore the earnings of its stockholders.[7] In Friedman's words, "The responsibility [of the corporation] is to conduct the business [in accordance with the desire of its shareholders] which generally will be to make as much money as possible while conforming to the basic rules of society, both those embodied in law and those embodied in ethical custom."[7] Acceptance of this view was reinforced in the corporate realm by paying corporate managers in company stock and stock options, which tied their (exceptionally large) salaries to the value of the stock of their corporations.

This narrow view has resulted in predatory capitalism, ridiculously high payments to corporate executives, and the widening gap between the rich and the poor. Moreover, in practice, as European economist Mariana Mazzucato has observed,

> Maximizing shareholder value has often involved loading companies with debt—a supposedly efficient model which leverages a company's capital base—with the risk that the company is dangerously exposed to unexpected turns of events, such as a pandemic or a market downturn.[8]

More recently, at least some corporate leaders have argued that predatory capitalism has run its course, and it is time to take seriously not only the interests of stockholders but also the interests of other stakeholders in the corporation, including employees, suppliers, customers, the environment, and even human rights and population health.[9] The disaster of climate change—and the contribution to it by many oil, gas, and coal corporations—is just one example in which corporate action to reduce pollution and rising temperatures can be beneficial for both the corporation's stockholders and its customers.

The public health goal is to make the social responsibility of corporations a reality rather than just a feel-good marketing slogan. This will require transforming the corporation from an instrument designed and run to make money while indifferent to polluting the planet and destroying the health of humans to an entity whose money-making must be consistent with preserving the health of the planet and its inhabitants. Central to this objective is to replace the current post-2008 system in which profits are kept by the owners of capital, and losses are socialized by being paid for by governments, most notably for corporations that are "too big to fail." Any sustainable system requires that both gains and losses are shared by corporations and governments. Sharing gains and losses will require a restructuring of corporate tax, including a minimum tax for all corporations, both domestic and multinational.[10] As one example, social responsibility of multinational pharmaceutical companies would require them to support (and even lead) the quest for effective vaccines against SARS-CoV-2, but also to meaningfully share their intellectual property in a way that maximizes its beneficial impact on the global population.

Only governments can regulate the activities of corporations, but instead of constraining destructive or monopolistic activities, governments have continued to use the artificial person construct to endow corporations with even more life-like qualities.

18.3 EMPOWERING CORPORATIONS WITH FREEDOM OF SPEECH AND RELIGION

Corporations historically communicate through advertising and branding. The goal is to increase sales and thus profits. Contemporary corporations continue to advertise (in a much more focused manner that threatens consumer privacy) but also have become widely involved in what we can call political speech, especially lobbying to reduce or eliminate regulation of their products or actions, to reduce or eliminate taxes for themselves and their shareholders, and to obtain government subsidies for themselves. Even *The Wall Street Journal* endorses corporate lobbying on issues that help the corporation produce more profits for shareholders. But both the *Journal* and the *Economist* worry about corporations going beyond corporate welfare (in both senses of the term) to support their own visions of a healthy society and a healthy planet.[11,12]

In one of the most controversial U.S. Supreme Court decisions in the past two decades, *Citizens United v. Federal Election Commission* (2010), the Court decided that corporations should be treated like real (natural) persons for the purposes of First Amendment free speech rights.[13] This is implausible on its face. As Justice John Paul Stevens noted in dissent, "Corporations have no consciences, no beliefs, no feelings, no thoughts, no desires. . . Their personhood often serves as a useful legal fiction. But they are not themselves members of 'We the People' by whom and for whom our Constitution was established." The majority of the Court, however, wrote as if treating artificial persons as real persons was simply a logical conclusion. In the Court's words, "The First Amendment does not allow political speech restrictions based on a speaker's corporate identity. . . Political speech does not lose First Amendment protection 'simply because its source is a corporation.'" But, of course, that conclusory statement "simply" begs the question (never answered by the Court), "Why not?" As Justice John Paul Stevens stated, "The conceit that corporations must be treated identically to natural persons in the political sphere is not only inaccurate but also inadequate to justify the Court's disposition of this case."

Legal philosopher Ronald Dworkin was even less kind:

> The argument that corporations must be treated like real people under the First Amendment is in my view preposterous. Corporations are legal fictions. They have no opinions of their own to contribute and no rights to participate with equal voice or vote in politics.[14]

Nonetheless, these "free speech" rights permit the corporation to lobby and lie on its own behalf. Big Oil's "hugely profitable public relations campaign" has been described as a campaign that "will likely cause more death and destruction than any lobbying effort in human history."[15,16]

Citizens United was followed 4 years later by *Burwell v. Hobby Lobby*, in which the major question was whether to expand the First Amendment rights of corporations by adding to their characteristics the ability to have religious beliefs.[17] The question was presented by regulations adopted under the Affordable Care Act that required that contraceptives be covered by corporation-sponsored health insurance plans. The corporation challenging this rule, Hobby Lobby, argued that following this requirement would violate its religious beliefs. Specifically, as summarized by the majority of the Court, "The owners of the businesses have religious objections to abortion, and according to their religious beliefs the four contraceptive methods at issue are abortifacients." The Court then went on to treat the "owners of the business" as if they were identical to the corporation (the artificial person) itself. Arguably, the Court had to do this to come out the way it did—because Justice Stevens in *Citizens United* is certainly correct in noting that "corporations have no consciences, no beliefs" and therefore can have no religious views.

Nonetheless, the artificial person fantasy continues to grow, as does the destructiveness of major corporations. The extraction of raw materials from the earth by corporations has caused massive climate change. Corporations are currently expanding their extraction agenda to include the collection of private information from citizens which has already resulted in devastating loss of privacy and identity. It is time to ask how the growing power of corporations and their insatiable appetite for the planets and its inhabitants' resources can be brought under democratic government control.

This question is vital now that, like Klara and the next generation of artificial people, corporations will soon take virtual control of the world economy, deciding among other things what further resources can be extracted, what more types of devastating pollution can be produced, what unhealthy and dangerous products can be created, what corporations can know and manipulate about us, and what price we will all pay for failing to take action as a global community.[18] As we witnessed with the insurrection at the U.S. Capitol on January 6, 2021, information corporations can literally ignite a violent attack on the government by propagating blatant lies (e.g., that the election was "stolen") that many members of the public cannot distinguish from truth.[19,20]

18.4 REFORMING THE CORPORATION

There are many steps that can (and should) be taken to reform corporations to transform them from destructive monsters to useful pets. The first is perspective. Corporations are not and cannot be (at least in the real world) people. Treating them as if they really have human attributes, such as political opinions, religious beliefs, and a conscience, treats the "big lie" of corporate personhood as a fact—which in turn makes meaningful regulation of the corporate form impossible, or at least incoherent.

There are millions of corporations in the world. Nonetheless, the ones that deserve our immediate public health attention are global (i.e., multinational) corporations because they have the widest and deepest influence on the planet and its inhabitants. It is an important initial step that all such corporations both join the United Nations Global Compact (approximately 10,000 have done so to date) and pledge to abide by its 10 principles, which should be made obligatory rather than purely voluntary. The purpose of the Global Compact, launched by the United Nations in 2000, is to provide a framework for more sustainable and responsible corporations.[21] It is founded on human rights and seeks to uphold the health of the planet and its inhabitant by endorsing 10 basic principles:

Human rights
1. Businesses should support and respect the protection of internationally proclaimed human rights; and
2. Make sure that they are not complicit in human rights abuses.
Labor
3. Businesses should uphold the freedom of association and the effective recognition of the right to collective bargaining;
4. The elimination of all forms of forced and compulsory labor;
5. The effective abolition of child labor; and
6. The elimination of discrimination in respect to employment and occupation.
Environment
7. Business should support a precautionary approach to environmental challenges;
8. Undertake initiatives to promote greater environmental responsibility; and
9. Encourage the development and diffusion of environmentally friendly technologies.

Anti-corruption

10. Businesses should work against corruption in all its forms, including extortion and bribery.

These principles were drafted to be purposefully vague, to garner corporate support. The time has come to begin worldwide monitoring and reporting on how individual corporations are doing and to adopt economic sanctions against corporations that are violating them. In short, it is time for a global organization that has been a "guide dog" to become a "watchdog." It may be a form of wishful thinking, but climate change sparked by fossil fuels may yet provide the incentive for governments to work together in a way that can transform private corporations by requiring them, under financial penalties, to curb and pay for their pollution and to take specific actions to help the planet and all its inhabitants. In the absence of world government, Nobel Prize winner in economics, William D. Nordhaus, has suggested that the time is right to form a "global compact" of countries that are on board with this agenda and are willing to work together on it. No country could be "forced" to be a member in this new government compact, but all members would agree to penalize countries and their corporations that refused to join and continued to pollute in unacceptable and destructive ways with embargos and other penalties.[22]

To cure the destructiveness of *Citizens United*, all corporate political activity, including both lobbying for special treatment by the government and campaigning and fundraising for political candidates, should be outlawed. Government regulatory agencies, especially those charged with protecting the environment such as the U.S. Environmental Protection Agency, should be strengthened.

Corporations are creatures of their charters and, as corporate attorney Robert Hinkley has previously recommended, the following words should be added to the purpose clause in all corporate charters: "But not at the expense of the environment, human rights, public health and safety, dignity of employees, and the welfare of the communities in which the company operates." I would add two additional explicit duties, the first a response to January 6 and the second to artificial intelligence-drive information collecting and disseminating algorithms: "[not at the expense of] democracy or invading the privacy and dignity of individuals."

To attempt to ensure that corporations work for all the inhabitants of the planet and not just for their shareholders, we need both a global minimum tax on corporate profits and the ability of governments to be paid for their contributions to research, infrastructure, and other public goods by acquiring and trading in the stock of specific corporations.

In other words, we went through a revolution in corporate liability during the last century (mostly concentrated on the safety of products and the rights of workers) that included abolition of child labor, worker safety regulations, and food and drug safety, and we are about to enter a second wave of corporate reform—this one going much deeper to take seriously both the human rights and public health obligations of global corporations.

The artificial person has been a destructive metaphor, but personhood is its myth rather than its reality. Klara's owner and companion is dying of an unidentified illness. Her mother agrees to a scheme to have Klara literally replace her dying daughter, Josie, as a substitute: Josie merged with the body and mind of Klara. Not to take our analogy too far, but would the duplicate Josie (the former Klara and Josie) be a real person or an artificial person? Or, in the words of the bioengineer/artist who is remodeling Klara to merge with Josie, when will we let go of our fantasy that there is more to humans, something like a soul or a heart, than the materials we are composed of? We want to keep believing that "there's something unreachable inside each of us. Something that's unique and won't transfer. But there's nothing like that, we know that now."

Whether we believe humans have a unique property (that we designate a "soul" or a "heart"), corporations have no such thing. Nonetheless, it can be useful to humans to use a life metaphor for corporations to help us think about how to use the corporate form to human advantage. One potentially fruitful way would be to treat the world's global corporations, together with the world's countries, as one giant organism—and ensure that that organism gets all the support it needs for the planet and its inhabitants to thrive—clean air, clean water, and a sustainable environment—and is protected from a slow death by pollution. Governments do not just have obligations to protect corporations; corporations (and the governments that regulate them) have obligations to protect the lives and health of us all.

REFERENCES

1. Galbraith JK. *The New Industrial State*. Princeton University Press; 1967.
2. Ishiguro K. *Klara and the Sun*. Knopf; 2021.
3. Winkler A. *We the Corporations: How American Businesses Won Their Civil Rights*. Norton; 2018.
4. Barrat J. *Our Final Invention: Artificial Intelligence and the End of the Human Era*. St. Martin's; 2013.
5. Keefe PR. *Empire of Pain: The Secret History of the Sackler Dynasty*. Doubleday; 2021.
6. Annas GJ. Corporations, profits, and public health. *Lancet*. 2010; 376: 583–584.
7. Friedman M. The social responsibility of business is to increase its profits. *The New York Times Magazine*. September 13, 1970.
8. Mazzucato M. *Mission Economy: A Moonshot Guide to Changing Capitalism*. Harper Business; 2021.
9. Salter AW. "Profit keeps corporate leaders honest. *Wall Street Journal*. December 9, 2020; A17.

10. Tankersley J, Rappeport A. Democrats push for higher taxes on global firms. *The New York Times*. April 6, 2021; 1A.
11. CEOs vs. shareholders. *Wall Street Journal*. April 7, 2021; A14.
12. The Political CEO. Economist. April 17, 2021; 11.
13. *Citizens United v. Federal Election Commission*, 558 U.S. 310 (2010).
14. Dworkin R. The "devastating" decision. *New York Review*. February 25, 2010; 39.
15. Rich N. *Losing Earth: A Recent History*. Farrar, Straus & Giroux; 2019.
16. Klinenberg E. The great green hope. *New York Review*. April 23, 2020; 55–58.
17. *Burwell v. Hobby Lobby*, 573 U.S. 682 (2014).
18. Perlroth N. *This Is How They Tell Me the World Ends: The Cyberweapons Arms Race*. Bloomsbury; 2021.
19. Zuboff S. The knowledge coup. *The New York Times*. January 31, 2021; SR3.
20. Zuboff S. *The Age of Surveillance Capitalism: The Fights for a Human Future at the New Frontier of Power*. Public Affairs; 2019.
21. Ruggie JG. *Just Business: Multinational Corporations and Human Rights*. Norton; 2013.
22. Nordhaus WD. *The Spirit of Green: The Economics of Collisions and Contagions in a Crowded World*. Princeton University Press; 2021.

CHAPTER 19

Industry Influence on Research

A Cycle of Bias

LISA BERO

1969: "The Tobacco Institute has probably done a good job for us in the area of politics and as an industry we also seem to have done very well in turning out scientific information to counter the anti-smoking claims"— Smoking and Health Proposal, Brown and Williamson.

1977: Research and scientific publication are key elements in the marketing strategy for drugs. The stated goal of Parke-Davis' "publication strategy" was to use research "to disseminate the information about [the use of a drug for an unapproved indication] as widely as possible through the world's medical literature."

2000: Per- and polyfluoroalkyl substances (PFAS) are a class of widely used chemicals that persist in the environment and accumulate in humans and animals. Manufacturers knew PFAS were "highly toxic when inhaled and moderately toxic when ingested" by 1970. In 2000, 3M announced it would no longer be manufacturing a PFAS-containing product because "it is too persistent in the environment and gets into our blood." A lawyer for 3M explained that "the plant recognizes it must get public first . . . better late than never."

2017: A survey of lead academic authors of pharmaceutical industry-funded drug trials found that only 33% (29 of 80) reported that they had the "final say" in the design of their studies.

Lisa Bero, *Industry Influence on Research* In: *The Commercial Determinants of Health.* Edited by: Nason Maani,
Mark Petticrew, and Sandro Galea, Oxford University Press. © Oxford University Press 2023.
DOI: 10.1093/oso/9780197578742.003.0019

19.1 INTRODUCTION

Public health policies should be built upon pillars of rigorous evidence. If the evidence base that informs these decisions is flawed or distorted, the entire foundation for systematic reviews, guidelines, health policy, clinical advice, and consumer information crumbles. For decades, tobacco, pharmaceutical, chemical, food, and other companies have used similar strategies to bias evidence to boost sales of their products, minimize regulation, and protect their profits. This chapter focuses on industry influence on the evidence base—the actual data that policy makers have available to inform their decisions. Chapter 8 describes multiple strategies that corporations use to influence evidence dissemination and use. This chapter describes how bias in bodies of evidence can be detected and how companies influence research agendas and the design, conduct, and publication of research to produce a biased body of evidence.

19.2 WHAT IS BIAS AND HOW IS IT DETECTED?

Empirical research demonstrates that pharmaceutical, tobacco, food, or chemical industry funding biases human studies toward outcomes that are favorable to the sponsor, even when controlling for other biases in the methods. Case studies describing specific pieces of research that have been manipulated by industry make a valuable contribution to the literature, but meta-research is a method used to identify biases across an entire body of evidence.

Meta-research—research on research[1]—examines the evidence across a topic area, not just individual studies. A bias is a "systematic error, or deviation from the truth, in results or inferences"[2] that can over- or underestimate the true effect. Although biases related to internal validity, such as appropriateness of randomization or proper control for confounding, can be detected in a single study, the impact of such biases on a research area can only be determined by examining multiple studies. For example, meta-research examining the association of the appropriateness of randomization in clinical trials with the magnitude of the intervention effect in groups of studies across different clinical areas has shown that inadequate randomization will overestimate efficacy estimates.[3] This means that the results of inadequately randomized trials on any therapeutic topic are probably exaggerated. Meta-research has been used to identify important biases in research that are not related to study methodology, such as publication bias, outcome reporting bias, and spin.[1]

19.3 META-RESEARCH AND FUNDING BIAS

Meta-research has also been used to detect funding bias in pharmaceutical, to-bacco, nutrition, chemical, and other research areas.[4–8] Meta-research can tell us not only the direction of industry influence on a body of research results but also its magnitude. For example, a Cochrane review included 75 studies examining the association between sponsorship and research outcomes of drug or device studies across different clinical areas. The number of studies with statistically significant efficacy results that favored the sponsor was approximately 27% higher among industry-sponsored studies compared with non-industry-sponsored studies. Industry-sponsored studies also more often had harm results (showing less harm) and conclusions that favored the sponsor's product.[5]

The distinction between the effects of industry sponsorship on research results (either their statistical significance or effect size) and conclusions is important. The conclusions of a research paper present the author's interpretation of the data and offer a form of influence, as the same data can be presented either more or less favorably. Biased conclusions are important because these may be disproportionately promulgated in lay and social media, or even affect the decisions of those who do not read beyond the conclusion. However, the actual numerical results of a study are arguably even more important because it is the data that are brought forward into systematic reviews and other types of evidence synthesis that are increasingly influential in policymaking.

The majority of meta-research studies examining industry bias have focused on the association of sponsorship with conclusions of studies. For example, a meta-research study included 12 studies that examined the association of research funding with outcomes of nutrition studies. Of the 12 studies, 8 examined the conclusions of studies and found that industry-sponsored studies were more likely to have favorable conclusions compared to non-industry-sponsored studies.[9] Two reports assessed the association of food industry sponsorship and the statistical significance of research results; neither found an association. One report examined effect sizes and found that studies sponsored by the food industry reported significantly smaller harmful effects of soft drink consumption compared to those not sponsored by the food industry. More recent meta-research studies examining the association of food industry sponsorship with the results and conclusions of studies of whole-grain or dairy foods and cardiovascular disease have reported similar findings.[9,10]

19.4 LIMITATIONS OF META-RESEARCH

It can be difficult to conduct meta-research to detect industry bias. For example, all research on a particular topic may be industry-funded; thus, there is no comparison group. In addition, a substantial proportion of studies in a sample may have missing, incomplete, or inaccurate disclosure of funding sources and author conflicts of interest. Due to these disclosure limitations, few meta-research studies have examined the association of author conflicts of interest only with research outcomes.[5,11,12] In addition, sample sizes or effect sizes of studies on a particular topic may be small, thus requiring large numbers of studies to detect differences between industry- and non-industry-funded studies. Finally, outcomes of studies may not be measured in the same way, so they cannot be grouped or compared. Despite these limitations, meta-research provides empirical evidence of funding bias across a variety of health research areas.

Although meta-research studies identify funding bias, they do not provide information on the mechanism by which the bias occurs. Additional types of research are needed to explain the observation of funding bias. It is important to understand how biases in results and conclusions can occur because the biases, and the methods used to reduce them, are the same regardless of the product being studied. This chapter investigates potential mechanisms of funding bias by supplementing meta-research with qualitative research from internal corporate documents and interview studies. These mechanisms are also explored in more depth in the case study examples presented in other chapters in this volume.

19.5 THE CYCLE OF BIAS

Research production is a cyclical process and is vulnerable to industry interference at every step, including (a) setting the research agenda and framing research questions, (b) designing the methods of the study, (c) conducting the study, and (d) publishing the study (Figure 19.1).

Research builds on previous research, so the impact of bias is magnified if the biases persist over time. Systematic reviews, although a rigorous method to synthesize evidence, can also perpetuate biases. If an entire evidence base on a particular question is biased, this needs to be accounted for in the systematic review by excluding the biased studies, not completing the synthesis of the evidence, or conducting subgroup analyses to explore differences between industry- and non-industry-funded studies.

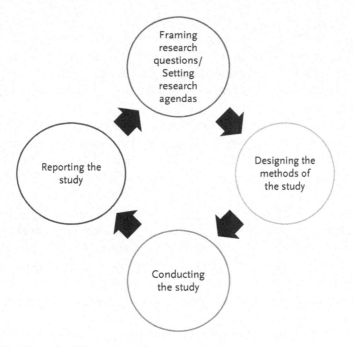

Figure 19.1 The cycle of bias in research.

19.5.1 Bias in Research Agendas

Formulating the research agenda and framing the research questions are the first steps in conducting research. One possible explanation for observed industry bias is that industry sponsors could influence research questions in ways that would enhance the benefits and minimize the harms of their products. In other words, sponsors may not ask a question or may fund researchers to ask questions that they do not want answered.

A scoping review of research studies that explored the influence of industry sponsorship on research agendas across different scientific fields identified 36 studies. The majority (19/36) examined medically related fields, but industry influence on research agendas was also examined for tobacco, food, plant or animal biotechnology, chemical, alcohol, and mining research. These studies used a variety of approaches and data sources, including qualitative analysis of internal industry documents, cross-sectional studies of published scientific papers, and surveys of researchers.

The scoping review identified two main strategies to influence research agendas. First, industry-funded research focused on products with commercial applications rather than public health topics.[13] For example, an analysis of randomized controlled trials of nutrition interventions to address obesity showed that 67% (n = 16/24) of the food industry-sponsored studies tested specific nutrients, whereas only 25% (n = 6/24) examined broader levels of dietary composition, such as whole foods.[12] Manufactured foods with specific nutrient profiles, compared with whole foods, are potentially more profitable for food companies.

Second, corporate sponsors established priority research agendas that favored the industry's legal and policy positions by funding research to distract from the harms of their products. The tobacco industry influenced the research agenda on the health effects of secondhand smoke by funding "distracting" research suggesting that other components of indoor air were more harmful than tobacco.[14] The sugar industry has used similar tactics to influence the dental research agenda.[15] Research funded by food companies might also distract from nutrition as a potential health problem, focusing on exercise.[16] Research on gambling, predominantly funded by the gambling industry, has focused on gambling as an individual problem or addiction that emphasizes individual treatment, rather than focusing on gambling as a public health issue (see Chapter 13).[17]

It is not surprising that industry funders support research that will enhance corporate profits and protect companies from litigation and regulation. However, industry influence over research agendas is a commercial determinate of health because such influence can affect policymaking by shaping the type of evidence available and the policy solutions considered.

19.5.2 Bias in Research Methods

Different study designs use different research methods to protect against bias. For example, randomized studies should use a truly random sequence generation, blind the researchers and study participants when possible, and measure outcomes accurately. Observational studies should include methods that minimize selection bias, confounding, and measurement bias.

However, differences in methods rarely explain the observed biases in results and conclusions of industry-sponsored studies versus non-industry-sponsored studies. For example, the Cochrane review demonstrating funding bias in drug trials found no difference between industry-funded and non-industry-funded drug studies in sequence generation, concealment of allocation, loss to follow-up, or selective outcome reporting.[5] This suggests that other factors, such as the use of unfair comparator doses or the failure to publish studies with unfavorable results, explain the different outcomes of industry- and non-industry-sponsored studies. Similarly, meta-research studies have shown that both industry- and non-industry-sponsored nutrition studies have similar and high risks of bias in their methods.[9,10]

Risk of bias tools do not capture influences on question formation, how the study is actually conducted, whether the full results and analyses are published, or a combination of these mechanisms. Furthermore, we may not be able to identify all mechanisms of bias. Thus, existing tools for assessing risk of bias are not sufficient for identifying the mechanisms of bias associated with funding source.[18]

19.5.3 Bias in How Research Is Conducted

Even if a study asks an important question and the methods are rigorous, bias can be introduced in the way the research is conducted. The observed bias in industry-sponsored studies could be due to what goes on behind the scenes of a research study. Analyses of industry documents provide insight into how industry scientists, lawyers, and executives manipulate research studies to achieve their desired outcomes.

Documents from pharmaceutical, tobacco, sugar, lead, vinyl chloride, chemical, and silicosis-generating industries (mining, foundries, sandblasting, and others) all describe similar strategies to manipulate research to obtain predetermined results.[19] One strategy is to control all aspects of the conduct and publication of a study. A tobacco industry study, created to refute the influential Hirayama paper[20] demonstrating that secondhand smoke was associated with lung cancer, is a comprehensive example of hidden industry interference in the design, data collection, analysis, and publication of research.[21]

Controlling how studies are conducted behind the scenes is a key part of an industry strategy to disseminate information that is favorable to their products. For example, scientific publication was a key part of the pharmaceutical industry's marketing strategy with the aim of flooding the scientific literature with research that maximized the benefits and minimized the harms of their products.[22]

19.5.4 Bias in What Gets Published (or Not)

Creating, conducting, and publishing favorable research allows industry to shape the body of evidence on a topic. Similarly, suppressing data, or not publishing studies, can skew the evidence available to policymakers, practitioners, and those who do evidence synthesis. In addition, the body of published evidence on a topic guides further research questions and primary research. Among industry-sponsored research, selective reporting of research is one possible explanation for the observed biases in bodies of evidence. Selective outcome reporting facilitates the suppression of research that does not favor the sponsor's product.

Biases in the publication of research are collectively known as "reporting biases" and can be introduced on three levels: analysis, outcome reporting, and entire study publications. Selective analysis reporting occurs when a study has multiple analyses, such as adjusted and unadjusted analyses or multiple subgroup analyses, and only some of these are published. Selective outcome reporting occurs when a study has multiple outcome measures, such as an outcome measured at multiple time points or efficacy and harm outcomes, and only some of these are published. Publication bias occurs when an entire study is not published. Evidence shows that these types of selective publication result in bodies of evidence that tend to overestimate efficacy or underestimate harms of the interventions or exposures being tested.

Reporting biases are identified by comparing the data and analyses in full study reports to the reports that are published. These comparisons have been used to investigate reporting biases across research funded by a variety of industries. Reporting biases have been identified by interviewing investigators,[23] comparing the full reports of drug studies submitted to regulatory databases with what is published in the scientific literature,[24] comparing data released as part of legal settlements with published research articles,[25,26] and comparing study protocols or data from trial registries with published research articles.[27]

Most of the data sources used to study reporting bias in pharmaceutical and tobacco research are not available for observational research, such as research on diet or alcohol. Therefore, meta-research and statistical methods have been used to estimate publication bias in these areas and have demonstrated reporting bias in the epidemiological literature examining the associations of tobacco, alcohol, diet, physical activity, and sedentary behavior with mortality.[28]

In summary, reporting biases have been detected across a variety of health fields. Reporting biases occur in industry-funded studies, but due to the prevalence of reporting biases among all studies, significant differences in the extent of reporting bias between industry- and non-industry-funded studies are not always detected. Nevertheless, reporting biases uniformly align with industry interests because they result in the published body of evidence being overwhelmingly positive for questions of efficacy but overwhelmingly negative for questions of harm.

19.6 WHAT CAN BE DONE ABOUT IT? BREAKING THE CYCLE OF INDUSTRY BIAS IN RESEARCH

Existing efforts to minimize industry influence are necessary but insufficient. No single solution will eliminate industry bias in research. However, given the evidence on industry bias, and the common mechanisms used by different industries, any suggestions for minimizing industry influence on research should be applied to all types of industry-sponsored research.

Technically it is (1) consortia of multiple industries or (2) consortia of industry and non-industry, where no single industry has influence over the topics of the funded research. More ambitious would be a call to action for funders to refocus on public health questions so that scientists can disengage from corporate influence. Incentives for investigators to seek industry funding at the structural level, such as having the amount of industry funding generated count toward tenure or promotion, should be eliminated. Instead, research practices that promote integrity should be rewarded.

When relationships with industry do exist, disclosure of funding sources and researcher conflicts of interest is necessary for transparency and to conduct the type of meta-research described in this chapter. However, disclosure does not eliminate bias. Although disclosures are increasingly required by journals, they remain inaccurate, incomplete, uninformative, and are still missing from many research articles.[29] Disclosure requirements need to be enforced, with penalties for nondisclosure, such as authors being banned from publication for a period of time. Public registries of investigator financial ties could improve disclosures of author conflicts of interests.[30]

Universities require contracts with sponsors that are aimed at protecting the integrity of the sponsored research. However, contracts cannot be relied on to prevent industry involvement in the cycle of research. Among industry-funded trials of drugs, which usually have more institutional oversight than other types of research, 92% of authors stated that the sponsor was involved in the design of the study, 73% in data analysis, and 87% in the reporting of study.[31]

The research community needs to recognize industry funding and financial ties of investigators as a source of bias and account for it when evaluating research findings. Funding source should be included as an independent item in tools for study evaluation. Then, the impact of funding bias can be assessed descriptively or by using subgroup analysis, comparing industry-funded to non-industry-funded studies. To improve transparency around funding, funding source should also be disclosed in the abstracts of papers, as recommended in the CONSORT guidelines for reporting randomized controlled trials.[32]

Bias in how research is conducted behind the scenes and what gets published can be reduced by enforcing open data policies for all. Industry-sponsored research should not be guaranteed secrecy due to considerations of commercial gain. The value of the information to public health should supersede the exclusivity of industry profits. Transparency throughout the entire research cycle is needed so that independent evaluators can determine if protocols have been followed and that all the data collected have been reported. This can be accomplished by more widespread participation in study registries, the publication of peer-reviewed protocols and registered reports, and open publication of data sets and analysis plans.

Eliminating industry influence on research will require a change in the culture of science. Scientists, industry executives and lawyers, and journal editors involved in the cycle of research use mechanisms of moral disengagement to eliminate the moral consequences of manipulating research.[33] Safeguards to protect against moral disengagement include encouraging diversity of opinion within an organization, collaboration across disciplines, and institutional protection of dissent within corporate structures. Another safeguard is for research publishers to monitor, publicize, and make transparent strategies utilized by industries to manipulate research. A further safeguard involves careful management of the conflicts of interest of those engaged in research. Cultural change has begun in some sectors. The *British Medical Journal* published a special series aimed at promoting independence from commercial influence in health that included empiric research, a call to action, and approaches to minimizing bias in the clinical research, practice, and education.[34]

REFERENCES

1. Bero L. Meta-research matters: Meta-spin cycles, the blindness of bias, and rebuilding trust. *PLoS Biol*. 2018; 16(4): e2005972.
2. Higgins JPT, Savović J, Page MJ, Elbers RG, Sterne JAC. Assessing risk of bias in a randomized trial. In: Higgins JPT, Thomas J, Chandler J, Cumpston M, Li T, Page MJ, Welch VA, eds. *Cochrane Handbook for Systematic Reviews of Interventions*. 2nd ed. Cochrane; 2021; 205–227.
3. Page MJ, Higgins JPT, Clayton G, Sterne JAC, Hróbjartsson A, Savović J. Empirical evidence of study design biases in randomized trials: Systematic review of meta-epidemiological studies. *PLoS One*. 2016; 11(7): e0159267.
4. Barnes DE, Bero LA. Why review articles on the health effects of passive smoking reach different conclusions. *JAMA*. 1998; 279(19): 1566–1570.
5. Lundh A, Lexchin J, Mintzes B, Schroll JB, Bero L. Industry sponsorship and research outcome. *Cochrane Database Syst Rev*. 2017; 2: Mr000033.
6. Lesser LI, Ebbeling CB, Goozner M, Wypij D, Ludwig DS. Relationship between funding source and conclusion among nutrition-related scientific articles. *PLoS Med*. 2007; 4(1): e5.
7. Huss A, Egger M, Hug K, Huwiler-Müntener K, Röösli M. Source of funding and results of studies of health effects of mobile phone use: Systematic review of experimental studies. *Environ Health Perspect*. 2007; 115(1): 1–4.
8. Shrader-Frechette K. Climate change, nuclear economics, and conflicts of interest. *Sci Eng Ethics*. 2011; 17(1): 75–107.
9. Chartres N, Fabbri A, Bero LA. Association of industry sponsorship with outcomes of nutrition studies: A systematic review and meta-analysis. *JAMA Intern Med*. 2016; 176(12): 1769–1777.
10. Chartres N, Fabbri A, McDonald S, Diong J, McKenzie JE, Bero L. Association of food industry ties with findings of studies examining the effect of dairy food

intake on cardiovascular disease and mortality: Systematic review and meta-analysis. *BMJ Open.* 2020; 10(12): e039036.

11. Hansen C, Lundh A, Rasmussen K, Hróbjartsson A. Financial conflicts of interest in systematic reviews: Associations with results, conclusions, and methodological quality. *Cochrane Database Syst Rev.* 2019; 8(8): Mr000047.

12. Fabbri A, Chartres N, Bero LA. Study sponsorship and the nutrition research agenda: Analysis of cohort studies examining the association between nutrition and obesity. *Public Health Nutr.* 2017; 20(17): 3193–3199.

13. Friedman L, Friedman M. Financial conflicts of interest and study results in environmental and occupational health research. *J Occup Environ Med.* 2016; 58(3): 238–247.

14. Barnes DE, Bero LA. Industry-funded research and conflict of interest: An analysis of research sponsored by the tobacco industry through the Center for Indoor Air Research. *J Health Polit Policy Law.* 1996; 21(3): 515–542.

15. Kearns CE, Glantz SA, Schmidt LA. Sugar industry influence on the scientific agenda of the National Institute of Dental Research's 1971 National Caries Program: A historical analysis of internal documents. *PLoS Med.* 2015; 12(3): e1001798.

16. Fabbri A, Holland TJ, Bero LA. Food industry sponsorship of academic research: Investigating commercial bias in the research agenda. *Public Health Nutr.* 2018; 21(18): 3422–3430.

17. Cassidy R, Loussouarn C, Pisac A. *Fair Game: Producing Gambling Research.* Goldsmiths University of London; 2013.

18. Bero LA. Why the Cochrane risk of bias tool should include funding source as a standard item. *Cochrane Database Syst Rev.* 2013; 2013(12): ED000075.

19. White J, Bero L. Corporate manipulation of research: Strategies are similar across five industries. *Stanford Law Policy Rev.* 2010; 21: 105.

20. Hirayama T. Non-smoking wives of heavy smokers have a higher risk of lung cancer: A study from Japan. *Br Med J (Clin Res Ed).* 1981; 282(6259): 183–185.

21. Hong M-K, Bero LA. How the tobacco industry responded to an influential study of the health effects of secondhand smoke. *BMJ.* 2002; 325(7377): 1413–1416.

22. Steinman MA, Bero LA, Chren MM, Landefeld CS. Narrative review: The promotion of gabapentin: An analysis of internal industry documents. *Ann Intern Med.* 2006; 145(4): 284–293.

23. Misakian AL, Bero LA. Publication bias and research on passive smoking: Comparison of published and unpublished studies. *JAMA.* 1998; 280(3): 250–253.

24. Rising K, Bacchetti P, Bero L. Reporting bias in drug trials submitted to the Food and Drug Administration: Review of publication and presentation. *PLoS Med.* 2008; 5(11): e217.

25. Vedula SS, Bero L, Scherer RW, Dickersin K. Outcome reporting in industry-sponsored trials of gabapentin for off-label use. *N Engl J Med.* 2009; 361(20): 1963–1971.

26. McHenry LB. The Monsanto Papers: Poisoning the scientific well. *Int J Risk Saf Med.* 2018; 29(3–4): 193–205.

27. Chan AW, Hróbjartsson A, Haahr MT, Gøtzsche PC, Altman DG. Empirical evidence for selective reporting of outcomes in randomized trials: Comparison of protocols to published articles. *JAMA.* 2004; 291(20): 2457–2465.

28. Rezende LFMd, Rey-López JP, Sá THd, et al. Reporting bias in the literature on the associations of health-related behaviors and statins with cardiovascular disease and all-cause mortality. *PLoS Biol.* 2018; 16(6): e2005761.

29. Grundy Q, Dunn AG, Bero L. Improving researchers' conflict of interest declarations. *BMJ*. 2020; 368: m422.
30. Dunn AG. Set up a public registry of competing interests. *Nature*. 2016; 533(7601): 9.
31. Rasmussen K, Bero L, Redberg R, Gøtzsche PC, Lundh A. Collaboration between academics and industry in clinical trials: Cross sectional study of publications and survey of lead academic authors. *BMJ*. 2018; 363: k3654.
32. Hopewell S, Clarke M, Moher D, et al. CONSORT for reporting randomized controlled trials in journal and conference abstracts: Explanation and elaboration. *PLoS Med*. 2008; 5(1): e20.
33. White J, Bandura A, Bero LA. Moral disengagement in the corporate world. *Account Res*. 2009; 16(1): 41–74.
34. Moynihan R, Macdonald H, Heneghan C, Bero L, Godlee F. Commercial interests, transparency, and independence: A call for submissions. *BMJ*. 2019; 365: l1706.

CHAPTER 20

The Global Technology Sector as a Commercial Determinant of Health

NORA KENWORTHY, KATERINI TAGMATARCHI STORENG, AND MARCO ZENONE

20.1 INTRODUCTION

Digital technology is becoming a central part of public health and health care provision. Digital technology companies are increasingly commercializing health sectors globally through data acquisition, market disruption, and product innovation.[1] Simultaneously, digital technologies influence population health in myriad indirect ways—for example, serving as essential conduits for information and misinformation, and contributing to growing polarization and extremism.[2–4] Despite these two intertwined phenomena, a climate of techno-optimism in global public health and medicine has allowed the technology sector to gain major footholds in health systems with little scrutiny or regulation.[5,6] In recent years, for example, the World Health Organization (WHO) has launched a Department of Digital Health, a Global Digital Health Strategy, and a Digital Clearinghouse—all geared toward approving and disseminating new health technologies.[7] In heavily market-oriented health systems such as the United States, the encroachment of digital technology into health provision and the private accumulation of health data has been particularly acute, but countries with more robust universal health systems, such as the United Kingdom, have not been spared this trend.[5] The COVID-19 pandemic has rapidly accelerated the expansion of Big Tech—the dominant American technology companies—into public health policy and practice, with the pandemic contributing to a vacuum of power and services that corporations have moved aggressively to exploit.[8] Despite these trends, the influence

Nora Kenworthy, Katerini Tagmatarchi Storeng, and Marco Zenone, The Global Technology Sector as a Commercial Determinant of Health In: The Commercial Determinants of Health. Edited by: Nason Maani, Mark Petticrew, and Sandro Galea, Oxford University Press. © Oxford University Press 2023. DOI: 10.1093/oso/9780197578742.003.0020 of the global technology sector as a commercial determinant of health has largely been overlooked.[9]

This chapter provides brief case studies from our research of three companies—Meta (formerly Facebook), Google, and GoFundMe—and the diverse impacts they are having on public health systems. Although in no way a comprehensive look at the technology sector as a contributor to commercial determinants of health, these three cases provide lessons about the strategies that technology companies use to transform and disrupt health systems and help clarify the longer term implications for population health that warrant further in-depth research.

20.2 FACEBOOK, MISINFORMATION, AND PUBLIC HEALTH PARTNERSHIP

Facebook, owned by Meta, is the largest social media platform in the world—with more than 2.7 billion active monthly users—making up the bulk of the 4.3 billion social media users worldwide.[10] The growth of such social media platforms has amplified the spread of health-related misinformation. Even prior to COVID-19, Facebook was a hub for the spread of conspiracy theories about vaccines, unproven treatments, and conditions such as autism, questioning scientific information and public health professionals' motivations.[11] In 2019, WHO labeled vaccine hesitancy a top 10 threat to global health,[12] and such hesitancy has only exacerbated during the pandemic. A July 2020 report found that misinformation about vaccines and other COVID-19 topics was viewed approximately 3.8 billion times on Facebook.[13]

The spread of misinformation on social media platforms is due primarily to platform design. Facebook algorithms match content to users based on their interests, creating "echo chambers" that reinforce user perspectives.[14] For example, a user who engages with anti-vaccine Facebook content is likely to have more anti-vaccine content suggested to them. Although Facebook does have limited policies to remove harmful social media posts, this often does not extend to misinformation unless it could contribute to what Facebook determines is "imminent harm."[15] The reluctance of Facebook and other social media platforms to moderate harmful content emerges from two interests, one political and the other financial. Politically, social media platforms prefer to be seen as "neutral" vessels for information,[11] not publishers, whom are held to higher standards for responsibility in many countries. To remain the dominant platform across numerous political and national contexts while avoiding regulation requires a careful maintenance of so-called neutrality, achieved largely through minimal moderation, particularly of powerful institutions and leaders. Financially, social media platforms are often built so that more controversial and extreme content generates the most interest, which in turn generates more ad revenue.

Despite Facebook's central role in contributing to the spread of vaccine misinformation, Meta positions itself as a trusted public health partner. As early as January 2020, WHO Director General Tedros Adhanom Ghebreyesus praised the company for "efforts to combat misinformation and rumors on #2019nCoV & direct users to reliable sources."[16] By February 2021, Meta's (then Facebook's) Head of Health, Kang-Xing Jin, announced the "largest worldwide campaign to help public health organizations share accurate information about COVID-19 vaccines and encourage people to get vaccinated."[17] As part of this campaign, Meta donated $120 million in advertising credit to WHO and committed to remove vaccine misinformation from its platforms. In separate events, prominent public health figures such as the Director of the U.S. National Institute of Allergy and Infectious Diseases, Anthony Fauci, appeared alongside Meta Chief Executive Officer Mark Zuckerberg to promote public confidence in vaccination programs.[18]

Although laudable at first glance, corporations such as Meta labeling themselves as part of the solution to industry-created public health problems from which they profit is a common strategy reported in the commercial determinant of health literature. Unhealthy commodities industries such as alcohol or tobacco have been said to "legitimize their presence in public health policy decisions" to preserve industry interests[19]—and there are reasonable grounds to argue that Meta acts with similar motivations.

However, in contrast to unhealthy commodities industries, public health advocates have little choice but to work with social media platforms to communicate with the public. Platforms exert significant power: Their organizational size, resources, and influence leave public health authorities with little control to intervene on public health issues such as misinformation. The lack of a well-functioning regulatory scheme allows Meta to leverage complete control over its platforms on any suggested public health action. As Lacy-Nichols and Marten argue, "Corporate actors excise power through both coercion and appeasement," where appeasement "neutralizes" criticism or industry opposition.[20] Through voluntary COVID-19 response efforts, Meta demonstrates an intentional strategy to nullify public criticisms. Efforts to influence public opinion are matched with efforts to subvert external regulation, including the creation of a Facebook "oversight board" to make summary judgments on whether content on the platform is permissible and also investment in "third-party" fact-checkers.[21] Meta uses its platform power to position itself as an altruistic public health partner while strategically retaining control over, and influence within, institutions tasked with protecting the public from the very public health harms it exacerbates.

20.3 GOOGLE AND THE COVID-19 RESPONSE

In addition to Meta's activities in managing misinformation, Amazon, Apple, Microsoft, and Google all contributed directly to the global pandemic response in ways that illustrate the sector's disruptive potential, whether advising governments on strategy, providing access to big data and computational analytics, or developing new technological solutions for infectious disease monitoring and control. Often, this involved novel partnerships with government bodies, such the U.S. Centers for Disease Control and Prevention, the UK National Health Service (NHS), and WHO.[22]

The most striking of Big Tech's early pandemic innovations was the Google–Apple Exposure Notification System (GAEN), established by the rival companies in May 2020. GAEN was intended as an alternative to governments' experiments with digital contact tracing, which privacy advocates had criticized for their reliance on centralized storage of personal information, which they feared could succumb to "mission creep" and result in widespread state surveillance. By early 2021, Google and Apple's system was in use in more than 50 countries, states, and regions as a "privacy-friendly alternative," and Google claimed GAEN was "saving lives at all levels of adoption."[23] This claim, however, was based not on empirical evidence but, rather, on unpublished results from a mathematical model that showed GAEN had "potential to meaningfully reduce the number of coronavirus cases, hospitalization and deaths."[24]

Many welcomed GAEN for its promise to protect privacy, despite mixed evidence about its ability to do so and its uncertain public health impact. Warnings that reliance on corporately controlled platforms and infrastructures had the potential to de-center the power of public health authorities while normalizing wide-scale digital surveillance[25] and reinforcing inequities[26] were largely ignored.

GAEN is only one of dozens of COVID-19 response endeavors spearheaded by Google and its parent company Alphabet Inc. during the pandemic. Other examples include using artificial intelligence for biomedical research and response efforts, leveraging big data and partnerships to assist with disease surveillance and, like Meta, offering millions in advertising credits to WHO, nonprofits, and government bodies to manage (mis)information. Google also donated directly to charitable relief efforts via Google.org, as part of a $100 million commitment. This included contributions to the COVAX Facility to provide access to vaccines in poor countries and direct relief to India's crisis.

Amid such largesse, one could lose sight of the extent to which Google and other Big Tech companies' assistance to the global pandemic response were not simply acts of corporate social responsibility but also served the companies' interests in diverse ways. For example, in offering pro bono assistance to' pandemic response, Big Tech corporations deflected attention from their own monopolistic business practices at a time when they faced unprecedented scrutiny, ingratiating themselves with the very governments grappling with how to regulate them. Ironically, while Google carried out its efforts under the auspices of its "AI for Good" initiative, its claims to social good were being made against a backdrop of pervasive and mounting critiques. These critiques included revelations about Google's mistreatment of women and minoritized employees—such as the treatment and firing of Timnit Gebru, one of the leaders of Google's ethical artificial intelligence (AI) team, for her co-authorship of a paper on the risks of using natural-language processing AI—and the numerous harms associated with its products, such as search algorithms that return racist results, for marginalized communities.[27,28]

The involvement of companies such as Google in public health responses should be seen as part of their broader expansionary logic, consolidating reliance on and demand for their devices, platforms, and data and contributing to an exponential revenue growth. Pandemic experiences fed into Google's strategy for "carving out" space in future health care markets,[8] raising questions about how it leverages data and cloud control for further market expansion. What will health care look like when the majority of health data are privately controlled and potentially sold to the highest bidder?

Crucially, Big Tech's involvement in public health responses raises critical questions about governance, notably the implications for broader concerns about achieving an appropriate balance between corporate and state control of the digital sphere.[22] There have been some quarters in which these companies' involvement has been criticized. In the United Kingdom, Google's management of COVID-19 data raised unease, especially given a pre-pandemic scandal that saw Google transferring identifiable NHS patient records without explicit consent for the purposes of developing a clinical alert app.[29] In France, GAEN was interpreted as part of a broader attack on the country's "digital sovereignty,"[30] while Latvia also questioned the legitimacy of tech giants "dictating" the public health policies of elected governments.[31] A Chatham House report on digital tech during the pandemic also questions what the imposition of policy by unaccountable companies says about the legitimacy of the resultant policy.[32]

As Latvia's presidential adviser on digital technology noted, these concerns are being raised for the first time during the pandemic—but certainly will not end as the pandemic wanes. In many countries, pandemic-era decisions allowed companies with documented histories of bias and harm to not only control data systems but also be in a position to profit from them and more powerfully negotiate for Big Tech interests in subsequent policy-making related to regulation, privacy, and data ownership. This undermines governments' ability to moderate or regulate these companies in the future, particularly with regard to harmful health effects. It is distressing that few decision-makers listened to concerns about the danger of unfettered tech company intrusion into pandemic response.[33,34] The speed and breadth of that intrusion—and the ways in which it was largely welcomed during the early period of crisis—indicate the severity of the regulatory challenges countries face with regard to new tech disruptions.

20.4 GOFUNDME: CROWDFUNDING AS DISRUPTIVE HEALTH CARE FINANCING?

Disruptive potential among tech companies also extends to newer, more seemingly beneficent, digital platforms than Meta and Google. Personal crowdfunding emerged in the wake of the 2008 financial crisis as a way for individuals to raise money for needs or projects from their online social networks. Companies such as GoFundMe, Kickstarter, Crowdfunder, and M-Changa invite users to create campaign pages and then promote them across social media. Crowdfunding originated as a means of financing business or creative projects, but appeals for medical needs are now the most common on platforms such as GoFundMe, which controls more than 90% of U.S. market share. Although it can look like an innocuous, even feel-good technological fix for inadequate health care coverage, crowdfunding's simple façade conceals complex ways in which it disrupts health access and contributes to health inequalities.[9] It creates a marketplace in which people compete for scarce funds, appealing to networks where existing wealth inequalities and social mores of deservingness shape campaign outcomes, reproducing and exacerbating structural inequities.[35,36] Campaigns are more common and perform better in areas with greater wealth and privilege.[37]

GoFundMe offers a for-profit, downstream intervention that at best addresses discrete, solvable problems, while individuals with complex, overlapping needs struggle to succeed.[9] Campaigns for preventative care are rare. Globally, as people turned to crowdfunding to cope with the severe economic and health impacts of COVID-19, many did not anticipate how low success rates were. Whereas even prior to 2020, only 10% of medical campaigns met their financial goals, in the first months of the pandemic, more than 40% of campaigns in the United States did not receive a single donation.[38] Campaigns in areas with higher education and income were more common, and earned more, contributing to disparities in access to crisis support.[38]

GoFundMe has exploited the COVID-19 crisis by strengthening its control over the crowdfunding marketplace and campaign outcomes. Increasingly, the site promotes consolidated campaigns for broad areas of need, such as "COVID-19 relief," that are run by GoFundMe.org, its nonprofit arm. Donations to these "causes," which leverage celebrity endorsements and corporate partnerships to garner interest, are distributed at GoFundMe's discretion. There is no transparency regarding how individual campaigns are selected or funds allocated. What began as a crowdfunding start-up has now become a social assistance organization—one with no oversight, which provides revenue and tax relief for a highly profitable private corporation.

Crowdfunding also powerfully influences public perceptions, undermining awareness of health inequalities. Algorithms ensure that users primarily interact with highly successful campaigns, rendering the vast majority of campaigns that do not achieve widespread success largely invisible.[39] Like Meta and Google, GoFundMe spends a great deal of money portraying itself as a beneficent and progressive organization helping those in need. Consequently, in the public imagination, personal crises and financial shortfalls are increasingly met with the suggestion, "Why don't you start a GoFundMe?"

The ubiquity of this seemingly easy fix to health system gaps diverts attention from the political determinants of health care and crowdfunding's role as a driver of disparities. As Snyder notes, crowdfunding campaigns "reduce pressure for systemic reforms" and normalize the idea that private fundraising is a partial solution to inadequate healthcare coverage.[36] As crowdfunding platforms expand throughout the world, they exploit, profit from, and contribute to health system gaps. Although it still represents a small portion of the tech sector involvement in health systems, crowdfunding offers important lessons about how disruption occurs and to what ends it is put. It also reminds us that the social dimensions of technology in the health sector—the way it shifts social mores, expectations, and political will—may be just as important as its more direct health impacts.

20.5 CONCLUSION

Digital technology firms are aggressively expanding into, and transforming, public health and health care markets throughout the world, a process accelerated by the COVID-19 pandemic.[8] Across the brief case studies discussed in this chapter, several themes emerge. First, while "disruption" is an often-invoked ethos of this sector, it is useful to pay attention to what is being disrupted. Although companies certainly disrupt existing markets, they also co-opt entire sectors and data flows, and they create new sectors, such as with GAEN and the digitalization of contact tracing.

Partnerships and claims of beneficence are key strategies of disruption, allowing corporations to capture negotiating power and create systems—whether for spreading information or collecting user data—upon which health systems must rely. Technology firms not only carry monopoly power over systems with extensive health impacts but also create, transform, and control systems that are necessary to protect the public's health. Many companies, aware of the public scrutiny and criticism they face, position their technology as a solution to problems they create and from which they benefit. There is an urgent need for scholars to critically examine these claims of interventions for "social good." This chapter calls for heightened awareness of technology companies' influence over social norms as well—about who should provide and protect health services, who is responsible for protecting health data, and what constitutes misinformation. Certainly, there are technologies that have brought great health benefits to society, and the tech sector is made up of many diverse actors. Technology is a powerful force determining human health in the 21st century, but techno-optimism will not protect health systems from its documented, and future, harms.

REFERENCES

1. Bustreo F, Jha S, Germann S. Global health disruptors: Fourth industrial revolution. *BMJ Opinion*. November 30, 2018. Accessed April 23, 2021. https://blogs.bmj.com/bmj/2018/11/30/global-health-disruptors-fourth-industrial-revolution
2. Vaidhyanathan S. *Antisocial Media: How Facebook Disconnects Us and Undermines Democracy*. Oxford University Press; 2018.
3. Noble SU, Tynes BM, eds. *The Intersectional Internet: Race, Sex, Class and Culture Online*. Lang; 2015.
4. Couldry N, Mejias U. *The Costs of Connection: How Data Is Colonizing Human Life and Appropriating It for Capitalism*. Stanford University Press; 2019. Accessed April 23, 2021. http://www.sup.org/books/title/?id=28816
5. Storeng KT, Fukuda-Parr S, Mahajan M, Venkatapuram S. Digital technology and the political determinants of health inequities: Special issue introduction. *Global Policy*. 2021; 12: 5–11.
6. World Health Organization. *Future of Digital Health Systems*. WHO Regional Office for Europe; 2019. Accessed April 23, 2021. https://www.euro.who.int/en/health-topics/Health-systems/digital-health/publications/2019/future-of-digital-health-systems-report-on-the-who-symposium-on-the-future-of-digital-health-systems-in-the-european-region-copenhagen,-denmark,-68-february-2019
7. Ghebreyesus TA. *Harnessing the Power of Digital Technology for a Healthier World*. UNCTAD; 2020. Accessed April 23, 2021. https://unctad.org/news/harnessing-power-digital-technology-healthier-world
8. Big tech in healthcare: Here's who wins and loses as Alphabet, Amazon, Apple, and Microsoft target niche sectors of healthcare. *Business Insider*. February 14, 2021. Accessed April 28, 2021. https://www.businessinsider.com/2-14-2021-big-tech-in-healthcare-report?r=US&IR=T
9. Kenworthy NJ. Crowdfunding and global health disparities: An exploratory conceptual and empirical analysis. *Glob Health*. 2019; 15(1): 71–84. doi:10.1186/s12992-019-0519-1
10. Global social media stats. Datareportal. Accessed June 22, 2021. https://datareportal.com/social-media-users
11. Wardle C, Singerman E. Too little, too late: Social media companies' failure to tackle vaccine misinformation poses a real threat. *BMJ*. 2021; 372: n26. doi:10.1136/bmj.n26

12. World Health Organization. Ten threats to global health in 2019. 2019. Accessed April 23, 2021. https://www.who.int/news-room/spotlight/ten-threats-to-global-health-in-2019

13. Avaaz. Facebook's algorithm: A major threat to public health. August 19, 2020. Accessed April 23, 2021. https://secure.avaaz.org/campaign/en/facebook_threat_health/

14. Cinelli M, De Francisci Morales G, Galeazzi A, Quattrociocchi W, Starnini M. The echo chamber effect on social media. *Proc Natl Acad Sci USA*. 2021; 118(9): e2023301118. doi:10.1073/pnas.2023301118

15. Clegg N. Combating COVID-19 misinformation across our apps. Facebook. March 25, 2020. Accessed April 23, 2021. https://about.fb.com/news/2020/03/combating-covid-19-misinformation

16. @DrTedros. It's time for facts, not fear. We appreciate @Google, @Facebook, @TencentGlobal, @Tiktok and @Twitter's efforts to combat misinformation and rumors on #2019nCoV & direct users to reliable sources. We ask all digital companies to step up and help the world beat this outbreak. Twitter. January 31, 2020. Accessed April 23, 2021. https://twitter.com/DrTedros/status/1223288483265089537

17. Jin K-X. Reaching billions of people with COVID-19 vaccine information. Facebook. February 8, 2021. Accessed April 23, 2021. https://about.fb.com/news/2021/02/reaching-billions-of-people-with-covid-19-vaccine-information

18. Isaac M. Facebook says it will remove coronavirus vaccine misinformation. *The New York Times*. December 3, 2020. Accessed April 23, 2021. https://www.nytimes.com/2020/12/03/technology/facebook-coronavirus-vaccine-misinformation.html

19. Knai C, Petticrew M, Mays N, et al. Systems thinking as a framework for analyzing commercial determinants of health: Framework for analyzing commercial determinants of health. *Milbank Q*. 2018; 96(3): 472–498. doi:10.1111/1468-0009.12339

20. Lacy-Nichols J, Marten R. Power and the commercial determinants of health: Ideas for a research agenda. *BMJ Glob Health*. 2021; 6(2): e003850. doi:10.1136/bmjgh-2020-003850

21. Facebook's third-party fact-checking program. Facebook Journalism Project. Accessed April 23, 2021. https://www.facebook.com/journalismproject/programs/third-party-fact-checking

22. Storeng KT, de Bengy Puyvallée A. The smartphone pandemic: How Big Tech and public health authorities partner in the digital response to COVID-19. Glob Public Health. 2021; 16(8–9): 1482–1498. doi:10.1080/17441692.2021.1882530

23. Hannon S. Exposure notifications: End of year update. Google. December 11, 2020. Accessed May 6, 2021. https://blog.google/inside-google/covid-19/exposure-notifications-end-year-update

24. Abueg M, Hinch R, Wu N, et al. Modeling the combined effect of digital exposure notification and non-pharmaceutical interventions on the COVID-19 epidemic in Washington state. *medRxiv*. Published online September 2, 2020. doi:10.1101/2020.08.29.20184135

25. Erikson SL. COVID-19 mobile phone apps fail the most vulnerable. *Glob Policy J*. Published online July 2020. https://www.globalpolicyjournal.com/articles/health-and-social-policy/covid-19-mobile-phone-apps-fail-most-vulnerable

26. French M, Guta A, Gagnon M, et al. Corporate contact tracing as a pandemic response. *Crit Public Health*. 2023; 32(1): 48–55. doi:10.1080/09581596.2020.1829549

27. Noble SU. *Algorithms of Oppression: How Search Engines Reinforce Racism*. New York University Press; 2018.

28. Metz C, Wakabayashi D. Google researcher says she was fired over paper highlighting bias in A.I. *The New York Times*. December 3, 2020. Accessed May 4, 2021. https://www.nytimes.com/2020/12/03/technology/google-researcher-timnit-gebru.html

29. Roberts S. Covid-19: The controversial role of big tech in digital surveillance. LSE. April 25, 2020. Accessed May 4, 2021. https://blogs.lse.ac.uk/businessreview/2020/04/25/covid-19-the-controversial-role-of-big-tech-in-digital-surveillance

30. Traçage numérique: Le moment est venu d'établir notre souveraineté numérique. *Le Monde*. April 25, 2020. Accessed May 4, 2021. https://www.lemonde.fr/idees/article/2020/04/25/tracage-numerique-le-moment-est-venu-d-etablir-notre-souverainete-numerique_6037729_3232.html

31. Ilves I. Why are Google and Apple dictating how European democracies fight coronavirus? *The Guardian*. June 16, 2020. Accessed May 4, 2021. http://www.theguardian.com/commentisfree/2020/jun/16/google-apple-dictating-european-democracies-coronavirus

32. The COVID-19 pandemic and trends in technology. Chatham House; 2021. Accessed May 4, 2021. https://www.chathamhouse.org/2021/02/covid-19-pandemic-and-trends-technology

33. McDonald S. Coronavirus: A digital governance emergency of international concern. Centre for International Governance Innovation; 2020. Accessed May 4, 2021. https://www.cigionline.org/articles/coronavirus-digital-governance-emergency-international-concern

34. Kind C. Exit through the app store? Patterns. 2020; 1(3): 100054. doi:10.1016/j.patter.2020.100054

35. Berliner LS, Kenworthy NJ. Producing a worthy illness: Personal crowdfunding amidst financial crisis. *Soc Sci Med*. 2017; 187: 233–242. doi:10.1016/j.socscimed.2017.02.008

36. Snyder J. Crowdfunding for medical care ethical issues in an emerging health care funding practice. *Hastings Cent Rep*. 2016; 46(6): 36–42.

37. van Duynhoven A, Lee A, Michel R, et al. Spatially exploring the intersection of socioeconomic status and Canadian cancer-related medical crowdfunding campaigns. *BMJ Open*. 2019; 9(6): e026365. doi:10.1136/bmjopen-2018-026365

38. Igra et al. Crowdfunding as a response to COVID-19: Increasing inequities at a time of crisis; 2021. https://doi.org/10.1016/j.socscimed.2021.114105

39. Kenworthy N. Like a grinding stone: How crowdfunding platforms create, perpetuate, and value inequities. *Med Anthropol Q*. 2021; 35(3): 327–345.

SECTION 5

Advancing Science and Scholarship

CHAPTER 21

Defining the Commercial Determinants of Health

JENNIFER LACY-NICHOLS,
CASSANDRA DE LACY-VAWDON, AND ROB MOODIE

21.1 INTRODUCTION

With the rise of the "corporation" throughout the 20th century, it is surprising that public health has been so slow to focus on commerce (i.e., the exchange of goods and services) as a determinant of health. This lag is particularly remarkable given that there are so many powerful and egregious examples of how the tobacco, alcohol, nuclear arms, chemical weapons, firearms, pharmaceuticals, and automobile industries have negatively affected health.[1] However, 30 years after the rise of the social determinants of health, the exploration of the commercial determinants of health (CDOH) has emerged in public health research. Figure 21.1 demonstrates the rapid growth and development of the terms used to describe this perspective during the past 15 years. The increased interest in the CDOH coincides with the overwhelming growth, consolidation, and power of corporations throughout the world. In 2000, 51 of the world's largest economies were corporations[2]; this had increased to 71 in 2018.[3] Corporate revenue is now comparable to (and often exceeds) national economies, giving corporations unprecedented market power that is easily (and often) translated into political influence.

Although (largely) uncritical literature praising the benefits of commerce abounds in business and marketing scholarship, and corporations are quick to promote the benefits that commerce generates for society, public health researchers have yet to measure the positive impact of commerce on health. In response to this gap, this chapter constructs a more nuanced approach

Jennifer Lacy-Nichols, Cassandra de Lacy-Vawdon, and Rob Moodie, *Defining the Commercial Determinants of Health*
In: *The Commercial Determinants of Health*. Edited by: Nason Maani, Mark Petticrew, and Sandro Galea,
Oxford University Press. © Oxford University Press 2023. DOI: 10.1093/oso/9780197578742.003.0021

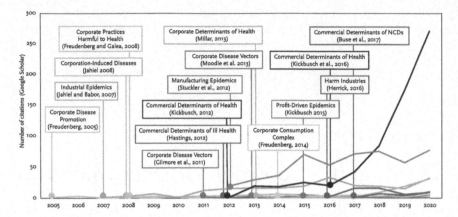

Figure 21.1 Emergence and use of commercial determinants of health terms from 2005 to the present. NCDs, noncommunicable diseases.

for CDOH research that presents an alternative narrative to the corporate rhetoric.

This new approach is needed because the existing frame of CDOH as the determinants of *ill* health risks siloing the public health community during a period when a productive and informed dialogue is needed to address the harms of unfettered capitalism and many of its commercial actors. We contend that it is particularly important and timely to start this conversation within public health because alcohol and ultra-processed food (UPF) corporations have leveraged the COVID-19 pandemic as a marketing opportunity to further embed themselves within society.[4]

This chapter develops this more nuanced approach to the CDOH by first unpacking existing definitions and argues for the need to acknowledge that some commercial activity is (directly or indirectly) health promoting. It then explores the existing models that demonstrate the complex relationships that exist between upstream drivers, commercial actors, and health outcomes to argue that researchers need to focus more on understanding the upstream drivers that enable commercial activities. We then problematize the public health understanding of the private sector by exploring the sheer diversity of commercial actors and activities that could be included within CDOH research. We conclude by theorizing what these new understandings mean for public health researchers and practitioners.

21.2 DEFINITIONS OF CDOH

Numerous definitions of CDOH have been proposed within the public health research since the CDOH term was introduced (Table 21.1). The first usage of phrases similar to CDOH occurred in 2013.[5,6] These definitions perform a tight balancing act, endeavoring to be broad enough to incorporate all core components but not so broad as to be ineffectual. These definitions differ in their breadth and framing of CDOH.

One of the key differences between CDOH definitions is how commercial actors are framed. Most commonly used definitions focus on the harms of commercial actors to health.[1,7-14] This is understandable given the significant contribution of industry actors within tobacco, alcohol, and UPF industries to increased global disease burdens and is also observable within commercial and industrial contributions to significant environmental risk factors such as air, water, and soil pollution and contamination. For example, Kickbusch et al.'s definition explicitly focuses on outcomes that are "detrimental to health."[8] This conceptualization of the CDOH strongly differs from the neutral framing of social determinants of health, in which conditions are recognized for their potential as risk and/or protective factors. Recognizing commercial sources of harm is an essential first step for public health to determine areas in which intervention is necessary to mitigate commercial harms and protect population health. However, a negative framing is reductive because it does not recognize that the harms and benefits within CDOH systems are complex, situational, and can occur simultaneously.[15] This initial framing of CDOH appears to be changing within Freudenberg's recent definition that explicitly acknowledges that business activities contribute to both health and disease.[16]

CDOH definitions also differ with regard to how they interpret "health." Some definitions are quite biomedical in nature, and this has led to much CDOH research focusing on noncommunicable diseases (NCDs).[9,14,17-19] Although the burden of disease attributable to NCDs is substantial, this narrower focus risks downplaying other social, legal, environmental, ethical, and economic drivers that affect health. For example, exposure to chemical hazards during production and the impact of poor employment practices on mental health are important externalities of business practices that deserve greater public health consideration. Similarly, environmental and planetary health has historically been left out of framings of CDOH, although there are now CDOH frameworks that incorporate human and planetary health.[20]

The nature of commercial actors (and their activities) is another parameter used to limit the scope of CDOH definitions. Existing definitions focus on "unhealthy commodities,"[21] "unhealthy commodity industries," the "risks inherent from the consumption of, or exposure to, commercial products,"[9] and "corporate entities as social structural diseases."[22] These definitions often focus on specific commodities (typically tobacco, alcohol, and UPFs), which is understandable considering public health's protracted battle with these industries. This focus has led to greater attention on larger, more powerful, and better resourced corporations (typically transnational businesses) without considering the diversity of actors involved in commerce. We acknowledge

Table 21.1 KEY CDOH DEFINITIONS

Reference	Year	Term and Definition
Wiist[22]	2006	Corporate entity: "A social structural determinant of disease." (p. 1370)
Jahiel and Babor[10]	2007	Industrial disease epidemics: "Diseases of consumers, workers and community residents caused by industrial promotion of consumable products, job conditions and environmental pollution, respectively, and to endemic as well as epidemic conditions. In each instance, public health-oriented policies run the risk of being opposed by industrial corporations in a health versus profit trade-off. . . . Industrial disease epidemics are driven at least in part by corporations and their allies who promote a product that is also a disease agent." (p. 1335)
Jahiel[24]	2008	Corporation-induced diseases: "Diseases of consumers, workers, or community residents who have been exposed to disease agents contained in corporate products." (p. 517)
Gilmore et al.[11]	2011	Industrial epidemics: "An epidemic emerging from the commercialization of potentially health-damaging products. . . . Adapting traditional public health constructs, it identifies the role of the host (the consumer), agent (the product, e.g. cigarettes, alcohol), environment and, crucially, the disease vector (the corporation)." (p. 2)
Stuckler et al.[21]	2012	Unhealthy commodities: These are "highly profitable because of their low production cost, long shelf-life, and high retail value. These market characteristics create perverse incentives for industries to market and sell more of these commodities." (p. 1)
Millar[5]	2013	Corporate determinants of health: "The business sector has an enormous effect on population health, health inequities and health care expenditures." (p. e327)
West and Marteau[6]	2013	Commercial determinants of health: "Factors that influence health which stem from the profit motive." (p. 686)
Moodie et al.[12]	2013	Industrial epidemics: "The vectors of spread are not biological agents, but transnational corporations. Unlike infectious disease epidemics, however, these corporate disease vectors implement sophisticated campaigns to undermine public health interventions." (p. 671)

Table 21.1 CONTINUED

Reference	Year	Term and Definition
Freudenberg[1]	2014	Corporate consumption complex: "A network of corporations, financial institutions, banks, trade associations, advertising, lobbying and legal firms, and others that promote what I call 'hyperconsumption,' a pattern of consuming that is directly linked to premature mortality and preventable illness or injury. . . . the corporate consumption complex threatens public health, democracy, and sustainable economic development." (p. xi)
Kosinska and Ostlin[7]	2016	Commercial determinants of health: "A good or a service where there is an inherent tension between the commercial and the public health objective." (p. 127)
Kickbusch et al.[8]	2016	Commercial determinants of health: "Strategies and approaches used by the private sector to promote products and choices that are detrimental to health." (p. e895)
Buse et al.[9]	2017	Determinants of noncommunicable diseases: "The risks inherent from consumption of, or exposure to, commercial products—such as ultra-processed foods and beverages, tobacco and alcohol." (p. 2)
Freudenberg[16]	2020	Commercial determinants of health: "The structures, rules, norms and practices by which business activities designed to generate wealth and profits influence patterns of health and disease across populations" (presentation).
Knai et al.[13]	2021	Unhealthy commodity industries: "Industries or groups of corporations where a significant share of their product portfolio comprises unhealthy commodities with high profit margins aimed at, and easily accessible to, large numbers of consumers." (p. 2)

that this approach risks encouraging a focus on siloed industries without considering how to challenge the broader systems within which commercial actors work.

CDOH definitions should seek to recognize the diversity and complexity of commercial actors contributing to health outcomes. This approach is used in the forthcoming *Lancet* series on CDOH, which frames the CDOH more in terms of the diverse means through which human health and inequalities are influenced by commercial forces, to overcome the issues identified in existing CDOH definitions. This definition explicitly acknowledges the influence of CDOH on health inequalities.

21.3 MODELS OF CDOH

Given the complexity evident within the CDOH definitions, several models have been designed to show the relationships between different commercial actors and health outcomes. By exploring the pathways through which commercial actors influence health outcomes, these models investigate the relationship between commercial characteristics, practices, strategies, and outcomes for health. These models demonstrate that there are broad upstream drivers, dynamics, and ideologies that create environments that encourage specific commercial characteristics and practices that influence exposure to risk factors and consumer behaviors as well as population health outcomes.

Most CDOH models are hierarchical in nature, where larger upstream drivers are shown to lead to health outcomes. These upstream drivers—referred to as "drivers,"[8] "political and economic system,"[23] "political factors,"[24] and "political economic and regulatory context"[25]—explain the broader contexts in which commercial actors exist as well as the conditions that enable their actions. Baum et al. argued that these upstream drivers exist at different levels, differentiating between global, national, and local contexts.[25]

Some models demonstrate that the relationship between commercial actors and their enabling environment is reciprocal.[23,26] This means that commercial actors benefit from ideologies and laissez-faire systems of governance while actively fostering these conditions. For example, Schram et al. proposed a model that recognizes the interrelationships between globalization, trade, investment, unbounded economic growth, and urbanization in driving unhealthy diets and contributing to NCDs.[26] These models differ from earlier models that were informed by epidemiological frameworks, which employed a more simplistic relationship between consumers and corporations.[24,26]

The corporate practices of commercial actors are outlined within these CDOH models. These are typically divided into political and market practices. Political practices are behaviors that seek to influence regulatory environments (e.g., lobbying, tax avoidance, and political donations), whereas market practices seek to influence consumption patterns through marketing, product design, and supply chain management. Madureira Lima and Galea discuss how these corporate practices are "vehicles of power" that commercial actors use to exercise power over government decision-making to minimize potential harm to their profits.[27]

Models also differ in how they represent the effects of commercial practices. Most models focus exclusively on negative health outcomes.[8,23,24,26,27] However, other models acknowledge that health outcomes exist on a spectrum from positive to negative[28] and incorporate considerations of equity, including the impact on environmental and social conditions,[25] within their assessment of impacts. In addition, Freudenberg and Galea's CDOH model complicates this by theorizing that corporations influence health behavior and norms and values which then leads to negative health outcomes.[23] These decisions around which outcomes to include within a CDOH model have significant consequences for which businesses are considered within research and potential counter-responses from public health.

Like the CDOH definitions, models seek to balance providing a simple and easily understandable representation with acknowledging the complexity of interactions between commercial actors and their surrounding systems. Likely due to its simplicity, Kickbusch et al.'s model[8] is the most commonly used model in CDOH research. We believe that this model misses some key upstream drivers, such as overarching ideology, facilitative regulation, and power dynamics. However, we recognize that these upstream drivers are more difficult to link to the direct effect of commercial actors and attempts to holistically capture all the commercial actors, mechanisms, relationships, and system-level dynamics contributing to population health are likely to create a framework that is ineffectual. As such, there must be a trade-off between comprehensiveness and ease of use of future CDOH models.

21.4 DEFINING THE PRIVATE SECTOR—A KEY ISSUE FOR CDOH SCHOLARSHIP AND PRACTICE DEFINITIONS

The term CDOH is currently used within public health without consideration of the complexity of the private sector. A number of terms and attributes are used to characterize the range of commercial actors within CDOH research, including terms that focus on the qualities of specific actors (e.g., transnational corporations, global corporations, large companies, vested interests, private companies, for-profit corporations, profit-driven actors, and powerful corporations).[8,12,29-31] These terms imply differences in size and geographic scale of commercial actors, whether actors are public or for-profit, and the power held by these actors. Currently, the diversity of commercial actors and forces that impact health and inequalities is not yet adequately understood by public health. Below, we discuss some of the challenges with conceptualizations of commercial actors within public health research.

Although obvious, the fact that commercial actors differ in size and geographic scale is often ignored within CDOH research. Size and scale of commercial actors can act as a proxy for their market power, with the understanding that market power can be used as political influence. Whereas Philip Morris International and ABInBev are both transnational corporations that are active throughout the world and have revenues the size of national economies, most commercial actors are small, locally owned, and operate with modest revenues. Lumping all these actors together is inappropriate. However, the question of how large a corporation must be to be explored within CDOH remains unclear. Potential factors that could be considered for inclusion in CDOH research include revenue, profits, employees, geographic footprint, whether to differentiate at national or global production scales, and supply chain size.

The diversity of goods and services provided by commercial actors also creates challenges for CDOH research. Manufacturers of "unhealthy" or "harmful" commodities (e.g., tobacco, alcohol, UPFs, gambling, and weapons) are easy to identify as part of the CDOH. However, most industries are far more ambiguous. Even actors that provide goods and services that appear neutral or health promoting (e.g., fruit and vegetable producers, education, or renewable energy) may engage in harmful business practices (e.g., exploitation of workers). In addition, larger commercial actors produce a mixture of health-harming and health-promoting goods and services (e.g., Coca-Cola Company produces water and sugary drinks).[29] This complicates how public health actors evaluate these corporations, which often promote their portfolio diversification as evidence of their "good" intentions. However, corporate social responsibility is typically a political strategy designed to improve corporate reputations, foster partnerships, and minimize the risk of government regulation.[11,32]

The distinction between public and private sectors has become increasingly murky. The key difference between corporations and governments is that governments are typically elected to act in the public interest and are subject to public accountability.[33] In contrast, corporations lack democratic accountability and are generally beholden to shareholder interests (typically short-term profits).[29] However, many previously publicly owned sectors (e.g., utilities, incarceration, and "public" transport) have become privatized during recent decades. Corporations have also increased their engagement with governments and nongovernmental organizations through the rise of public–private partnerships. Furthermore, the rise of state-owned enterprises (especially in China) further complicates the distinction between public and private sectors. This blurring of private and public enterprises makes it more difficult for researchers to define the private sector.

The complexities of characterizing commercial actors highlight the limitations of the reductive understanding of the private sector found in much of the CDOH research. It is important that conceptualizations of CDOH do not ignore specific sectors or industries that impact health through less direct and visible pathways (e.g., the finance industry).[25] Public health must take these missing components into account (even when they are difficult to research and/or change) in order to work to develop a more comprehensive understanding of how the private sector impacts on health.

21.5 WHERE TO FROM HERE?

This chapter has explored the complexity and nuances within CDOH. As we have argued, definitions and models of CDOH walk a tight line of balancing comprehensive and easily understandable knowledge. We have argued that a nuanced understanding of CDOH offers theoretical and strategic benefits to public health. This understanding recognizes that few (if any) commercial actors are exclusively health promoting or health harming, and it acknowledges the range of upstream drivers that influence CDOH and the complexity of the private sector. Although the commercial world is complex, it is crucial for public health to remember that good practice does not excuse bad practice (or harmful goods and services). Understanding and disaggregating the attributes of commercial actors will enable public health as well as policymakers and regulators to undertake a more informed approach to managing conflicts of interests, partnerships, and other forms of engagement with private sector actors.

As evidence continues to emerge, the field will move toward a more nuanced and integrated understanding of CDOH that reflects how commercial actors influence health in negative and positive ways and how commercial activities interact with and amplify other activities. That is not to say that we should be underestimating population harms. For instance, industries such as firearms, opioids, fossil fuels, and others present immediate and significant threats to global health and should be researched and regulated as such. These industries should thereby be prioritized for regulation and immediate action. Similarly, there is no implication that we should be attempting to balance positive and negative CDOH outcomes, implying that good practices or outcomes can compensate for bad, or that we should be ranking commercial actors based on assessments of these.

New CDOH research is increasingly recognizing the enormous diversity of the private sector. We expect that future work will be based on a newly developed CDOH definition and conceptual framework developed by the *Lancet* working group, including an analytic framework of commercial actors that illustrates how commercial actors have both negative and positive traits and that practical trade-offs are faced when interacting with such actors. It is our view that adding greater nuance to discussions of CDOH will enable stakeholders to make better informed decisions about commercial actors while making it more difficult for the commercial sector to criticize or dismiss public health for taking broad-brush, black-and-white approaches and being out of touch with the complex realities of modern business. This definition and framework will help public health understand the nature and extent of the harms (and benefits) these actors generate, the contexts in which they exist, and potential solutions that could minimize harms and maximize benefits to population health. It may also help to identify other commercial actors and sectors not yet on the public health radar but whose market and political practices warrant scrutiny.

Although there has been expansion in funded research into CDOH, in many countries it is still difficult to attract funding that is commensurate with the magnitude of the problem. We think that future funding needs to be focused on the following:

- Continuing the detailed documentation of the practices and behaviors of commercial actors that harm and/or promote health
- Developing models that communicate the impact of CDOH to key stakeholders, including policymakers, regulators, and investors
- Deconstructing the mythology that champions the private sector vis-à-vis the public sector to counteract attacks on corporate taxation and regulation
- Understanding how public health intersects and aligns with other social movements[34]

This research agenda will help public health develop tactical solutions that can be implemented without being captured and/or stymied by commercial actors. These include (but are not limited to) increasing government monitoring as well as designing "non-gameable" ratings of corporate effects on health and a composite index to measure CDOH as risk factors for NCDs. In addition, public health could seek to leverage one sector against another (e.g., tobacco-free portfolios or divestment from fossil fuel and weapons industries) to weaken the political power of harmful commercial entities.[35] Unless society has a dramatic global shift away from capitalism, the solutions to the harmful impacts of commercial actors will be commercial in nature. This highlights the importance for public health to develop a deeper understanding of the diversity of commercial actors, their practices, and the context that enables them. This knowledge will help us fight against the harmful effects of commerce and be better able to harness the benefits of commerce to promote health.

REFERENCES

1. Freudenberg N. *Lethal But Legal: Corporations, Consumption, and Protecting Public Health*: Oxford University Press; 2014.
2. Anderson S. *Top 200: The Rise of Corporate Global Power*: Diane Publishing; 2008.
3. Babic M, Fichtner J, Heemskerk EM. States versus corporations: Rethinking the power of business in international politics. *Int Spectator*. 2017; 52(4): 20–43.
4. Collin J, Ralston R, Hill SE, Westerman L. *Signalling Virtue, Promoting Harm: Unhealthy Commodity Industries and COVID-19*. NCD Alliance, SPECTRUM; 2020.
5. Millar JS. The corporate determinants of health: How big business affects our health, and the need for government action! *Can J Public Health*. 2013; 104(4): e327–e329.
6. West R, Marteau T. Commentary on Casswell (2013): The commercial determinants of health. *Addiction*. 2013; **108**(4): 686–687.
7. Kosinska M-K, Ostlin P-O; World Health Organization. Building systematic approaches to intersectoral action in the WHO European Region. *Public Health Panorama*. 2016; 2(2): 124–129.

8. Kickbusch I, Allen L, Franz C. The commercial determinants of health. *Lancet Glob Health*. 2016; 4(12): e895–e896.
9. Buse K, Tanaka S, Hawkes S. Healthy people and healthy profits? Elaborating a conceptual framework for governing the commercial determinants of non-communicable diseases and identifying options for reducing risk exposure. *Global Health*. 2017; 13(1): 34.
10. Jahiel RI, Babor TF. Industrial epidemics, public health advocacy and the alcohol industry: Lessons from other fields. *Addiction*. 2007; 102(9): 1335–1339.
11. Gilmore AB, Savell E, Collin J. *Public Health, Corporations and the New Responsibility Deal: Promoting Partnerships with Vectors of Disease?* Oxford University Press; 2011: 2–4.
12. Moodie R, Stuckler D, Monteiro C, et al. Profits and pandemics: Prevention of harmful effects of tobacco, alcohol, and ultra-processed food and drink industries. *Lancet*. 2013; 381(9867): 670–679.
13. Knai C, Petticrew M, Capewell S, et al. The case for developing a cohesive systems approach to research across unhealthy commodity industries. *BMJ Glob Health*. 2021; 6(2): e003543.
14. Knai C, Petticrew M, Mays N, et al. Systems thinking as a framework for analyzing commercial determinants of health. *Milbank Q*. 2018; 96(3): 472–498.
15. de Lacy-Vawdon C, Vandenberg B, Livingstone C. Recognising the elephant in the room: The commercial determinants of health. *BMJ Glob Health*. 2022; 7(2): e007156.
16. Freudenberg N. *The Commercial Determinants of COVID-19: Implications for Public Health Practice and Policy*. Milken Institute School of Public Health, George Washington University and CUNY Urban Food Policy Institute; 2020.
17. Collins T, Mikkelsen B, Axelrod S. Interact, engage or partner? Working with the private sector for the prevention and control of noncommunicable diseases. *Cardiovasc Diagn Ther*. 2019; 9(2): 158.
18. Kickbusch I. A game change in global health: The best is yet to come. *Public Health Rev*. 2013; 35(1): 2.
19. Smith K, Dorfman L, Freudenberg N, et al. Tobacco, alcohol, and processed food industries: Why do public health practitioners view them so differently? *Front Public Health*. 2016; 4: 64.
20. Sula-Raxhimi E, Butzbach C, Brousselle A. Planetary health: Countering commercial and corporate power. *Lancet Planet Health*. 2019; 3(1): e12–e13.
21. Stuckler D, McKee M, Ebrahim S, Basu S. Manufacturing epidemics: The role of global producers in increased consumption of unhealthy commodities including processed foods, alcohol, and tobacco. *PLoS Med*. 2012; 9(6): e1001235.
22. Wiist WH. Public health and the anticorporate movement: Rationale and recommendations. *Am J Public Health*. 2006; 96(8): 1370–1375.
23. Freudenberg N. *Corporate Practices: Macrosomial Determinants of Population Health*. Springer; 2007: 71–104.
24. Jahiel RI. Corporation-induced diseases, upstream epidemiologic surveillance, and urban health. *J Urban Health*. 2008; 85(4): 517.
25. Baum FE, Sanders DM, Fisher M, et al. Assessing the health impact of transnational corporations: Its importance and a framework. *Global Health*. 2016; 12(1): 1–7.
26. Schram A, Labonté R, Sanders D. Urbanization and international trade and investment policies as determinants of noncommunicable diseases in sub-Saharan Africa. *Prog Cardiovasc Dis*. 2013; 56(3): 281–301.

27.   Madureira Lima J, Galea S. Corporate practices and health: A framework and mechanisms. *Global Health*. 2018; 14(1): 21.
28.   Rochford C, Tenneti N, Moodie R. Reframing the impact of business on health: The interface of corporate, commercial, political and social determinants of health. *BMJ Glob Health*. 2019; 4(4): e001510.
29.   McKee M, Stuckler D. Revisiting the corporate and commercial determinants of health. *Am J Public Health*. 2018; 108(9): 1167–1170.
30.   Maani N, Collin J, Friel S, et al. Bringing the commercial determinants of health out of the shadows: A review of how the commercial determinants are represented in conceptual frameworks. *Eur J Public Health*. 2020; 30(4): 660–664.
31.   Lima JM, Galea S. The Corporate Permeation Index-A tool to study the macrosocial determinants of non-communicable disease. *SSM Popul Health*. 2019; 7: 100361.
32.   Herrick C. The post-2015 landscape: Vested interests, corporate social responsibility and public health advocacy. *Sociol. Health Illn*. 2016; 38(7): 1026–1042.
33.   Fuchs D, Kalfagianni A, Havinga T. Actors in private food governance: The legitimacy of retail standards and multistakeholder initiatives with civil society participation. *Agric Hum Values*. 2011; 28(3): 353–367.
34.   Freudenberg N. At What Cost: Modern Capitalism and the Future of Health: Oxford University Press; 2021.
35.   Lacy-Nichols J, Marten R. Power and the commercial determinants of health: Ideas for a research agenda. *BMJ Glob Health*. 2021; 6(2): e003850.

CHAPTER 22

Assessing Power Structures

JOANA MADUREIRA LIMA

22.1 INTRODUCTION

As in a game of chess, power lies not just in the playing pieces but in the configuration of forces, and each set of moves and counter moves presents fresh possibilities to prize open the seams of a historical bloc.[1(p807),2]

Public health scholars have studied the playing pieces of corporate influence on population health for decades. As a result of this work, the field has now documented the pathways through which commercial interests influence policy and societal attitudes.[3,4] To understand the *configuration of forces*, however, it is useful to take a step back from thinking of the state and the private sector as separate entities, with the latter using its financial resources, status, and access to coax or bribe the former into taking the "right" policy and operational decisions. In practice, what we see is a penetration of the private sector, or in some cases simply a pro-private mindset, into the state, such that the interests of the "public" and the interests of shareholders come to be blurred and taken for each other. As Miller and Harkins argue, "It is no longer enough to think about corporations only as attempting to influence policy. Much decision-making power has been directly devolved to them while corporations are increasingly internal to the state."[5] Indeed, corporations are increasingly integral to most societal processes.

This chapter discusses how corporate power drives this internalization process through the lens of Steven Lukes' overarching theory of power,[6] Doris Fuchs' theory of corporate power,[7] and the following typology of power:

Joana Madureira Lima, *Assessing Power Structures* In: *The Commercial Determinants of Health*. Edited by: Nason Maani, Mark Petticrew, and Sandro Galea, Oxford University Press. © Oxford University Press 2023. DOI: 10.1093/oso/9780197578742.003.0022

- Instrumental power or Lukes' first dimension of power: A has power over B because it uses its resources to get B to do something B would not do otherwise.
- Structural power or Lukes' second dimension of power: A has power over B because B depends on A. B can anticipate A's desires, which A does not have to voice explicitly, and does not act in any way that could go against A's interests.
- Discursive power or Lukes' third dimension of power: A has power over B because B has interiorized A's interests as their own and does not conceive of a reality where A's interests are not B's own interests.

This three-dimensional view of power is well placed to systematically study commercial determinants of population health because processes underpinning these determinants are complex and varied. Unidimensional analyses are bound not to tell the whole story.

22.2 INSTRUMENTAL POWER

This one-dimensional view of power involves a focus on behaviour in the making of decisions on issues over which there is an observable conflict of (subjective) interests, seen as express policy preferences, revealed by political participation.[6]

Instrumental power can be traced back to specific resources of corporate and other commercial actors. Corporate actors use these resources to directly influence decision-makers such as politicians and regulators to remove any obstacles (e.g., regulations) to profit-making. These resources may be financial as well as nonfinancial (i.e., organizational capacities, human resources, and access to decision-makers).[7]

The political environment is the dominant vehicle for this face of power, which can be exerted through quid pro quo tactics such as lobbying and political party campaign donations and/or tactics such as revolving doors, which give the private sector access to regulators. It can also be exerted through extralegal practices such as opposition intimidation. In Mexico, civil society advocates, public health policymakers, and government employees advocating for the doubling of a pioneering 2014 soda tax were at the center of an intimidation campaign. Spyware that is sold exclusively to governments to fight terrorism was used to harass them, raising questions about whether these tools are being used to advance the soda industry's commercial interests.[8] Similarly, in Colombia, advocates for a legislative proposal for a 20% tax on sugary drinks reported a campaign of threats to their physical safety urging them to stop their efforts as the proposal was heading for Colombia's Legislature.[9]

A transnational corporation or a government acting to protect corporate interests may influence policy adoption in a given country by threatening to take investment elsewhere, what Dolowitz and Marsh call "direct coercive policy transfer."[10] When Uzbekistan's tobacco industry was privatized in 1994, British American Tobacco established a production monopoly. The Uzbek health authorities planned to ban tobacco advertising and smoking in public places and introduce health warnings. British American Tobacco responded by delaying completion of its investment until the decree was replaced with a voluntary advertising code that resulted in ubiquitous advertising throughout the country.[11,12] This type of power can also be exerted by states protecting their industries. The U.S. government, for example, threatened punitive trade measures and the withdrawal of military support from Ecuador when, in 2018 at the World Health Organization World Health Assembly, Ecuador proposed a resolution to encourage breastfeeding, a move that would threaten profits of the U.S.-based infant formula industry. The attempts of health advocates to find another sponsor for the resolution among poor countries in Africa and Latin America were hampered as countries backed off, citing fears of retaliation.[13]

The COVID-19 pandemic opened many opportunities for the exertion of instrumental power by health sector industries. Much like the reality of instrumental power more broadly, however, this most often required collusion between both the private and the public sector. The urgency in decision-making in the early days of the COVID-19 pandemic meant that transparency and oversight in public procurement were cast aside in countries throughout the world. In the United Kingdom, the government handed out thousands of contracts for services to fight the spread of the virus to a select few companies with connections to the party in government, some of them in a secretive "V.I.P. lane."[14] Of the 1,200 published central government contracts awarded in the first 7 months of the response ($22 billion worth), approximately $5 billion went to politically connected companies.[2,14] Some had former ministers and government advisers on staff. Others donated to the party in government. A number of these companies had a record of tax evasion, fraud, corruption, and human rights abuses.[14]

Similar concerns were raised by professional associations and academics regarding potential conflicts of interest of members of the UK government's Scientific Advisory Group of Experts and members of the Vaccine Taskforce, created to expedite research to produce a vaccine. The chair of the taskforce, married to a government minister, was on leave from their role as a managing partner in a life sciences venture capital firm.[15] The government's Chief Scientific Adviser and Head of the Taskforce had $800,000 worth of shares in a pharmaceutical company with which the UK government had signed a coronavirus vaccine deal for an undisclosed sum, securing 60 million doses of an untested treatment that was still being developed.[15] Similarly, in the United

States, the vaccine taskforce, called Operation Warp Speed, was being directed by a former executive of a top pharmaceutical company. This executive had been criticized by senators for failing to disclose his pharmaceutical company investment, which could amount to unresolved conflicts of interest.[16]

In the leaked words of a senior executive of a company that delivers services on behalf of the UK government, COVID-19 is "going a long way in cementing the position of the private sector companies in the public sector supply chain."[17] "Cementing" is an uncannily apposite term for the process of legitimization of the private sector as the default partner in health taking place in the past four decades, replacing government procurement and delivery of services. This model of public–private partnerships (PPPs) has a weak evidence base for its cost efficiency and cost-effectiveness.[18] Yet, as illustrated in the following sections, it was adopted, exported, and woven into the national and international policy discourse as a desirable attribute of health financing and health service delivery.

22.3 STRUCTURAL POWER

The bias of the system is not sustained simply by a series of individually chosen acts, but also, most importantly, by the socially structured and culturally patterned behaviour of groups and practices of institutions, which may be manifested by individual's inactions.[6]

Fuchs describes this second dimension of power as the influence that the dependence of governments and political elites on private sector profitability—that is, dependence on tax revenues, employment, and export goods that help incumbents get re-elected—has on political agendas and policy options. This is in contrast to instrumental power, whereby power is operationalized through direct action over a perceived threat. This rule-setting power of business has become a focal point in the discussion on global governance in the context of self-regulation, PPPs, and the emergence of "private authority."[7] In the case of the breastfeeding resolution presented above, the structural power of the baby formula industry would mean that there would be no need for the baby formula industry to lobby the government to dissuade Ecuador from proposing it. The government, aware of the economic importance of that industry, would have anticipated the risk to the bottom line posed by the resolution and taken pre-emptive action.

Dolowitz and Marsh discuss another form of structural power—indirect coercive policy transfer—whereby externalities, functional interdependence, economic constraints, competition between countries, and the emergence of international consensus fostered by supranational institutions may all influence policy adoption.[10] Holden uses this concept to frame his study of how the British government developed a health care industrial strategy that included the export of the PPP model to developing and eastern European countries.[19] This export laid the basis for the winning of consultancy, construction, and other contracts by British firms. The analysis reveals the deployment of the UK Department for International Development, international financial institutions such as the World Bank (WB), and private sector consultancies to influence governments in these target countries. At the time, these countries were undergoing substantial shifts in economic and governance models, and international pressure pushed them toward adopting the British Private Finance Initiative model.[19]

Lesotho's PPP, designed to replace the country's main public hospital, is another example of indirect coercive policy transfer mediated via the emergence of an international consensus fostered by supranational institutions. The Queen 'Mamohato Memorial Hospital was built through a PPP signed in 2009 with technical assistance from the International Finance Corporation (IFC), the arm of the WB focused exclusively on the private sector in developing countries.[20] The PPP was described as opening a new era for private sector involvement in health care in Africa, and the model was to be replicated throughout the continent. Instead, as revealed in an analysis by Oxfam, the Ministry of Health in one of the poorest and most unequal countries in the world was locked into an 18-year contract that, in 2014, was already using more than half of the government's health budget (51%) while providing high returns (25%) to the private partner.[21] This diversion of scarce public funds from primary health care services in rural areas, where three-fourths of the population live, compromises funding of, access to, and equity in health service delivery, and ultimately universal health coverage. Despite the poor quality of its advice to the government of Lesotho, which, by its own admission, did not have the technical capacity to design and manage the contract, the IFC has not been held to account.[21] In addition, the Independent Evaluation Group—a unit within the WB—is marketing this health PPP as a success internationally, despite its unsustainable costs.[22]

These instances of structural power cannot be analyzed in isolation. They were enabled by a political and ideological environment in public and policy spheres that was conducive to framing PPPs as the only viable option for health financing, management, and service delivery. Theories of discursive power help us understand the process by which this came to be.

22.4 DISCURSIVE POWER

Is it not the supreme and most insidious exercise of power to prevent people from having grievances by shaping their perceptions, cognitions and preferences in such a way that they accept their role in the existing order of things? . . . To assume that the absence of grievance equals genuine consensus is simply to rule out the possibility of false or manipulated consensus.[6]

Fuchs builds on Lukes' third dimension of power, which she calls discursive power: the ability to shape norms and ideas in public discourse, cultural values, and institutions. This type of power precedes the formation and articulation of interests in the political process by constituting and framing policies, actors, and societal norms in a way that legitimizes corporate actors as partners in health policy to advance corporate interests.[7]

For example, both Big Food and Big Tobacco, when faced with regulations of their products, promoted the image of the "nanny state" curtailing individual freedom to choose what to eat, drink, or smoke.[23] This reframed the idea of health protection negatively as a reduction of personal freedom and legitimized opposition to these regulations. An analysis of the "third face of power" should thus consider the socialization of politicians and the public into accepting "truths" about desirable policies and political developments.[7]

Control over the research agenda is a key tactic for framing discourse. One systematic literature review found that papers in favor of PPPs were substantially less likely to document the evidence underpinning their position compared to papers against it. Furthermore, it found that where conflicts were declared, absence of conflicts was more frequent in critics of PPPs than in supporters (86% vs. 17%).[24] A subsequent review had similar findings: Evaluations that were favorable to the use of PPPs in health promotion were more frequently classed as "not independent" and of poor quality and were more common when the PPP involved a private partner with conflicting financial interests.[25] Evaluations done by the WB, International Monetary Fund, and European Investment Bank—organizations with a record of promoting PPPs—have found evidence of PPPs not yielding the expected outcome, instead resulting in a significant rise in government fiscal liabilities.[18] Yet they are an omnipresent policy tool in global health. In the late 1970s and early 1980s, as neoliberal ideologies influenced public policy and attitudes, relationships began to change and influential international organizations championed a greater role for the private sector.[26] In the austerity drive that characterized the aftermath of the last financial crisis, PPPs have been heralded as an effective way to address a growing resource gap in global health. They have contributed to the emergence of a complex global health governance architecture in which private solutions relying on market mechanisms are generally privileged over public approaches.[27] It could be argued that all three dimensions of power are at play here. Instrumental power of corporations allows them to fund research, and their structural power makes researchers whose universities or international organizations depend on corporate funding more likely to produce results in favor of PPPs.[24,25] The biased research agenda is consonant with the ideology of supranational organizations: Discourse is shaped, and a new truth accepted. Power is at its most effective when all its dimensions are present, exerted through a variety of complementary, synergetic tactics.

This trend is far from abating, with the ever more prominent role of philanthrocapitalism in promoting private sector involvement in global health. Although philanthrocapitalism is personified in individuals, these individuals have accrued their fortunes via their corporations and their corporate behavior. It is therefore important to include them in discussions of corporate discursive power. McGoey argues that philanthrocapitalism is simply a new version of Adam Smith's proposition that individual self-interest, allowed to operate under free market conditions, will "naturally" bring about the common good.[28] In her words,

> What may be most new about philanthrocapitalism is the very explicitness of the self-interested motives underlying large-scale charitable activities . . . the explicitness of the belief that as private enrichment purportedly advances the public good, increased wealth concentration is to be commended rather than questioned."[28]

These beliefs can reverberate top down through philanthropic financing of supranational organizations such as the WB, the Global Alliance for Vaccines and Immunization, or the Global Fund.

The Bill and Melinda Gates Foundation, for example, has an outsized influence in setting international health policy priorities. This is problematic because the funders' priorities are often driven by personal interests and not necessarily aligned with the health policy priorities of the recipient country.[29] So-called intellectual monopoly capitalism, which captures intellectual property owners' preference to avoid competition, has been defined as a hallmark of 21st-century capitalism.[30] Bill Gates' personal belief in the role of patents as motors for innovation in medicines and medical technology[31] is an example of discursive power in the perpetuation of intellectual monopoly capitalism.

Public funding, unlike private funding, has been especially critical for vaccine research, where the failure rate of product development is as high as 94%, and has enabled the rapid development of many COVID-19 vaccines. Public funding accounted for 97.1–99.0% of the funding toward research and development of the technology underpinning the SARS-CoV-2 vaccine carried out at Oxford University.[32] In what seemed like a gesture of good stewardship of public investment, in April 2020 Oxford University promised to donate the rights to its coronavirus vaccine to any drugmaker.[33]

True to his belief in intellectual monopoly capitalism, Bill Gates encouraged Oxford to sell exclusive rights to its vaccine to AstraZeneca instead of allowing it to be open-sourced.[34] AstraZeneca's confidential coronavirus vaccine deal with Oxford University allows it to make as much as 20% on top of the cost of goods for manufacturing the vaccine. AstraZeneca has pledged to sell the vaccine "at cost" during the pandemic, eschewing profits, but is yet to say how much the vaccine costs to make.[34] This stance is at odds with that of WHO, which in February 2021 called for a waiver of COVID-19 vaccine patents.[35]

This is discursive power at its best. Actors with perceived legitimacy are linked to ideas that place the corporate sector as the only way to advance health goals, shaping the narrative in the way of business as usual. In other words, the model whereby manufacturers get exclusive rights is perpetuated, and the unique opportunity posed by the pandemic to change the economics of vaccine development, and indeed drug development, is lost. The dominant discourse about vaccine pricing is once again that it is a matter of good will as opposed to a matter of public good.

22.5 CONCLUSION

Taken together, the examples in this chapter illustrate how the instrumental, structural, and discursive power of commercial interests converge to shape the status quo. They show that a particular exercise of power might be multi-dimensional, exerted through multiple vehicles and tactics. Revolving doors between the public and the private sector may place commercial actors in a position to deliver health services and goods to populations (instrumental power), but this tactic may also be used to export this model to other jurisdictions to increase the client base (structural power). At the same time, private actors who have established themselves as legitimate players in global health use their power to portray the public sector as inefficient, and thus illegitimate, and shape the narrative in a way that consolidates their power and that of their ideology (discursive power).

A future research agenda on power and commercial actors should recognize these dimensions while exploring the role of non-corporate actors, namely by the national and international institutions that are designed to be stewards of population health, in promoting corporate narratives.

REFERENCES

1. Levy DL, Egan D. A neo-Gramscian approach to corporate political strategy: Conflict and accommodation in the climate change negotiations. *J Manag Stud*. 2003; 40(4): 803–829. doi:10.1111/1467-6486.00361
2. United Kingdom Government. Response to article published by the *New York Times* on UK government procurement. 2021. https://www.gov.uk/government/news/response-to-article-published-by-the-new-york-times-on-uk-government-procurement

3. Mialon M, Swinburn B, Sacks G. A proposed approach to systematically identify and monitor the corporate political activity of the food industry with respect to public health using publicly available information. *Obes Rev*. 2015; 16(7): 519–530. doi:10.1111/obr.12289

4. Madureira Lima J, Galea S. Corporate practices and health: A framework and mechanisms. *Glob Health*. 2018; 14(1): 21.

5. Miller D, Harkins C. Corporate strategy, corporate capture: Food and alcohol industry lobbying and public health. *Crit Soc Policy*. 2010; 30(4): 564–589. doi:10.1177/0261018310376805

6. Lukes S. *Power: A Radical View*. 2nd ed. Palgrave Macmillan; 2005.

7. Fuchs D. Commanding heights? The strength and fragility of business power in global politics. *Millenn J Int Stud*. 2005; 33(3): 771–801. doi:10.1177/03058298050330030501

8. Perlroth N. Spyware's odd targets: Backers of Mexico's soda tax. *The New York Times*. 2017. https://www.nytimes.com/2017/02/11/technology/hack-mexico-soda-tax-advocates.html

9. Ritchel M, Jacobs A. She took on Colombia's soda industry. Then she was silenced. *The New York Times*. 2017. https://www.nytimes.com/2017/11/13/health/colombia-soda-tax-obesity.html

10. Dolowitz D, Marsh D. Who learns what from whom: A review of the policy transfer literature. *Polit Stud*. 1996; 44(2): 343–357. https://doi.org/10.1111/j.1467-9248.1996.tb00334.x

11. Gilmore AB, Collin J, McKee M. British American tobacco's erosion of health legislation in Uzbekistan. *Br Med J*. 2006; 332(7537): 355–358. doi:10.1136/bmj.332.7537.355

12. Gilmore AB, McKee M, Collin J. The invisible hand: How British American Tobacco precluded competition in Uzbekistan. *Tob Control*. 2007; 16(4): 239–247. doi:10.1136/tc.2006.017129

13. Jacobs A. Opposition to breast-feeding resolution by U.S. stuns world health officials. *The New York Times*. 2018. https://www.nytimes.com/2018/07/08/health/world-health-breastfeeding-ecuador-trump.html

14. Bradley J, Gebrekidan S, McCann A. Waste, negligence and cronyism: Inside Britain's pandemic spending. *The New York Times*. 2021. https://www.nytimes.com/interactive/2020/12/17/world/europe/britain-covid-contracts.html

15. Thacker PD. Conflicts of interest among the UK government's COVID-19 advisers. *BMJ*. 2020; 371: m4716. doi:10.1136/bmj.m4716

16. Select Subcommittee on the Coronavirus Crisis of the United States Congress. Documents reveal potential unresolved conflicts of interest among top operation warp speed advisors. September 22, 2020. https://coronavirus.house.gov/news/press-releases/documents-reveal-potential-unresolved-conflicts-interest-among-top-operation

17. Geoghegan P. Cronyism and clientelism. *London Rev Books*. 2020. https://www.lrb.co.uk/the-paper/v42/n21/peter-geoghegan/cronyism-and-clientelism

18. Jomo K, Chowdhury A, Sharma K, Platz D. Public–private partnerships and the 2030 Agenda for Sustainable Development: Fit for purpose? DESA Working Paper No. 149. February 2016. https://www.un.org/esa/desa/papers/2016/wp148_2016.pdf

19. Holden C. Exporting public–private partnerships in healthcare: Export strategy and policy transfer. *Policy Stud*. 2009; 30(3): 313–332. doi:10.1080/01442870902863885

20. International Finance Corporation. IFC supports Lesotho's infrastructure development through public–private partnerships. 2011. Accessed January 22, 2021. https://pressroom.ifc.org/all/pages/PressDetail.aspx?ID=23118

21. Marriott A. A dangerous diversion. Oxfam. 2014. https://www.oxfam.org/en/research/dangerous-diversion

22. Independent Evaluation Group. World Bank Group support to public–private partnerships: Lessons from experience in client countries, Fy 02–12. 2014. https://ieg.worldbankgroup.org/sites/default/files/Data/reports/ppp_eval_updated2_0.pdf

23. Magnusson RS. Case studies in nanny state name-calling: What can we learn? *Public Health*. 2015; 129(8): 1074–1082. doi:10.1016/j.puhe.2015.04.023

24. Hernandez-Aguado I, Zaragoza GA. Support of public–private partnerships in health promotion and conflicts of interest. *BMJ Open*. 2016; 6(4): 1–11. doi:10.1136/bmjopen-2015-009342

25. Parker LA, Zaragoza GA, Hernández-Aguado I. Promoting population health with public–private partnerships: Where's the evidence? *BMC Public Health*. 2019; 19(1): 1–8. doi:10.1186/s12889-019-7765-2

26. Buse K, Harmer AM. Seven habits of highly effective global public–private health partnerships: Practice and potential. *Soc Sci Med*. 2007; 64(2): 259–271. doi:10.1016/j.socscimed.2006.09.001

27. Ruckert A, Labonté R. Public–private partnerships (PPPs) in global health: The good, the bad and the ugly. *Third World Q*. 2014; 35(9): 1598–1614. doi:10.1080/01436597.2014.970870

28. McGoey L. Philanthrocapitalism and its critics. *Poetics*. 2012; 40(2): 185–199. doi:10.1016/j.poetic.2012.02.006

29. Stuckler D, Basu S, McKee M. Global health philanthropy and institutional relationships: How should conflicts of interest be addressed? *PLoS Med*. 2011; 8(4): e1001020. doi:10.1371/journal.pmed.1001020

30. Sell SK. What COVID-19 reveals about twenty-first century capitalism: Adversity and opportunity. *Development*. 2020; 63(2–4): 150–156. doi:10.1057/s41301-020-00263-z

31. New W, Saez C. Bill Gates calls for "vaccine decade"; Explains how patent system drives public health aid. Intellectual Property Watch. 2011. Accessed July 12, 2021. https://www.ip-watch.org/2011/05/17/bill-gates-calls-for-vaccine-decade-explains-how-patent-system-drives-public-health-aid

32. Cross S, Rho Y, Reddy H, et al. Who funded the research behind the vaccine? *medRxiv*. Published online 2021. https://doi.org/10.1101/2021.04.08.21255103

33. Hancock J. Oxford's COVID vaccine deal with AstraZeneca raises concerns about access and pricing. *Fortune*. 2020. https://fortune.com/2020/08/24/oxford-astrazeneca-covid-vaccine-deal-pricing-profit-concerns

34. Cookson C, Donato PM. Vaccine deal allows AstraZeneca to take up to 20% on top of costs. *Financial Times*. 2020. https://www.ft.com/content/e359159b-105c-407e-b1be-0c7a1ddb654b

35. Dr Tedros Adhanom Ghebreyesus. Waive COVID vaccine patents to put world on war footing. World Health Organization. 2021. Accessed February 20, 2021. https://www.who.int/news-room/commentaries/detail/waive-covid-vaccine-patents-to-put-world-on-war-footing

CHAPTER 23

Rethinking Conflict of Interest

From Individual to Structural Understandings

JEFF COLLIN, ROB RALSTON, AND SARAH HILL

23.1 INTRODUCTION

The United Nations Sustainable Development Goals reflect broad political commitments to governance via public–private partnerships, multi-stakeholder platforms, and corporate social responsibility to advance health policy objectives. Such mechanisms are based on an assumption that commercial sector interests can be aligned with public goals,[1] to which commercial determinants of health perspectives pose a particularly stark challenge in relation to non-communicable diseases (NCDs). Because NCDs are substantially driven by unhealthy commodity industries,[2] increasingly extensive interactions between such commercial actors and health researchers, nongovernmental organizations, and health agencies are likely to be characterized by complex and potentially conflicting interests.

NCD governance is thus positioned on a fault line in which management of conflict of interest is both urgent and increasingly contested.[3] Whereas tobacco control is defined by a distinctive model of health governance that recognizes a fundamental conflict of interest with the tobacco industry,[4] in other contexts the recognition and management of such conflicts remain nascent. This is partly a function of variation and uncertainty in how conflict of interest is understood. Debates have been characterized by diverse conceptions of "conflict," "interest," and "conflict of interest" across multiple disciplines and diverse corporate, medical, legal, and governmental contexts.[5,6] Alongside this conceptual ambiguity, discussions about conflict of interest in

Jeff Collin, Rob Ralston, and Sarah Hill, *Rethinking Conflict of Interest* In: *The Commercial Determinants of Health*. Edited by: Nason Maani, Mark Petticrew, and Sandro Galea, Oxford University Press. © Oxford University Press 2023. DOI: 10.1093/oso/9780197578742.003.0023

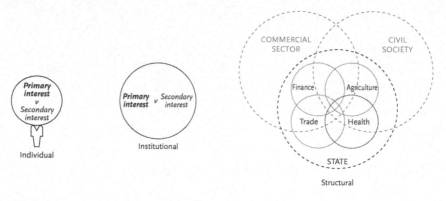

Figure 23.1 Individual, institutional, and structural conceptions of conflict of interest.

health governance have become highly polarized and often serve as a light-ning rod for broader debates about the role of the private sector in public health.[7] Commercial actors have complicated these debates by seeking to shape discourse and practice around conflicts of interest in health, downplay-ing the role (and regulation) of conflicts involving tobacco, alcohol, and ultra-processed food manufacturers.[8–10]

As a step toward more effective management of conflict of interest in health policy and research, it is helpful to unpack the diverse ways in which such con-flicts have been conceptualized both within and beyond health governance. Drawing on work on managing conflicts of interest in nutrition policy,[3] we ex-amine different conceptions of conflict of interest and how such conceptions can inform different approaches to health governance. Our account is organ-ized around a threefold typology encompassing individual, institutional, and structural understandings (Figure 23.1).

23.2 INDIVIDUAL CONFLICTS

Both in academic literature and in policy contexts, the concept of conflict of interest is most commonly addressed at the level of the *individual*, denoting tensions across *different roles*, *objectives*, or *interests* held by the person con-cerned. The most widely cited definition in health contexts is from Thompson, who characterizes conflict of interest as "a set of conditions in which profes-sional judgement concerning a primary interest (such as a patient's welfare or the validity of research) tends to be unduly influenced by a secondary interest (such as financial gain)."[11]

This definition frames conflicts as occurring at an individual level, with the practitioner (or researcher) experiencing tension in which private interests may distract from professional roles or obligations. Here, the obligations of health professionals to their patients, or of health researchers to advancing knowledge, are given a moral weight as primary interests and differentiated from lesser secondary interests.[12,13] Thompson's definition principally focuses attention on intrapersonal rather than interpersonal dimensions of conflict; that is, he is concerned with the idea that a person's professional obligations may be compromised by their interests in another (often personal) sphere, rather than with tensions between the interests of different groups or sectors.[14]

Thompson's definition continues to shape debates and practices around conflict of interest in health. Individualized understandings underpin most policies for managing conflict of interest, such as disclosure and recusal across research and policymaking contexts.[15] Some approaches have expanded on Thompson's definition, including a distinction between *actual* and *perceived* conflict of interest. Operationalizing this distinction draws upon long-standing practice in jurisprudence, which emphasizes the need to manage the *appearance* (as well as the actual existence) of partiality or bias in decision-making.[6]

The comparative significance of *financial* and *nonfinancial interests* is among the more contentious aspects of contemporary debates.[16] The existence of financial incentives is sometimes presented as necessary and integral to conflict of interest.[17] Some scholars envisage conflict only where the financial incentive is significant, with Thompson going so far as to suggest there is a value floor below which no meaningful conflict exists.[11] Others contend that gifts of negligible value (e.g., pharmaceutical company "freebees") can influence recipients' behavior (e.g., by influencing doctors' prescribing practices).[18] Saver is among those who emphasize the salience of nonfinancial interests as sources of conflict, suggesting that incentives relating to career advancement, social relationships, or personally held values can influence professionals' behavior.[19] By contrast, Bero and Grundy warn that a focus on such interests tends to divert attention from those conflicts arising from financial interests, which they position as both more important and demonstrably more likely to result in biased outcomes.[13]

The debate concerning financial versus nonfinancial interests is compounded by commercial actors' attempts to influence such discussions. The Brussels Declaration, for example, was presented as establishing ethical principles across science, society, and policy, but its content was shaped by and advanced objectives of unhealthy commodity industries.[20,21] Significantly, the Declaration frames conflicts associated with commercial sector financing as relatively benign in comparison with the personal interests of advocates or researchers:

> In fact, commercial conflicts of interest are fairly easy to deal with if they are properly declared and the relationship between the science and the marketing made explicit. Ideological, personal or academic conflicts of interest, on the other hand, are much harder to detect or deal with.[20]

This strategic "muddying of the waters"[13] highlights the merit of maintaining a primary focus on financial interests in health governance because such interests are readily identified and their impacts on decision-making have been extensively demonstrated.[13,16] Financial conflicts arising from for-profit private sector actors are likely to be particularly significant for NCD governance.[15]

23.3 INSTITUTIONAL CONFLICTS

In engaging with tensions beyond individual interests, scholars, civil society, and health organizations have paid increasing attention to the concept of *institutional conflict of interest*. As defined by the U.S. Institute of Medicine, "Institutional conflicts of interest arise when an institution's own financial interests or the interests of its senior officials pose risks to the integrity of the institution's primary interests and missions."[22]

This definition essentially takes the idea of individual conflict of interest and applies it at the level of an organization. Rather than an individual person experiencing tension between their primary (e.g., professional) and secondary (e.g., personal) interests,[11] the conflict is now envisaged as operating between an *organization's* primary interest (e.g., its duty to deliver quality health care) and its secondary interest(s) (e.g., need to remain financially solvent or to retain experienced staff). Besides extrapolating from the individual to the organizational level, this conception does little to unpack what is "institutional" about such interests[23] or how these might be distinguished from individual interests. Thus, the distinction between individual and institutional conflicts of interest often remains underspecified. For example, one analysis of institutional conflicts of interest in global health philanthropy suggests such conflicts are common but fails to define or discuss the term "institutional"[24]— despite highlighting the inadequacy of individual disclosure mechanisms for managing conflicts at the institutional level.

Where organizations do seek to manage institutional conflicts of interest, policies typically refer to official mandates as articulating "primary interests." This is exemplified by the World Health Organization's (WHO) Framework for Engagement with Non-State Actors:

> All institutions have multiple interests, which means that in engaging with non-State actors WHO is often faced with a combination of converging and conflicting interests. *An institutional conflict of interest is a situation where WHO's primary interest as reflected in its Constitution may be unduly influenced by the conflicting interest of a non-State actor* in a way that affects, or may reasonably be perceived to affect, the independence and objectivity of WHO's work. [Emphasis added][25]

The distinction between an organization's primary interest and conflicting secondary interests *may* be workable for institutions such as WHO that have a clear overarching purpose or a mission embedded in a formal mandate. This approach works less well for organizations such as governments and universities in which public health objectives do not necessarily take primacy over other goals and agendas. In such cases, the organization is likely to have multiple primary objectives with no agreed hierarchy to guide prioritization in addressing conflicts.

In many contexts, organizational policies adopted to manage institutional conflict of interest are rather narrow in scope, with institutional definitions serving to exclude or downplay the significance of wider tensions. This approach is evident in the governance of key health-related partnerships, including the Scaling Up Nutrition initiative: "An organizational or institutional conflict arises when pursuit of an organization's interests, whether 'private' or secondary, has the effect of compromising, interfering with, or *taking precedence over the joint endeavor*."[26]

By narrowing the scope of relevant conflicts, such definitions can accommodate collaborations or partnerships viewed by participants as compatible with the specific activities of "the joint endeavor" but that are highly problematic from a broader public health perspective. This is exemplified in the Global Fund's partnerships with alcohol giants SAB Miller and Heineken.[27,28] When criticized by local health advocates and researchers for collaborating on an HIV/AIDS intervention in South Africa,[27] Global Fund officials defended its partnership with SAB Miller by emphasizing the importance of generating resources to tackle HIV/AIDS, malaria, and tuberculosis. In asserting that they did not recognize any conflict of interest in this case, this defense noted that the Global Fund "does not endorse the actions, practices or policies of any corporation or industry beyond the field of the fight against these three diseases."[29] By defining relevant conflicts in such narrow terms, this approach privileges support for specific program activities over wider tensions with alcohol as a key structural driver of HIV transmission and with its broader impacts on regional and global health.[27,28]

23.4 STRUCTURAL CONFLICTS

A more expansive—or structural—understanding of conflict of interest derives from the sociology of collective action.[30] This approach pays particular attention to the circumstances in which conflicts arise, recognizing that conflicts reflect the context or structure of particular situations rather than the preferences of individuals.[31] Friedberg notes that conflicts are likely when actors have roles in more than one "sphere of action."[30] In other words, actors (whether individual or organizational) typically engage in a diverse range of relational contexts, and they may have divergent goals and resources across these different fields.[32] Conflicts are likely to arise at the intersection of these fields of activity or policy spheres, and particularly where actors can draw on resources from one field (e.g., a commercial enterprise) to generate advantages in another field (e.g., a health governance platform).[30]

In contrast with individual or institutional conceptions, a structural understanding acknowledges the existence of multiple overlapping spheres of action—such as a government's health and financial sectors—each of which has its own logic and goals. Rather than locating the conflict or tension *within* a particular individual or organization, a structural approach acknowledges the likelihood of tension *at the point of interaction* between different spheres of action, given their diverse logics and goals.[30] For example, governments may simultaneously be committed (within the health sector) to reducing the harmful use of alcohol and (within the financial sector) to promoting economic growth via a successful domestic alcohol industry. Similarly, an individual might be part of a research community committed to the advancement of health-related knowledge and director of a research unit whose employees depend on the individual's ability to attract grants. Rather than categorizing interests as intrinsically "primary" or "secondary," this definition recognizes the existence of diverse interests that dominate in different contexts and compete where those contexts come into contact with one another.

A structural understanding of conflict of interest has broad implications for identifying and managing such conflicts in health research and governance. This approach questions scope for a straightforward application of a normative hierarchy that can differentiate between primary and secondary interests. Instead, a structural approach recognizes the existence of diverse goals and mandates that—in particular situations—will overlap and thereby come into tension with one another, requiring decision-makers to actively adjudicate between competing or conflicting interests. A structural understanding assumes particular importance given the contemporary dominance of multisectoral approaches to NCDs and health governance[1-4] because it identifies such platforms as entailing (and requiring management of) conflicts inherent in operating across policy spheres.

In the context of health governance, an "essentialist orientation" (centered narrowly on individual and role-focused understandings of conflict of interest) fails to take adequate account of the extent to which diverse goals may be viewed as legitimate in different contexts.[30] Such a narrow perspective leads to the development of policies and procedures that focus on practices such as transparency, recusal, or disclosure[15] but do not adequately address core challenges facing health actors tasked with engaging external actors. A broader, structural understanding of conflict of interest is necessary to move beyond narrow debates about what does or does not constitute such a conflict and to develop the tools needed for effective health governance.

23.5 TOWARD MORE EFFECTIVE GOVERNANCE OF CONFLICT OF INTEREST

A structural approach offers substantive advantages for efforts to manage conflicts of interest in health policy and research. Such an approach extends our understanding of relevant conflicts beyond the immediate confines of the specific organizational context, thus providing a basis for understanding and addressing the kinds of concerns evident in recent attempts to delineate appropriate terms of engagement between actors across public health and the commercial sector (Table 23.1). It is consistent, for example, with Galea and McKee's governance tests for proposed partnership approaches,[33] including appraising the harmful impact of products and services and broader corporate conduct beyond the immediate confines of the specific initiative. Similarly, a structural approach fits with the "3P" assessment proposed by Brazil's National Cancer Institute, which assesses the *products*, *policies*, and *practices* of private sector entities and their alignment with or divergence from health goals.[34]

In recognizing the significance of conflicts at the intersections of different spheres of action, the structural understanding provides the most promising route for addressing conflicts of interest associated with collaborative forms of governance, including multi-stakeholder platforms and public–private partnerships. This allows for examination of broad tensions between public health and other goals, with conflicts of interest likely to be particularly significant amid the shifting and interdependent roles of state and non-state actors. Indeed, conflicts of interest appear inherent to (and perhaps inseparable from) the structure of such situations and interactions. A structural view implies that conflict of interest cannot be simply eliminated but must instead be identified and managed in order to protect health-related goals from other competing interests. In many contexts, this implies a fundamental challenge to the partnership model (as reflected in the principles outlined in Table 23.1). As Friedberg notes, "The risk of conflict of interest is inseparable from collective action"[30]—meaning its identification and management comprise a key challenge for governance processes. This points to the need to develop rules and codes that can check and manage such risks without imposing excessive opportunity costs via procedural overkill.

Perhaps most important in the current context, this structural understanding of conflict of interest is the one that resonates most closely with contemporary debates about the role of non-state actors in health governance. The recognition that diverse actors embody conflicting logics of action is consistent, for example, with the long-standing identification of a fundamental conflict of interest between the tobacco industry and public health.[4] Positioning conflict as a problem of strategic action draws attention to the inequitable distribution of resources, opportunities, and costs between

Table 23.1 EXAMPLES OF PRINCIPLES FOR ASSESSING PROPOSED
PARTNERSHIPS BETWEEN HEALTH ACTORS AND CORPORATE ACTORS,
REFLECTING A STRUCTURAL UNDERSTANDING OF CONFLICT OF INTEREST

Galea and McKee's "Five Tests"	Brazil National Cancer Institute's "3Ps"
1. Are the core products and services provided by the corporation health-enhancing or health-damaging?	*Products*: Do the corporation's products cause damage to population health?
2. Does the corporation promote the health and well-being of its own employees and contractors?	*Practices*: Does the corporation engage in practices that undermine health? For example:
3. Are the corporation's practices (including CSR) subject to independent audit?	Advertising and promotion to increase unhealthy consumption
4. Does the corporation make contributions to the public commons?	Lobbying against measures that would protect or promote health
5. Does the corporation's proposed input give it influence in development (cf. implementation) of health-related policies and programs?	*Policies*: Do the corporation's policies indicate it is endeavoring to increase health-damaging consumption at a population/global level?

Adapted from Galea & McKee[33] and Gomes.[34]

public health actors and commercial partners, as identified in analyses of
voluntary agreements in NCD policies.[2] An emphasis on understanding the
complex intersections of spheres of action and competing logics mirrors
tensions evident in leading philanthropies with investments in producers
of unhealthy commodities.[24,31] It also highlights the need for new tools to
identify and manage conflict of interest in complex settings, building on
experiences in developing WHO's tool for managing conflict of interest in
nutrition policy.[3]

Such approaches have the potential to more clearly articulate and protect
public health objectives in the context of competing (and often more powerful) interests. In seeking to extend governance of conflict of interest beyond selected unhealthy commodity industries, they can inform strategies
to both enhance policy coherence across different spheres of public policy[4]
and support efforts to regulate the commercial determinants of health.

REFERENCES

1. Collin J, Hill SE, Kandlik Eltanani M, Plotnikova E, Ralson R, Smith KE. Can
    public health reconcile profits and pandemics? An analysis of attitudes to com-
    mercial sector engagement in health policy and research. *PLoS One*. 2017;
    12(9): e0182612.

2. Moodie R, Stuckler D, Monteiro C, et al. Profits and pandemics: Prevention of harmful effects of tobacco, alcohol, and ultra-processed food and drink industries. *Lancet.* 2013; 381: 670–679.

3. Ralston R, Hill SE, Gomes FD, Collin J. Towards preventing and managing conflict of interest in nutrition policy? An analysis of submissions to a consultation on a draft WHO tool. *Int J Health Policy Manag.* 2021; 10(5): 255–265.

4. Collin J. Tobacco control, global health policy and development: Towards policy coherence in global governance. *Tob Control.* 2012; 21(2): 274–280.

5. Peters A. Conflict of interest as a cross-cutting problem of governance. In: Peters A, Handchin L, eds. *Conflict of Interest in Global, Public and Corporate Governance.* Cambridge University Press; 2012: 3–38.

6. Peters A. Managing conflict of interest: Lessons from multiple disciplines and settings. In: Peters A, Handchin L, eds. *Conflict of Interest in Global, Public and Corporate Governance.* Cambridge University Press; 2012: 357–421.

7. Richter J. WHO reform and public interest safeguards: An historical perspective. *Social Med.* 2012; 6(3): 141–150.

8. Brandt A. Inventing conflicts of interest: A history of tobacco industry tactics. *Am J Public Health.* 2012; 102(1): 63–71.

9. Hannum H. Conflicting interests, but not necessarily conflicts of interest. ICAP Review 4. International Center for Alcohol Policies. 2009. Accessed November 25, 2021. https://citeseerx.ist.psu.edu/viewdoc/download?doi=10.1.1.632.2697&rep=rep1&type=pdf

10. Mialon M, Ho M, Carriedo A, Ruskin G, Crosbie E. Beyond nutrition and physical activity: Food industry shaping of the very principles of scientific integrity. *Global Health.* 2021; 17: Article 37. https://doi.org/10.1186/s12992-021-00689-1

11. Thompson DF. Understanding financial conflicts of interest. *N Engl J Med.* 1993; 329(8): 573.

12. Lundh A, Lexchin J, Mintzes B, Schroll JB, Bero L. Industry sponsorship and research outcome. *Cochrane Database Syst Rev.* 2012; 12: MR000033. https://doi.org/10.1002/14651858.MR000033.pub3

13. Bero LA, Grundy Q. Why having a (nonfinancial) interest is not a conflict of interest. *PLoS Biol.* 2016; 14: e2001221. https://doi.org/10.1371/journal.pbio.2001221

14. MacCoun RJ. Conflicts of interest in public policy research. In: Moore DA, Cain DM, Loewenstein G, Bazerman MH, eds. *Conflicts of Interest: Challenges and Solutions in Business, Law, Medicine, and Public Policy.* Cambridge University Press; 2005: 233–262.

15. World Health Organization. Addressing and managing conflicts of interest in the planning and delivery of nutrition programmes at country level. Report of a technical consultation convened in Geneva, Switzerland, on October 8–9, 2015. 2016. Accessed November 25, 2021. https://apps.who.int/iris/bitstream/handle/10665/206554/9789241510530_eng.pdf?sequence=1&isAllowed=y

16. Grundy Q, Mazzarello S, Bero L. A comparison of policy provisions for managing "financial" and "non-financial" interests across health-related research organizations: A qualitative content analysis. *Account Res.* 2020; 27(4): 212–237.

17. Tereskerz PM, Moreno J. Ten steps to developing a national agenda to address financial conflicts of interest in industry sponsored clinical research. *Account Res.* 2005; 12(2): 139–155.

18. Katz D, Caplan A, Merz J. All gifts large and small: Toward an understanding of the ethics of pharmaceutical industry gift-giving. *Am J Bioeth.* 2010; 10(10): 11–17.

19. Saver RS. Is it really all about the money? Reconsidering non-financial interests in medical research. *J Law Med Ethics*. 2012; 40(3): 467–481.

20. Brussels Declaration: Ethics & principles for science & society policy-making. Presented at the American Association for the Advancement of Science's annual meeting, Boston, February 17, 2017. Accessed November 25, 2021. https://www.sci-com.eu/main/docs/Brussels-Declaration.pdf

21. McCambridge J, Daube M, McKee M. Brussels Declaration: A vehicle for the advancement of tobacco and alcohol industry interests at the science/policy interface? *Tob Control*. 2019; 28(1): 7–12.

22. Lo B, Field MJ, eds. *Conflict of Interest in Medical Research, Education, and Practice*. National Academies Press. 2009. Accessed November 25, 2021. https://www.ncbi.nlm.nih.gov/books/NBK22942/pdf/Bookshelf_NBK22942.pdf

23. Rodwin MA. Conflicts of interest, institutional corruption, and pharma: An agenda for reform. *J Law Med Ethics*. 2012; 40(3): 511–522.

24. Stuckler D, Basu S, McKee M. Global health philanthropy and institutional relationships: How should conflicts of interest be addressed? *PLoS Med*. 2011; 8(4): e1001020. https://doi.org/10.1371/journal.pmed.1001020

25. World Health Assembly. Framework for engagement with non-state actors. WHA69.10. May 28, 2016. Accessed November 25, 2021. https://www.who.int/about/collaborations/non-state-actors/A69_R10-FENSA-en.pdf

26. Global Social Observatory. Engaging in the SUN movement: Preventing and managing conflicts of interest. Reference Note. Global Health Observatory/ Scaling Up Nutrition. March 2014. Accessed November 25, 2021. http://docs.scalingupnutrition.org/wp-content/uploads/2014/05/COI_Reference_Notes_20140322_ENG_web.pdf

27. Matzopoulos R, Parry C, Corrigall J, Myers J, Goldstein S, London L. Global Fund collusion with liquor giant is a clear conflict of interest. *Bull World Health Organ*. 2012; 90: 67–69.

28. Marten R, Hawkins B. Stop the toasts: The Global Fund's disturbing new partnership. *Lancet*. 2018; 391(10122): 735–736.

29. Bampoe V, Clancy A, Sugarman M, Liden J, Lansang MA. Response from the Global Fund. *Bull World Health Organ*. 2012; 90(1): 70.

30. Friedberg E. Conflict of interest from the perspective of the sociology of organised action. In: Peters A, Handchin L, eds. *Conflict of Interest in Global, Public and Corporate Governance*. Cambridge University Press; 2012: 39–53.

31. Burch T, Wander N, Collin J. Uneasy money: The Instituto Carlos Slim de la Salud and conflict of interest in global health. *Tob Control*. 2010; 19: e1–e9. http://dx.doi.org/10.1136/tc.2010.038307

32. Dubois V. The fields of public policy. In: Hilgers M, Mangez E, eds. *Bourdieu's Theory of Social Fields: Concepts and Applications*. Routledge; 2012: 199–220.

33. Galea G, McKee M. Public–private partnerships with large corporations: Setting the ground rules for better health. *Health Policy*. 2014; 115(2): 138–140.

34. Gomes FS. Conflict of interest in food and nutrition. *Cad Saúde Pública*. 2015; 31(10): 1–8.

CHAPTER 24

Assessing the Health Impacts of the Commercial Determinants of Health

LUKE N. ALLEN

24.1 INTRODUCTION

This chapter introduces readers to a core element of commercial determinants of health (CDOH): understanding how we assess the ways that commercial activities impact human health. As the old axiom goes; "You can't manage what you don't measure," and robust scientific evidence on the impact of commercial activity fundamentally shapes action in this field. Policies such as sugar taxes, tobacco graphic warnings, and gambling restrictions all operate on the premise that they will constrain harmful impacts. This chapter guides readers through an overview of where those assumptions come from and the different methodological tools that CDOH researchers can use to assess the relationships between corporate actions and health outcomes.

24.2 WHY ASSESS THE IMPACT OF COMMERCIAL DETERMINANTS OF HEALTH?

Assessing and addressing the commercial determinants is a multidisciplinary venture, and the corpus of CDOH evidence is the result of myriad researchers probing, documenting, and synthesizing the different ways that corporate activity influences human behavior, environments, and health outcomes. This body of evidence is used for advocacy, prioritizing policy activities, and directing future research.

Luke N. Allen, *Assessing the Health Impacts of the Commercial Determinants of Health* In: *The Commercial Determinants of Health*. Edited by: Nason Maani, Mark Petticrew, and Sandro Galea, Oxford University Press. © Oxford University Press 2023. DOI: 10.1093/oso/9780197578742.003.0024

Without efforts to assess the health impacts of commercial activity, we would not understand the scale of the problem. Nor would we understand the inequitable distribution of the problem—that is, which groups are most affected. And we would not understand how the problem is changing over time. Rigorous, reliable, and accurate research is the means of identifying the most pernicious problems and directing effective action.

To date, most CDOH research that has examined the health impact of commercial practices has focused on quantifying harms or assessing harm mitigation strategies. However, it is important to start with an appreciation that the health impacts of commercial activities are rarely black and white.

24.3 NUANCE IN COMMERCIAL IMPACTS ON HEALTH

The reader may be familiar with Nestlé's breaches of milk formula marketing guidelines,[1] Philip Morris taking Australia to court to challenge the implementation of regulations on plain packaging of tobacco,[2] and the Scotch Whisky Association's powerful opposition to minimum unit pricing measures.[3] However, these high-profile "David versus Goliath" scandals belie the complexity of assessing the health impact of corporate actions. Even the most nefarious business practices may inadvertently benefit human health in one way or another (e.g., by providing stable employment), and the trade-offs of particular policy choices for health and health equity deserve careful consideration.

When thinking about the health impact of commercial actors, we often go straight to products: These might include cigarettes, alcohol, processed foods, and sugary drinks. Although it is relatively simple to determine the health impact of an individual product, it is much more difficult to gain a holistic understanding of how a given corporate actor influences health. For a start, many markets are so consolidated that major transnational corporations hold expansive portfolios of healthy *and* unhealthy products. For instance, Coca-Cola sells more than 500 different brands, and more than one-fourth of its revenue comes from fruit juices, dairy, and water.[4] Even for companies that only sell single products (e.g., China Tobacco), their overall health impact is mediated through myriad avenues, including their hiring and employment practices; the amount of tax they pay; how environmentally friendly their waste management practices are; the way the workers and communities in their supply chains are treated; as well as more distal contributions to infrastructure, education, gender equity, or political funding.

Baum and colleagues have developed an overarching analytical framework that can be used to assess the health impacts of corporate actions on health across the full scope of a given company's structures and practices.[5] Their approach uses a health equity perspective and was designed for application in low- and middle-income countries, specifically focusing on transnational corporations. Although it was developed with reference to food and non-alcoholic beverage and extractive industries, the general principles can be applied to other sectors. Their model leans on traditional health impact assessments by incorporating social, economic, and environmental factors that combine to determine overall impact. The entire model rests on the collection and analysis of data.

This overarching framework helps us train our sights on the specific elements of commercial activity that influence health while keeping a broader view of how any given element "fits in" with the overall picture. A panoply of data-gathering methods are required to assess overall impact. The next section considers the different methodological approaches that can be used for this task and how they relate to CDOH.

24.4 HOW DO WE GATHER DATA ON THE HEALTH IMPACT OF THE CDOH?

We have established that corporate activity influences the environment and human behavior in complex and nuanced ways. As such, the traditional *evidence-based medicine* paradigm and the "pyramid of research methods"[6]—originally developed to help choose the most methodologically robust method for assessing the effectiveness of clinical interventions—are not dominant in our field. However, evidence-based medicine's relentless focus on using the right method to answer a carefully articulated research question retains value. For some areas of enquiry, the "PICO" formulation can offer a helpful framework (which population, intervention, comparator, and outcomes are we interested in?), but many other CDOH questions do not fit this mold; for instance, what strategies have alcohol companies used to circumvent bans on sports advertising in the Premier League? On a deeper level, it is important to remember that the PICO approach is tied to a hierarchy of evidence for effectiveness; it is not a hierarchy of research methods. The important thing is to be as clear as possible about the phenomena being studied.

Once the research question has been formulated with as much precision as possible, the next step is to select the most appropriate research method. Because CDOH research encompasses public health, economics, psychology, anthropology, biology, and a number of other disciplines, it would not be practical to present an exhaustive list of all the different study types that can be used with their relative strengths and weaknesses here. Instead, it is helpful to rehearse the key questions that determine the overarching approach: Will the investigator assign the exposure? Will there be a comparison group? Are the researchers aiming to quantify something or understand why it occurs?

A great deal of CDOH research is qualitative work in which the investigators do not assign exposures or use comparison groups. This research has its roots in early analyses of tobacco industry strategies, and modern methods have been extended to news coverage, social media content, and assessing the ways that mis/information spreads across social networks.

Experimental methods are those in which the investigators assign the exposure. This branch of the research taxonomy has been overshadowed by observational analytic work, in which CDOH researchers seek to evaluate the impact of exposures that have not been assigned by the research team, using non-exposed populations as comparators. Examples include interrupted time series analyses to understand the impact of Tonga's sugar-sweetened beverage tax[7] and comparative work examining the impact of Berkeley, California's soda tax on consumption patterns in exposed and non-exposed neighborhoods.[8] The common feature is that CDOH researchers commonly aim to assess the impact of independent corporate actors and therefore have little or no influence over the decisions made by those entities. A compounding issue is access to commercially sensitive data; sales figures, corporate strategies, ingredient formulations, and profit margins are often confidential or proprietary.

24.5 CORPORATE CHALLENGES TO CDOH RESEARCH

It is understandable that commercial actors may not want to share their industry secrets, especially with public health advocates; however, corporate actors can also actively make life difficult for researchers who threaten to expose harmful practices and threaten their reputations and bottom lines. The tobacco industry provides plentiful examples of systematic efforts to undermine the credibility of studies, institutions, methodologies, and even individual scientists.[9,10] Corporations also wield visible, hidden, and invisible power over policymakers and funding agencies, including the ability to influence which issues are acceptable for public debate.[11-13]

In terms of funding, as the field of CDOH is growing in recognition, increasing opportunities are being made available, but the environment remains challenging. The UK Prevention Research Partnership, the Global Alliance for Chronic Diseases, and the research funding arms of major disease-specific charities (e.g., the British Heart Foundation) are good examples of grant-making bodies in the United Kingdom.

Data access remains a stubborn issue for CDOH researchers, but there are two main approaches that can be used. The first is to use qualitative interviews with company representatives to directly assess the inner machinations of corporate activity. This can often be enhanced by interviewing other stakeholders—such as consumers, industry representatives, and policymakers—in order to build up a rich picture of corporate activity situated within its sphere of influence. Where corporate representatives are not keen to engage with researchers directly, we need to rely on other—more distal— proxy measures. These include annual financial reports from publicly traded companies, tax returns, industry body reports, repositories provided by data analytics firms such as Kantar,[14] and state and international data repositories such as the International Trade Centre database.[15] These data can be used to indirectly track corporate activity in the social, economic, and physical spheres.

A more expensive approach involves gathering primary data from retailers, consumers, and the digital and physical environment to assess consumption patterns, corporate behaviors, and biological outcomes using tools such as surveys, recall diaries, and anthropomorphic measurements. Araya and colleagues provide one such example, using 24-hour dietary recall to assess intake of ultra-processed foods among preschoolers and then examining the association between intake, socioeconomic status, and body mass index.[16] These primary studies can be collated to generate internationally comparable estimates of consumption patterns and the associated epidemiological burden, such as the Global Burden of Disease systematic analysis of dietary risk from 195 countries.[17] As with qualitative interviews, it can be helpful to use multiple data sources to triangulate when distal proxies are being used.[18] Content analysis is an aligned approach whereby researchers use systematic methods to organize and analyze documents and media to understand meanings and relationships of words, concepts, and themes.[19,20] A good example is the recent analysis of alcohol industry–funded corporate social responsibility websites and communication materials.[21]

24.6 RANDOMIZED CONTROLLED TRIALS AND EPISTEMOLOGICAL PARADIGMS

Randomized controlled trials (RCTs) are commonly held up as the gold standard research approach, but they are not always the most appropriate means of answering a given research question, especially for CDOH research.[22,23] RCTs are the best tool in our arsenal for providing (almost) bias-free estimates of mean effect; however, they are costly, time-consuming, designed for testing interventions—which is not always relevant for CDOH research—and only ethical when there is clinical equipoise. RCTs tell us more about central tendencies than who benefits from interventions, and the use of healthy volunteers and the ubiquitous trade-off between internal and external validity (commonly driven by ethics boards) severely limit generalizability to real-life populations. As mentioned previously, researchers often have little or no influence over the interventions that are being evaluated, such as sugar taxes, salt policies, or tobacco tax changes. These interventions are better served by quasi-randomized controlled methods.

Randomization still has its place, and it has been used by CDOH researchers such as Theresa Marteau.[24,25] However, the minority of CDOH research questions require an RCT approach. Funding panels can sometimes struggle to accept that non-RCT evidence is valid and worthwhile, and it is helpful to recap the underlying epistemological and epidemiological tenets that support RCTs' dominance.

First, RCTs occupy the top rung of evidence of effectiveness hierarchies because they can probe the causal nature of associations. By randomizing participants, both known and unknown confounders are equalized between intervention and control arms (given a sufficiently large n) so that the only variable not held constant is the intervention. However, as Hume argued in the 18th century, causality is only ever deduced, it is never empirically observed (even with an RCT).[1] Although RCTs certainly offer stronger evidence that an association is causal, we need to be wary of denigrating non-RCTs purely on this basis.

Second, RCTs are generally underpinned by a positivist/realist worldview—a paradigm that is commonly associated with quantitative approaches. The focus here is on careful and precise value-free measurements of an objective reality that is independent of actors. The other end of the spectrum is occupied by constructionism/relativism, which hold opposing ontological, epistemological, and axiological positions: that the world is subjectively constructed by social actors; knowledge is embedded in value and culture; and the aim of research is to effect real-world change through contextual interpretation, acknowledging values as an inevitable part of research. Most qualitative research is grounded in a constructionist worldview.

It is important to revise these concepts because epistemological paradigms are foundational to how and why different methods are selected and used, and how their findings are interpreted. This applies across all fields of scientific enquiry. We need to ask whether the researchers are seeking to fastidiously elicit an unbiased population mean effect size that can be generalized to other populations (e.g., What is the association between vaping and lung disease?) or seeking to understand the perceptions, values, and actions of different groups (e.g., How and why is Philip Morris advocating for a "smoke-free world"?). Because CDOH research is a quintessentially mixed-methods endeavor, it commonly leans on more balanced philosophical paradigms such as critical realism ("There is an objective external reality but human influence on knowledge is inevitable") and pragmatism, which is a philosophical position encompassing a heterogeneous set of approaches that all seek to combine quantitative and qualitative methods while holding their fundamental differences in tension.

24.7 REALISM

An increasingly popular research paradigm is the "realism" originally advanced by Pawson and Tilley,[26] asserting that there is a social reality that cannot be directly measured because it is processed through our minds, culture, and language, but it can be known indirectly. Realism moves beyond mean differences to ask what works for whom, in which circumstances, how, and why?[27] Realist reviews and evaluations aim to unpack the relationships between context, mechanism, and outcomes to explain why certain interventions or policies succeed or fail. Ensuing explanations constitute a form of "middle-range theory"—that is, they involve abstraction but are "close enough to observed data to be incorporated in propositions that permit empirical testing,"[28] imbuing impressive explanatory power.

Working from a realist/pragmatist epistemological paradigm, and seeking to use methods that provide the most robust explanatory power, while operating within the ethical, funding, and data availability constraints common to the CDOH field has led many researchers to modeling and quasi-experimental designs for assessing the impact of specific corporate activities on health outcomes. For example, a recent systematic review exploring the impact of regional trade agreements on consumption of unhealthy commodities uncovered six bivariate analyses, four multivariate analyses, and one natural experiment design.[29] Natural experiments compare exposed and unexposed populations determined by policymakers (rather than the researchers) and explore impact on outcomes. Schram and colleagues provide an example of a natural experiment design, assessing trade liberalization and sugar-sweetened beverage sales in Vietnam and the Phillipines.[30] Because regional confounding factors cannot be perfectly measured and balanced, this approach is probably most powerfully used when a new policy or intervention is introduced in a stepwise manner across similar populations. Looking to the other methods, Allen and colleagues have combined publicly available policy data with composite indices for corporate permeation[31] and corporate financial influence[32] in order to understand the association between industry latent power and policymaking processes.[33] During the past few years, the authors' work has moved from regression analyses[34] toward structural equation modeling approaches, which is indicative of a broader shift in the field, because the latter approach allows researchers to develop complex path models with direct and indirect effects. Matching is another modeling approach that allows researchers to pre-process observational data in order to form quasi-experimental contrasts by reducing imbalances in covariates between exposed and unexposed groups.[35] Modeling can also draw on established relative risk ratios (e.g., between daily salt intake and hypertension[36]) to simulate the epidemiological impact of counterfactual policy implementation scenarios, such as reformulating salt, fat, and sugar content.[37,38]

24.8 COMPLEXITY

Most of the approaches discussed above are designed to examine relatively simple associations between a given aspect of corporate activity and one or more health outcomes, using methods situated at various positions along the epistemological spectrum, with the aim of probing causality and maximizing explanatory power. A third and final axis to consider is complexity. The opening section of this chapter emphasized the extensive and nuanced impact that corporations exert, and although Baum and colleagues' framework helpfully categorizes these multiple facets,[5] complexity arises when we try to assess corporate impact across multiple domains or when we assess a single issue with enough intellectual honesty to acknowledge that corporate actors operate within complex adaptive systems, characterized by nonlinearity, path dependencies, feedback loops, variable outcomes, emergence, and numerous interacting stakeholders and components (see also Chapter 2).[39,40] A number of complexity science approaches can be used to evaluate interventions ("events in complex systems"[41]), including agent-based modeling, network analysis, and system dynamic modeling.[42,43] Although all interventions are arguably complex if they take place in the real world, the decision to use complexity-informed approaches should be made on the basis of whether the research question demands it.[44] However, in situations in which a more "simple" approach is used—such as bivariate analysis—I strongly recommend eschewing undergirding linear logic models and theories of change (commonly presented as a series of arrows pointing from left to right) in favor of causal loop diagrams that are able to identify multiple competing agents, feedback loops, and interdependencies. Example of the latter are provided in Knai and colleagues' overviews of using systems and complexity perspectives in CDOH research.[45,46] By their very nature, complexity and systems approaches also offer powerful conceptual frameworks that can be used to synthesize CDOH research findings in order to attempt global impact assessments at the whole, company, or industry level.

24.9 PUTTING IT ALL TOGETHER

Corporations impact health through a wide spectrum of activities, and a multitude of different methods are required in order to assess corporate actions and design and test effective interventions. The basic toolkit of methods presented above can be used and adapted in disciplines ranging from biomedicine to psychology, economics, and political science. The important thing is to choose the correct tool for the job and to understand the strengths and limitations of each approach.

There is an increasing recognition that understanding complex corporate influences requires a mix of different methods, particularly the combination of quantitative (counting what is happening) with qualitative methods (speaking to and observing people, and analyzing documents to understand *why*). Often, in combining these approaches, the total is greater than the sum of the parts, particularly where data are limited; for instance due to commercial confidentiality or if there is a lack of funding due to political pressure.

The history of CDOH research is overflowing with examples of industry interference, and an important aspect of capacity building is developing resilience against overt and covert corporate subversion. Documentation and exposure of these tactics can help convince funders and policymakers of the need for structures and processes that insulate research communities from the most damaging industry practices.

In terms of future research priorities, there is already a significant amount of evidence on the direct health harms of tobacco, alcohol, and free sugars. There are fewer data on the holistic role of corporate entities and on gambling, fossil fuels, firearms, and other profit-driven risk factors. We need more work on how corporate practices spread unhealthy commodities, the global distribution of risk, and the specific impact of corporate practices in low- and middle-income countries, especially regarding the efficacy of policy interventions to constrain CDOH. Finally, we need holistic approaches to assessing health impacts of entire corporations, leaning on a paradigm of complex adaptive systems that can help us bring it all together.

NOTE

1. For an ironic example of deductive reasoning applied to the broader issue of common methodological flaws in RCT design, see Krauss' "Why All RCTs Produce Biased Results" (based on a sample of the 10 most cited RCTs).[22]

REFERENCES

1. Zelman NE. The Nestle infant formula controversy: Restricting the marketing practices of multinational corporations in the Third World. *Transnatl Law*. 1990; 3(2): 697–758.
2. Mitchell AD, Studdert DM. Plain packaging of tobacco products in Australia: A novel regulation faces legal challenge. *JAMA*. 2012; 307(3): 261–262. doi:10.1001/jama.2011.2009
3. Patterson C, Katikireddi SV, Wood K, Hilton S. Representations of minimum unit pricing for alcohol in UK newspapers: A case study of a public health policy debate. *J Public Health*. 2015; 37(1): 40–49. doi:10.1093/pubmed/fdu078
4. The Coca-Cola Company. Strategy. Coca-Cola Company. n.d. Accessed January 29, 2021. https://investors.coca-colacompany.com/strategy

5. Baum FE, Sanders DM, Fisher M, et al. Assessing the health impact of trans-national corporations: Its importance and a framework. *Global Health*. 2016; 12(1): 27. doi:10.1186/s12992-016-0164-x

6. Sackett DL, Straus SE, Richardson WS, Rosenberg W, Haynes RB. *Evidence-Based Medicine: How to Practice and Teach EBM*. 2nd ed. Churchill Livingstone; 2000.

7. Teng A, Puloka V, Genç M, et al. Sweetened beverage taxes and changes in beverage price, imports and manufacturing: Interrupted time series analysis in a middle-income country. *Int J Behav Nutr Phys Act*. 2020; 17(1): 90. doi:10.1186/s12966-020-00980-1

8. Lee MM, Falbe J, Schillinger D, Basu S, McCulloch CE, Madsen KA. Sugar-sweetened beverage consumption 3 years after the Berkeley, California, sugar-sweetened beverage tax. *Am J Public Health*. 2019; 109(4): 637–639. doi:10.2105/AJPH.2019.304971

9. Grüning T, Gilmore AB, McKee M. Tobacco industry influence on science and scientists in Germany. *Am J Public Health*. 2006; 96(1): 20–32. doi:10.2105/AJPH.2004.061507

10. Drope J, Chapman S. Tobacco industry efforts at discrediting scientific knowledge of environmental tobacco smoke: A review of internal industry documents. *J Epidemiol Commun Health*. 2001; 55(8): 588–594. doi:10.1136/jech.55.8.588

11. Lukes S. *Power: A Radical View*. Vol. 9. Macmillan; 2005. doi:10.2307/2065624

12. McKee M, Stuckler D. Revisiting the corporate and commercial determinants of health. *Am J Public Health*. 2018; 108(9): 1167–1170. doi:10.2105/AJPH.2018.304510

13. Madureira Lima J, Galea S. Corporate practices and health: A framework and mechanisms. *Global Health*. 2018; 14(1): 21. doi:10.1186/s12992-018-0336-y

14. Kantar. Understand people, inspire growth. n.d. Accessed July 27, 2021. https://www.kantar.com

15. International Trade Centre. International trade statistics 2001–2020. 2021. Accessed July 27, 2021. https://www.intracen.org/itc/market-info-tools/trade-statistics

16. Araya C, Corvalán C, Cediel G, Taillie LS, Reyes M. Ultra-processed food consumption among Chilean preschoolers is associated with diets promoting non-communicable diseases. *Front Nutr*. 2021; 8: 601526. doi:10.3389/fnut.2021.601526

17. Afshin A, Sur PJ, Fay KA, et al. Health effects of dietary risks in 195 countries, 1990–2017: A systematic analysis for the Global Burden of Disease Study 2017. *Lancet*. 2019; 393(10184): 1958–1972. doi:10.1016/S0140-6736(19)30041-8

18. Denzin NK. *Sociological Methods: A Sourcebook*. McGraw-Hill; 1978.

19. Hsieh H-F, Shannon SE. Three approaches to qualitative content analysis. *Qual Health Res*. 2005; 15(9): 1277–1288. doi:10.1177/1049732305276687

20. Elo S, Kääriäinen M, Kanste O, Pölkki T, Utriainen K, Kyngäs H. Qualitative content analysis: A focus on trustworthiness. *SAGE Open*. 2014; 4(1): 2158244014522633. doi:10.1177/2158244014522633

21. Petticrew M, Maani N, Pettigrew L, Rutter H, Schalkwyk MCV. Dark nudges and sludge in Big Alcohol: Behavioral economics, cognitive biases, and alcohol industry corporate social responsibility. *Milbank Q*. 2020; 98(4): 1290–1328. doi:10.1111/1468-0009.12475

22. Krauss A. Why all randomised controlled trials produce biased results. *Ann Med*. 2018; 50(4): 312–322. doi:10.1080/07853890.2018.1453233

23. American Psychological Association. The pitfalls of randomized controlled trials. 2010. Accessed July 27, 2021. https://www.apa.org/monitor/2010/09/trials

24. Lee I, Blackwell AKM, Scollo M, et al. Cigarette pack size and consumption: An adaptive randomised controlled trial. *BMC Public Health*. 2021; 21(1): 1420. doi:10.1186/s12889-021-11413-4

25. Reynolds JP, Kosīte D, Rigby Dames B, et al. Increasing the proportion of healthier foods available with and without reducing portion sizes and energy purchased in worksite cafeterias: Protocol for a stepped-wedge randomised controlled trial. *BMC Public Health*. 2019; 19: 1611. doi:10.1186/s12889-019-7927-2

26. Pawson R, Tilley N. *Realistic Evaluation*. SAGE; 2021.

27. Wong G, Greenhalgh T, Westhorp G, Buckingham J, Pawson R. RAMESES publication standards: Realist syntheses. *BMC Med*. 2013; 11(1): 21. doi:10.1186/1741-7015-11-21

28. Merton RK. *On Theoretical Sociology: Five Essays, Old and New*. Free Press; 1967.

29. Barlow P, McKee M, Basu S, Stuckler D. The health impact of trade and investment agreements: A quantitative systematic review and network co-citation analysis. *Global Health*. 2017; 13(1): 13. doi:10.1186/s12992-017-0240-x

30. Schram A, Labonte R, Baker P, Friel S, Reeves A, Stuckler D. The role of trade and investment liberalization in the sugar-sweetened carbonated beverages market: A natural experiment contrasting Vietnam and the Philippines. *Global Health*. 2015; 11: 41. doi:10.1186/s12992-015-0127-7

31. Lima JM, Galea S. The Corporate Permeation Index—A tool to study the macrosocial determinants of non-communicable disease. *SSM Popul Health*. 2019; 7: 100361. doi:10.1016/j.ssmph.2019.100361

32. Allen LN, Wigley S, Holmer H. Assessing the association between corporate political influence and implementation of policies to tackle commercial determinants of non-communicable diseases: A cross-sectional analysis of 172 countries. *Social Sci Med*. March 2022; 9297: 114825.

33. Allen LN, Wigley S, Holmer H. Implementation of non-communicable disease policies from 2015 to 2020: A geopolitical analysis of 194 countries. *Lancet Glob Health*. 2021; 9(11): e1528–e1538.

34. Allen LN, Nicholson BD, Yeung BYT, Goiana-da-Silva F. Implementation of non-communicable disease policies: A geopolitical analysis of 151 countries. *Lancet Glob Health*. 2020; 8(1): e50–e58. doi:10.1016/S2214-109X(19)30446-2

35. Stuart EA. Matching methods for causal inference: A review and a look forward. *Stat Sci Rev J Inst Math Stat*. 2010; 25(1): 1–21. doi:10.1214/09-STS313

36. He FJ, Li J, MacGregor GA. Effect of longer term modest salt reduction on blood pressure: Cochrane systematic review and meta-analysis of randomised trials. *BMJ*. 2013; 346: f1325. doi:10.1136/bmj.f1325

37. Breda J, Allen LN, Tibet B, et al. Estimating the impact of achieving Turkey's non-communicable disease policy targets: A macro-simulation modelling study. *Lancet Reg Health Eur*. 2021; 1. doi:10.1016/j.lanepe.2020.100018

38. Goiana-da-Silva F, Cruz-e-Silva D, Allen L, et al. Modelling impacts of food industry co-regulation on noncommunicable disease mortality, Portugal. *Bull World Health Organ*. 2019; 97(7): 450–459. doi:10.2471/BLT.18.220566

39. Craig P, Dieppe P, Macintyre S, Michie S, Nazareth I, Petticrew M. Developing and evaluating complex interventions: The new Medical Research Council guidance. *BMJ*. 2008; 337: a1655. doi:10.1136/bmj.a1655

40. Greenhalgh T, Papoutsi C. Studying complexity in health services research: Desperately seeking an overdue paradigm shift. *BMC Med*. 2018; 16(1): 95. doi:10.1186/s12916-018-1089-4

41. Hawe P, Shiell A, Riley T. Theorising interventions as events in systems. *Am J Community Psychol*. 2009; 43(3–4): 267–276. doi:10.1007/s10464-009-9229-9

42. Xue H, Slivka L, Igusa T, Huang TT, Wang Y. Applications of systems modelling in obesity research: Systems modelling review. *Obes Rev*. 2018; 19(9): 1293–1308. doi:10.1111/obr.12695

43. Hunter RF, Wickramasinghe K, Ergüder T, et al. National action plans to tackle NCDs: Role of stakeholder network analysis. *BMJ*. 2019; 365: l1871. doi:10.1136/bmj.l1871

44. Petticrew M. When are complex interventions "complex"? When are simple interventions "simple"? *Eur J Public Health*. 2011; 21(4): 397–398. doi:10.1093/eurpub/ckr084

45. Petticrew M, Knai C, Thomas J, et al. Implications of a complexity perspective for systematic reviews and guideline development in health decision making. *BMJ Glob Health*. 2019; 4(Suppl 1): e000899. doi:10.1136/bmjgh-2018-000899

46. Knai C, Petticrew M, Mays N, et al. Systems thinking as a framework for analyzing commercial determinants of health. *Milbank Q*. 2018; 96(3): 472–498. doi:10.1111/1468-0009.12339

CHAPTER 25

Assessing the Economic Impacts of Corporations

MARTIN MCKEE

25.1 A FALSE NARRATIVE

Those whose interests may be harmed by public health regulations—typically the manufacturers of harmful commodities such as tobacco, alcohol, or junk food—often frame such measures as being harmful to economic activity. In the competition for influence on public policy, they present issues as a trade-off between health and the economy. In this chapter, I challenge this narrative, presenting evidence that better health is—like education, knowledge, and infrastructure—a contributor to economic growth, while asking how these industries, and the public relations companies they enlist in their support, produce the findings they use to justify their arguments.

First, however, as this chapter is written in the midst of a pandemic, it is relevant to reflect on the arguments that have characterized the response to this global crisis. When the novel coronavirus swept across the world in early 2020, political leaders were faced with a choice. When would they introduce restrictions on movement, such as closures of schools, shops, and factories? With very few exceptions on both sides, the public health community was urging them to do so rapidly while sectors that would be most affected, such as retail and manufacturing, were urging delay. A widespread view was that they had to make a choice between health and the economy.[1]

Of course, it has now become clear that this was a false dichotomy. Those countries that failed to act decisively to reduce the entry of cases and spread of infection suffered some of the worst economic outcomes.[2] The experience of the Nordic countries illustrates this well. Exceptionally, and controversially,

Martin McKee, *Assessing the Economic Impacts of Corporations* In: *The Commercial Determinants of Health*. Edited by: Nason Maani, Mark Petticrew, and Sandro Galea, Oxford University Press. © Oxford University Press 2023. DOI: 10.1093/oso/9780197578742.003.0025

Sweden adopted a light touch approach. Although many Swedes did limit their movement[3] and some restrictions were imposed, in general the policy response was much less stringent than in Norway and Finland. Yet when the final account of 2020 was calculated, it was clear that Sweden had fared worse in both deaths and economic performance.[4]

This should have been no surprise. No country is immune to changes in the global economy, so even if Sweden sought to keep its markets open, it still had to trade with other countries that did not. In addition, as became increasingly clear during the pandemic, the public were frequently ahead of their governments, restricting their movement before they were instructed to do so. A very small, if often highly vocal minority, encouraged by corporate-funded libertarian U.S. organizations,[5] clamored for the right to put themselves and others at risk. However, they were the exceptions. The historical record reinforced this message. A study of 43 U.S. cities during the 1918 influenza pandemic found that those that imposed restrictions on social interactions earlier and retained them longer experienced a stronger subsequent economic recovery.[6]

It is not just in the COVID-19 pandemic that arguments have been advanced that politicians must choose between health and the economy. Perhaps the best-known example is that advanced over many years by the tobacco industry, claiming that anti-smoking policies would damage employment.[7] In countries such as the United Kingdom, the companies invested great effort in cultivating relationships with Members of Parliament with tobacco factories in their constituencies. Others were targeted with the argument that reduced smoking would harm tax receipts. Perhaps the most notorious example was a campaign by Philip Morris in the Czech Republic that estimated the benefit, in terms of savings on provision of health care, to those dying prematurely as a result of smoking. It argued that "public finance saved between 943 mil. CZK and 1,193 mil. CZK (realistic estimate:1,193 mil. CZK) from reduced healthcare costs, savings on pensions and housing costs for the elderly—all related to the early mortality of smokers."[8] At the time, $1 was equal to 38,5 CZK. By calculating that the premature death of every smoker would save about $1,000, Philip Morris hoped to persuade the Czech government to reject tobacco control measures.

The company did eventually apologize, saying "We understand that this was not only a terrible mistake, but that it was wrong. . . . To say it's totally inappropriate is an understatement."[9] However, it was also misleading. A detailed critique has been published elsewhere, concluding that rather than saving the Czech state budget $150 million per year, it would actually cost it at least $373 per year.[10] It is, however, useful to examine how this flawed analysis came to be, as it demonstrates the ways that economic analysis can be used to further commercial interests in relation to health.

Some of the reasons were related to the data used. The authors used outdated estimates of smoking-attributable mortality, a low figure for smoking-related deaths during productive ages, and inconsistent application of inflation adjustments. Others were methodological. First, it excluded some important costs linked to the state budget, such as the loss of income tax from smokers unable to work because of illness or who had retired early or benefits paid to their dependents. Second, it ignored the loss of production by smokers who died or of productivity by those who fell ill. It also ignored the contribution that retired people make to the economy—for example, through unpaid work or caring for children, thus allowing parents to work. Nor did it take account of how money not spent on cigarettes would have been spent on something else, which if domestically produced rather than imported could have generated more economic growth. This is important because the industry often argues that anything that reduces its sales will be bad for others, such as small retailers or tobacco farmers, groups it seeks to mobilize in its support. Yet it ignores evidence that the retail profit margin on tobacco products is much lower than that on other items that small retailers sell—6.6% in a UK study compared with 24.1% on other products—so a shift in sales would benefit the retailer.[11] Finally, the presentation of the calculations was confusing and impossible to replicate while there were apparent mistakes.

This example illustrates the need for caution in interpreting economic analyses where those funding them have a vested interest in the result. The tobacco industry long claimed that restrictions on smoking in bars and restaurants would reduce takings, yet a systematic review found that all studies finding that this was the case were funded by the industry, and they were significantly more likely to have methodological weaknesses than those finding the opposite.[12]

Of course, the tobacco industry is not alone in arguing that the cost of measures that would improve health would harm the economy, typically through loss of employment or tax revenue. Others include the sugar-sweetened beverage[13] and alcohol industries.[14] A 2017 analysis critically evaluated claims that the UK alcohol industry contributed positively to the economy, finding little evidence in support and setting out the substantial costs of alcohol-related harms.[15]

These and other industries collaborate to influence the debate on scientific methods—for example, by pressing for standards that would make it virtually impossible to demonstrate the harms associated with their products—and to argue for their inclusion in policy debates despite known problems with research they fund.[16] These industries have been especially vociferous in arguing that the research they fund—overtly or, in some cases, covertly—should be interpreted devoid of context. Yet there is now a wealth of scholarship challenging this view,[17-19] showing how, in examples such as the smoking ban described above, the most important determinant of the results obtained is the source of the funding used to produce them.

25.2 THE CONTRIBUTION OF HEALTH TO THE ECONOMY

If we reject the narrative of health versus the economy, what is the association between the two? It is both intuitive and borne out by a wealth of evidence that economic growth, providing it is inclusive and the benefits are shared, contributes to better health.[20,21] People and families spared the constant struggle to survive can gain access to the prerequisites for health, including food and shelter. Public authorities have the resources needed to create healthy environments and improve health care.

The association running from health to economic growth is perhaps less obvious, at least in high-income countries where much work is sedentary. In low- and middle-income countries, where work, and thus income, is especially dependent on physical strength, in agriculture and extractive industries especially, it is more clear, and it was set out in detail in 2000 in the publication of the Commission on Macroeconomics and Health.[22]

One part of the evidence is historical. Economic historians have identified health as a major contributor to economic growth. In 1994, Fogel attributed approximately 30% of income growth in the United Kingdom between 1780 and 1980 to improvements in health and nutrition.[23] A 2001 study by Arora, examining 10 industrialized countries from the late 1800s on, reached broadly similar conclusions.[24] Other studies have examined a larger sample of countries, both high- and low- or middle-income, in the post-war period.[25,26] Although there are several methodological challenges, most found similar results, especially in low- and middle-income countries. A 1996 study of approximately 100 countries, between 1960 and 1990, found that lower initial gross domestic product (GDP), better initial levels of health and education, low fertility, lower government consumption, the rule of law, terms of trade, and low inflation were the most powerful predictors of subsequent economic growth.[25] Life expectancy, the health measure used in the study, had a larger effect than even education. Holding other factors constant, a rise in life expectancy from 50 to 70 years would raise the growth rate by 1.4 percentage points per year. Importantly, the authors identified a positive feedback loop, with economic development encouraging further improvement in health. A more recent study in a similar number of countries over the same period, but including additional variables, reached a similar conclusion.[26] It estimated that a 1-year improvement in life expectancy contributed an increase of 4% in GDP. Another study found that the introduction of public health systems in Europe between 1820 and 2010 was associated with subsequent increased economic growth, mediated through better health.[27] There are a few contrary results, but these can generally be explained by issues related to data and methods.[28,29] A recent study that addressed the outstanding methodological challenges found a clear association between lower disease burden and economic growth.[30]

A major study undertaken for the European Commission in 2006 examined the pathways through which health contributed to economic growth.[31] Its starting point was the potential bidirectional relationship between health and economic development, and thus the scope for positive feedback, whereby investments in health and the economy are mutually reinforcing. While noting the question of whether associations found in low-income countries could be extrapolated to higher income settings, it noted how, although living conditions differ, even in some of the wealthiest countries there are communities in which health indicators are similar to those in low-income countries, including well-known studies comparing Glasgow, Scotland, with India[32] and comparing areas of New York with Bangladesh.[33]

Four main pathways have been identified through which health could contribute to economic growth. First, people in better health may be more productive. The relevant research has typically sought to capture this by comparing hourly wages. Second, healthier people might be more likely to participate in the labor force, measured by hours worked each week or by remaining in the labor force until or beyond the official retirement age rather than exiting it prematurely—for example, on grounds of ill health or early retirement. Third, those in better health, who could expect to live a longer life, might be more likely to invest in their education, and thus their potential to contribute to growth. Finally, such people might be more likely to invest in capital for the future—for example, in small and medium enterprises such as family businesses that would bring later rewards to themselves and society. Concerning the third and fourth mechanisms, it has been shown that those living in disadvantaged circumstances may believe, based on what they see in their communities, that they are unlikely to live a long and healthy life. As a consequence, their time preferences do not encourage investment in a future they believe that they are unlikely to experience.[34]

There is evidence in support of all of these mechanisms. Turning first to productivity, a German study using data from 1995 to 2005 found that increased satisfaction with one's health was associated with higher hourly wages of men and women.[35] An earlier U.S. study highlighted the importance of context. Poor health was associated with 6.2% lower total earnings, but African American males were more likely to exit the labor force or work fewer weeks, whereas White males were more likely to remain in work but with lower hourly wages.[36] Mental ill health can have particularly serious consequences over prolonged periods.[37] However, when interpreting these studies, it is important to take account of the settings in which they were undertaken, and in particular the link between employment and health insurance coverage in the United States.

There is considerable evidence that people in poor health are more likely to leave the labor force. An Irish study found that men with a chronic illness or disability that severely hampered their daily activities were 61% less likely to be in employment. The corresponding figure was 52% for women, controlling for age, education, and marital status.[38] However, a U.S. study found considerable differences by race and gender, with African Americans, who are already disadvantaged in labor markets, experiencing disproportionately worse outcomes that the White population.[39] Those experiencing a health shock in middle age are especially likely to leave the labor force,[40] with the impact increasing after the first year following the onset of illness. Other research has found that those in poor health are more likely to retire earlier, in one study by 1–3 years,[41] although again this varies by gender. Men caring for a chronically ill wife were more likely to retire early, whereas women caring for a chronically ill husband were more likely to remain in work.[41]

The evidence that good health leads to better educational outcomes is more limited, with challenges determining the direction of causality and potential confounding. However, some longitudinal research does point to the importance of this relationship. An example is an American study finding that adolescents in poor health are less likely to complete secondary education and enter higher education.[42] The fourth pathway, which considers the association between health and savings, is also dominated by literature from the United States, in particular examining the role of ill health on bankruptcy.[43]

Finally, if we take a narrower health system perspective, there is compelling evidence that public health interventions, especially population-level ones that industries frequently oppose, achieve a very high return on investment, often more than 40-fold.[44]

25.3 CONCLUSION

The narrative promoted by some industries that restrictions on their activity will damage the economy does not stand up to scrutiny. The evidence that they draw on is often misleading, and indeed we know that they have sought to influence the methods used in research in ways that favor their interests. The wider narrative that there is a trade-off between health and the economy is equally problematic. Like education, knowledge, and infrastructure, health is an important driver of economic growth, acting through multiple pathways. This means that products that damage health will, all else being equal, be expected to harm the economy. If those who manufacture these products wish to suggest otherwise, they have a high bar to cross.

REFERENCES

1. McKee M, Stuckler D. If the world fails to protect the economy, COVID-19 will damage health not just now but also in the future. *Nat Med*. 2020; 26(5): 640–642.

2. Oliu-Barton M, Pradelski BSR, Aghion P, et al. SARS-CoV-2 elimination, not mitigation, creates best outcomes for health, the economy, and civil liberties. *Lancet*. 2021; 397(10291): 2234–2236.

3. Vannoni M, McKee M, Semenza JC, Bonell C, Stuckler D. Using volunteered geographic information to assess mobility in the early phases of the COVID-19 pandemic: A cross-city time series analysis of 41 cities in 22 countries from March 2nd to 26th 2020. *Global Health*. 2020; 16(1): 85.

4. Gordon DV, Grafton RQ, Steinshamn SI. Statistical analyses of the public health and economic performance of Nordic countries in response to the COVID-19 pandemic. *medRxiv*. 2020; 2020.11.23.20236711.

5. Greenhalgh T, McKee M, Kelly-Invirng M. The pursuit of herd immunity is a folly—so who's funding this bad science? 2020. Accessed May 17, 2021. https://www.theguardian.com/commentisfree/2020/oct/18/covid-herd-immunity-funding-bad-science-anti-lockdown

6. Correia S, Luck S, Verner E. Pandemics depress the economy, public health interventions do not: Evidence from the 1918 flu. SSRN. 2020. March 3, 2020. https://papers.ssrn.com/sol3/papers.cfm?abstract_id=3561560

7. Warner KE, Fulton GA, Nicolas P, Grimes DR. Employment implications of declining tobacco product sales for the regional economies of the United States. *JAMA*. 1996; 275(16): 1241–1246.

8. A. D. Little International. Public balance of smoking in the Czech Republic. Report to Philip Morris CR. 2001. Accessed June 19, 2021. https://web.archive.org/web/20111001035336/http://hspm.sph.sc.edu/courses/Econ/Classes/cba cea/czechsmokingcost.html

9. Fairclough G. Philip Morris apologizes for report touting benefits of smokers' deaths. *The Wall Street Journal*. 2013. Accessed May 14, 2021. https://www.wsj.com/articles/SB996102070519922105

10. Ross H. Critique of the Philip Morris study of the cost of smoking in the Czech Republic. *Nicotine Tob Res*. 2004; 6(1): 181–189.

11. ASH. ASH research shows corner shops don't need tobacco to be profitable. 2016. Accessed May 17, 2021. https://ash.org.uk/media-and-news/press-releases-media-and-news/ash-research-shows-corner-shops-dont-need-tobacco-to-be-profitable/#:~:text=For%20retailers%2C%20average%20profit%20margins,24.1%25%20for%20all%20other%20products

12. Scollo M, Lal A, Hyland A, Glantz S. Review of the quality of studies on the economic effects of smoke-free policies on the hospitality industry. *Tob Control*. 2003; 12(1): 13–20.

13. Campbell N, Mialon M, Reilly K, Browne S, Finucane FM. How are frames generated? Insights from the industry lobby against the sugar tax in Ireland. *Social Sci Med*. 2020; 264: 113215.

14. Zatonski M, Hawkins B, McKee M. Framing the policy debate over spirits excise tax in Poland. *Health Promot Int*. 2018; 33(3): 515–524.

15. Bhattacharya A. *Splitting the bill: Alcohol's impact on the economy*. Institute of Alcohol Studies; 2017.

16. McCambridge J, Daube M, McKee M. Brussels Declaration: A vehicle for the advancement of tobacco and alcohol industry interests at the science/policy interface? *Tob Control*. 2019; 28(1): 7.

17. Diethelm PA, Rielle JC, McKee M. The whole truth and nothing but the truth? The research that Philip Morris did not want you to see. *Lancet*. 2005; 366(9479): 86–92.

18. Laverty AA, Diethelm P, Hopkinson NS, Watt HC, McKee M. Use and abuse of statistics in tobacco industry-funded research on standardised packaging. *Tob Control*. 2015; 24(5): 422–424.
19. Barnes DE, Bero LA. Industry-funded research and conflict of interest: An analysis of research sponsored by the tobacco industry through the Center for Indoor Air Research. *J Health Polit Policy Law*. 1996; 21(3): 515–542.
20. Lange S, Vollmer S. The effect of economic development on population health: A review of the empirical evidence. *Br Med Bull*. 2017; 121(1): 47–60.
21. McKee M, Kluge H. Include, invest, innovate: Health systems for prosperity and solidarity. *J Health Serv Res Policy*. 2018; 23(4): 209–211.
22. World Health Organization. *Report of the Commission on Macroeconomics and Health*. World Health Organization; 2002.
23. Fogel RW. *Economic Growth, Population Theory, and Physiology: The Bearing of Long-Term Processes on the Making of Economic Policy*. National Bureau of Economic Research; 1994.
24. Arora S. Health, human productivity, and long-term economic growth. *J Econ Hist*. 2001; 61(3): 699–749.
25. Barro R. *Health and Economic Growth*. World Health Organization; 1996.
26. Bloom DE, Canning D, Sevilla J. *The Effect of Health on Economic Growth: Theory and Evidence*. National Bureau of Economic Research; 2001.
27. Strittmatter A, Sunde U. Health and economic development—Evidence from the introduction of public health care. *J Popul Econ*. 2013; 26(4): 1549–1584.
28. Cervellati M, Sunde U. Life expectancy and economic growth: The role of the demographic transition. *J Econ Growth*. 2011; 16(2): 99–133.
29. Bleakley H. Health, human capital, and development. *Annu Rev Econ*. 2010; 2(1): 283–310.
30. Rocco L, Fumagalli E, Mirelman AJ, Suhrcke M. Mortality, morbidity and economic growth. *PLoS One*. 2021; 16(5): e0251424.
31. Suhrcke M, McKee M, Stuckler D, Arce RS, Tsolova S, Mortensen J. The contribution of health to the economy in the European Union. *Public Health*. 2006; 120(11): 994–1001.
32. Marmot M. The health gap: The challenge of an unequal world: The argument. *Int J Epidemiol*. 2017; 46(4): 1312–1318.
33. McCord C, Freeman HP. Excess mortality in Harlem. *N Engl J Med*. 1990; 322(3): 173–177.
34. Wilson M, Daly M. Life expectancy, economic inequality, homicide, and reproductive timing in Chicago neighbourhoods. *BMJ*. 1997; 314(7089): 1271–1274.
35. Jäckle R, Himmler O. Health and Wages Panel data estimates considering selection and endogeneity. *J Hum Resour*. 2010; 45(2): 364–406.
36. Luft HS. The impact of poor health on earnings. *Rev Econ Statistics*. 1975; 57(2): 43–57.
37. Bartel A, Taubman P. Some economic and demographic consequences of mental illness. *J Labor Econ*. 1986; 4(2): 243–256.
38. Gannon B, Nolan B. Disability and labour market participation. 2003. Accessed May 5, 2021. https://ideas.repec.org/p/esr/wpaper/hrb04.html
39. Chirikos TN, Nestel G. Further evidence on the economic effects of poor health. *Rev Econ Statist*. 1985; 67(1): 61–69.
40. Hagan R, Jones AM, Rice N. Health and retirement in Europe. *Int J Environ Res Public Health*. 2009; 6(10): 2676–2695.
41. Sammartino FJ. The effect of health on retirement. *Soc Sec Bull*. 1987; 50: 31.

42. Haas SA, Fosse NE. Health and the educational attainment of adolescents: Evidence from the NLSY97. *J Health Soc Behav.* 2008; 49(2): 178–192.
43. Himmelstein DU, Warren E, Thorne D, Woolhandler S. Illness and injury as contributors to bankruptcy. *Health Aff.* 2005; Suppl Web Exclusives: W5-63–w5-73.
44. Masters R, Anwar E, Collins B, Cookson R, Capewell S. Return on investment of public health interventions: A systematic review. *J Epidemiol Community Health.* 2017; 71(8): 827.

CHAPTER 26

Prioritizing Research on the Foundational Drivers of Corporate Policy Influence

WILLIAM H. WIIST

26.1 INTRODUCTION

This chapter "nudges" commercial and corporate determinants of health (CDOH) researchers to metaphorically look "below the surface" to the "root causes" and to move further "upstream" to the "cause of causes" of CDOH. The chapter proposes that CDOH research prioritize three corporate political tactics used in democracies, amounting to legal corruption, that provide the foundation of laws, policies, and regulations that enable all other CDOH strategies and tactics. The chapter provides guidance for making such research theory-based, using tried and tested social science methods and data sources. The United States is presented as a case study to stimulate CDOH researchers of other countries or different political systems to likewise seek out foundational tactics of corporate influence on policy and identify or develop research data sources. Acknowledging that some corporations provide beneficial products or operate with little detrimental effect, the chapter's perspective is polemically oppositional[1] to the pervasive influence and dominating power of for-profit corporations.

26.2 HISTORY OF CORPORATIONS IN THE UNITED STATES

History is important because it conditions our consciousness and helps motivate our desire to bring about change. The history of corporate influence and

William H. Wiist, *Prioritizing Research on the Foundational Drivers of Corporate Policy Influence* In: *The Commercial Determinants of Health.* Edited by: Nason Maani, Mark Petticrew, and Sandro Galea, Oxford University Press.
© Oxford University Press 2023. DOI: 10.1093/oso/9780197578742.003.0026

power in the United States is well documented,[2] and understanding that history helps identify and illuminate contemporary corporations' strategies and tactics and also strategies and tools for change. CDOH researchers could benefit from recalling the history of tactics used by the early textile, mining, railroad, asbestos, and lead industries and from relying on, but moving beyond, contemporary corporate historical analyses that already identified most, if not all, of the corporate "playbook"[3] and tactics.[4,5]

26.3 THE ORIGINS AND HISTORY OF U.S. CORPORATE POWER AND INFLUENCE

A CDOH researcher would not consider unusual a description of an industry or corporation whose product globally dominates; with wealthy elite male ownership and management; of fluctuating financial conditions; financed by banks or investors in New York and London; closely integrated with transportation industries; supported by government subsidies and financing, accommodating policies, and laws; supported by elected officials invested in the industry and by sympathetic judges; geographically expanding by usurping public resources; surveilling, systematically monitoring, and recording daily productivity of workers in specialized jobs; mechanized to reduce labor costs; reliant on women's and children's labor; compensating workers with unhealthful housing and inadequate food, resulting in high rates of morbidity and mortality; restricted site egress enforced by armed private guards; supervision with severe discipline; worker rebellions; specialized publications promoting efficiency; "would be" entrepreneurs eager to become owners or suppliers; use of military might, including invasion to ensure industry survival; an organization that dominates conditions in a country; and/or one founded on and perpetuating a specific ideology.

This description is not of a contemporary online order fulfillment warehouse or a U.S. electronics or garment firm sited in a low-income country. It describes the first dominant industry in North America—18th and 19th centuries' enslaved encampment cotton agriculture that, although not a single corporation, was the forerunner of today's modern factory.[6] It was a transnational industry powered by cruel and abhorrent industrial commodification of human beings: the enslavement, purchase, transport, and sale of Africans and their descendants, who individually and communally, as Black Americans, now embody its traumatic vestiges and experience continuation of disparities, inequalities, and injustice. Like contemporary corporations, the industry was based in the constitution, the law, policy, and regulation that resulted from the industry's influence on legislators and the executive branch, sympathizers in government policymaking positions, the judiciary, and from money.

The description illustrates that the types of strategies, tactics, and ideologies by which contemporary U.S. industries and corporations operate are not new. The North American British colonies founded in the 1600s were chartered corporations (e.g., Virginia and Massachusetts) with enslaved Africans transported to the colonies by corporate-owned ships. Although framers of the U.S. polity espoused ideals of liberty and democracy drawn from ancient Europe, corporations and enslavement also originated in 15th- to 18th-century European dualistic ideologies encoded into philosophical, governing, religious, and scientific documents.[7,8] Those codes expressed the right to subjugate nature; to take, own, and "make productive" "vacant" and "unsettled" land (*terra nullius*) occupied by Indigenous Peoples; and to conquer by violence. They concocted a hierarchy of "race" (racism) in which light-colored skin supposedly indicated biological, intellectual, and social "superiority" (White supremacy) of people who, by natural right, could dominate, suppress, own, and kill people of darker skin deemed to be "things" that were "inferior," "subhuman," "without souls," and "lazy." The codes also created patriarchy, private property, an elite economic class, and wage labor. The ideologies were mainly designed to serve personal and political economic interests, and corporations through their strategies and tactics became for-profit vectors spreading the ideologies. In the late 1800s' U.S. "gilded age," corporate monopolies and their owners wielded power over government and enriched themselves by the continued exploitation of laborers and the environment. Later, corporations built on two world wars to grow their political and economic power. More recently, the ideologies "evolved" into the neoliberal financialized foundation of globalization that granted today's short-term stock share-boosting corporations' agency over governments and other institutions, societies, and the natural environment.[9] And, through each era, imbricated with corporations, the ideology of institutional, structural, and interpersonal White supremacy continued.

Although in the United States during the 1700s and 1800s corporations were controversial, state governments and court rulings began creating and chartering the artificial entity of the corporation and endowing it with privileges and authorizations. An expansion of corporate rights began based on a false but perpetuated notion that corporations are "persons,"[10] with the rights held by human citizens to sue and be sued; diversify and be integrated with other corporate units; own stock; initiate and sign contracts; equal protection under the law; due process; freedom from unreasonable searches; jury trial in criminal and civil cases; compensation for government takings; freedom from double jeopardy; commercial speech; political speech; freedom of religion; sue governments for loss of anticipated profits; shareholders subordinate to management; shareholders with limited liability; and unlimited life span. Many of these rights resulted from rulings of the U.S. Supreme Court, especially those on the 1st Amendment (free speech) and the 14th Amendment (intended to ensure rights of the formerly enslaved but used many more times for corporate rights).[2] Every CDOH strategy and tactic, and every corporate practice, policy, procedure, product, or service, is founded on government laws and regulations based on the rights granted to the "artificial person," the "juristic person"—that is, the corporate entity. For example, corporate marketing, advertising, public relations, research publications, and political activities are based on the corporate right to commercial and political speech.

26.4 RECOMMENDATIONS FOR THREE CDOH POLICY RESEARCH PRIORITIES

Within the complex system of corporate strategies and tactics, not all have equal influence. Underlying the laws, policies, and regulations governing corporations are three corporate tactics on which all other CDOH strategies and tactics are founded. With those three tactics, U.S. corporations wield legally corrupt power and influence over government disproportionate to that of individual human persons and their advocacy organizations, or other institutions. Corporations use the three tactics to try to counter the democratic power of the citizen vote. Those three tactics should be the primary focus of CDOH researchers who study countries with democratically elected governments. In countries with other forms of government or with weak or incomplete institutionalization of democracy, researchers may first need to determine the underlying source of corporate influence (e.g., bribery).

Centering research on the three priority tactics would eliminate repetitive "siloed" industry research to identify CDOH tactics, provide a cohesive conceptual rationale, and foster more efficient use of research and advocacy resources. The three are also more proximal than other CDOH tactics to policy solutions for corporations' role in the critical public health issues of wealth inequality, climate change, and systemic racism and sexism.

Most important, CDOH research on the three tactics is critical because they are corporations' fundamental attacks on democracy's essential promise of liberty and freedom. Democracy is the best system of governance humans have yet designed to facilitate freedom of expression; participation in governance; ensure social, political, economic, and health equality, justice, and peace; protect nature; pursue happiness; reap the fruits of one's efforts; and avoid authoritarianism, tyranny, exploitation, and bondage. CDOH research on the three priorities can make an important contribution to protecting democracy and facilitating the realization of democracy's potential.

The three priority tactics are

- corporate election campaign donations to legislative, executive, and judicial candidates from corporate funds and from corporate executives and board

members (but could also include donations from individuals who became wealthy from corporate compensation or stock, and donations from corporate charitable foundations and from philanthropic foundations predominantly founded on and/or existing on corporate-derived funding);
- corporate lobbying of elected and appointed government officials and bureaucrats; and
- the "reverse revolving door" of corporate political appointees to positions in government policy and decision-making positions and in regulatory agencies, commissions, committees, boards, and as legislative staff.

Corporations focus the three tactics on the legislative and executive branches but also indirectly influence the judiciary by influencing executive branch appointments of judges and at the state level where many judges are elected and campaign donations lead to pro-business rulings.[11]

26.5 RESEARCH ON ELECTION CAMPAIGN CONTRIBUTIONS, LOBBYING, AND THE REVERSE REVOLVING DOOR

Political scientists, economists, legal scholars, and others have conducted research on the influence of corporate political activity, often with inconsistent, contingent, and sometimes contradictory results.[12] A detailed review of that research is beyond the scope of this chapter, and only a few affirmative generalizations are provided. However, because corporate wealth provides disproportionate power and the public believes that campaign money corrupts politics[13] although research results are mixed, more information is provided about campaign donations. Little empirical public health research about the three tactics has been conducted.[14]

26.5.1 Election Campaign Donations

Every election cycle, billions of dollars are raised and spent on campaigns, and the amounts continue to grow. Election campaign donations can be made to candidates, political parties, political action committees (PACs) and super PACs, and certain not-for-profit organizations. Corporate campaign contributions are important because elections are a direct threat to corporations' dominance of government policymaking. The 2010 U.S. Supreme Court ruling in the *Citizens United v. FCC* case allows corporations an unlimited amount of independent spending directly from their corporate treasury.[10]

Campaign contributions give access to politicians[13] and friendly relations that can lead to corporate benefits and give the appearance of quid pro quo corruption, so legislators prefer low-visibility influence, which may account for research results being divided about the influence of contributions.[15] Only positive associations are presented here.

Campaign donations and resulting expenditures seem to determine election winners.[16] Companies that give more to candidates receive more government contracts and show increased profits.[17] Those that receive the most corporate PAC money are more likely to vote favorably toward the contributing industry.[18] Contributions lead to congressional votes that support pro-business spending and non-expenditure programs.[19] Although one-third of congressional roll call votes show the effect of campaign contributions,[18] money is more likely to influence a legislator earlier and in less scrutinized aspects of the legislative process than voting. Industry money mobilizes supportive congressional committee members' participation in activities to promote industries' position on bills.[20] Corporate lobbyists' contributions to a member of a congressional committee that developed the Affordable Care Act legislation ("Obamacare") increased the bill's similarity to the contributor's preferences.[21] Contributions also serve as a "signal" to government regulators that enforcement against a company may be costly.[22] The greater a corporation's political expenditures, the fewer citations for safety violations by the Occupational Safety and Health Administration.[22] Members of congress who vote against environmental policies receive increased campaign contributions from fossil fuel industries,[23] and the more contributed, the less the likelihood that members will vote pro-environment.[24] Corporations also expend large amounts of campaign money to defeat direct democratic processes (e.g., ballot initiatives).[25]

26.5.2 Lobbying

Lobbyists are individuals or firms paid to represent a client's interests on government legislation and regulations and/or the public. Most lobbyists represent corporations rather than other organizations. In the United States, those who meet certain requirements are required by law to register with Congress (10,000–14,000 do so), but the number of lobbyists in Washington, DC, is probably 20,000[26] to 100,000[27] because some avoid registration. Lobbying disclosure laws are, in general, unenforced. Corporations may have in-house lobbyists, often in a government affairs office, or they may contract with an external lobbying firm and/or join an industry membership association that lobbies. Many members of Congress and Congressional staff become lobbyists after they leave government. Each year, corporations spend unprecedented billions (more than PAC donations) lobbying the government, including spending by the pharmaceutical and health products industries, hospital organizations, and health professions' organizations. The election campaign donations lobbyists provide give them access to elected government officials.

The targets of lobbying efforts are often members of Congress who chair or are members of committees that have budget and regulatory oversight of the industry the lobbyist represents. Elected officials and their staff have come to view lobbyists as expert advisors, so there are many leverage points within the complex processes of Congress for the passage of legislation where lobbyists assert influence. They meet with legislators and staff members, propose bills, draft bills, provide legislation templates, submit comments on legislation, and testify at hearings. They also lobby the President, political appointees to regulatory agencies, and bureaucrats who write rules and enforce regulations. Although lobbying does not guarantee results, it bends policy toward preferences of corporate interests.[28]

26.5.3 Reverse Revolving Door

The term *reverse revolving door* ("reverse revolvers") refers to the more than 4,000 political appointments a President makes from the private sector (many from corporations) to decision-making or policymaking positions in government regulatory agencies, commissions, boards, and committees. Former lobbyists hired to staff congressional committees are also reverse revolvers. An example of a reverse revolver is the executive of GlaxoSmithKline and board member of the pharmaceutical and biotechnology company Moderna who was appointed by the President to be the chief adviser for Operation Warp Speed, the group that vetted potential coronavirus vaccines and treatments and decided whether they should receive federal funding. Corporate stock returns improve when an industry official is appointed to a government position.[29]

Reverse revolvers may continue to identify with industry peers and carry their corporate worldview (e.g., profit motivation, reduce regulation, and lower corporate taxes) into their government positions. Those predispositions can bias their actions in favor of business at the expense of public welfare ("corporate capture"). They are likely to make decisions favorable to specific industries or companies with the award of contracts and with less strict regulatory scrutiny and enforcement, sometimes for the possibility of future industry employment. Agency regulators are likely to adopt policies close to the preferences of those with political oversight.

26.6 METHODS AND DATA RESOURCES FOR RESEARCH ON THE THREE PRIORITIES

26.6.1 Research Methods

Commercial determinants of health researchers need to build upon research about corporate political activity and related concepts conducted by political science, policy studies, public administration, economics, law, sociology, business, linguistics and discourse analysis, anthropology, history, and neuropsychology. They also need to become familiar with journal publications in those fields and, when reviewing the evidence, conduct literature searches using field-specific terminology such as "non-market strategies," "interest groups," "regulatory capture," "political agency," "rent-seeking," "free rider," and "social distance."

CDOH researchers also need to use theory to help structure research ideas, test plausibility, explain causality, and interpret results. They can integrate traditional public health biological, behavioral, and social epidemiology theories with social science theories used specifically to study corporate political activity[30] while incorporating perspectives from critical race theory, feminist theory, and Indigenous Peoples' theories.

To advance the CDOH research agenda,[31] researchers need to draw upon social sciences methodologies[32] and combine them with those of public health, such as policy surveillance (see http://publichealthlawresearch.org/content/policy-surveillance-program). Methods used to study corporate political activity include the Herfindhal Index, a measure of the inclusion of corporate preferences in laws and regulations, and the Scholes–Williams event-study method for examining a company's performance when a former employee is in a government position. Social network analysis has been used to study connections between regulators and corporations and also the disproportionate power relations between transnational corporations. Innovations in text analysis software have facilitated analysis of legislative documents. Monetary decision-making tasks (e.g., trust game/investment game) and brain scans (functional magnetic resonance imaging [fMRI]) have elucidated the areas of the brain in which processing of the psychological aspects of the revolving door occurs. Both fMRI and electroencephalography, as well as other physiological response measures to psychological tests, have been used to study the activation of specific regions of the brain by political attitudes and the effects of ideological preferences on judgment and behavior.[33]

Because of the uniqueness and expanse of accumulated knowledge in the social science research on the three priority tactics, CDOH researchers need to work in interdisciplinary teams. Effective interdisciplinary collaborative research necessitates researchers' willingness to spend time in team training and planning to build trust and gain understanding of differing viewpoints, theories, ideology, frameworks, methods, and data sources, as well as learning how to deal with potential power conflicts, personalities, and institutional processes and procedures that create barriers to interdisciplinary research.

26.6.2 Research Data Sources

There are challenges to data collection and reliability, but some data sources about election campaign financing, lobbying, and the reverse revolving door used in quantitative research have previously been identified[14(p177–178)] and are supplemented here for the U.S. context.

Lobbyist.info is an online subscription-based database of lobbyist registrations, names of lobbyists and lobbying firms, their backgrounds, contact information, and clients. *FollowTheMoney* provides data about sources and amounts of election campaign donations to state legislators. The Mercatus Center database (*RegData*) contains industry-specific U.S. federal regulations (and those of other countries) that can be combined with regulatory data from other data sets available through *QuatGov*. The U.S. Office of Personnel Management database identifies senior-level government appointees and regulators, and the Government Accountability Office maintains a database of temporarily filled executive positions. The Congressional *Yellow Book* identifies staff responsibilities. The Office of Information and Regulatory Affairs provides an overview of the federal regulatory actions, and the U.S. Independent Regulatory Commissioner Data Base is also available online. The Center for Economic and Policy Research's *Agency Spotlight* and proprietary databases about corporate employees such as *BoardEx* are potential sources for revolving door research. The University of California San Francisco Industry Documents Library is a searchable digital archive of documents from the tobacco, pharmaceutical, chemical, food, and fossil fuel industries.

Varieties of Democracy (V-Dem) provides data sets with 350 indicators for democracies in 177 countries from 1900 to the present. The International Institute for Democracy and Electoral Assistance provides searchable databases about political finance regulations. Transparency International makes available the database it uses for country rankings by public sector corruption (*Corruption Perceptions Index*). A proprietary source, *Opencorporates*, makes available (free for public benefit projects) databases of corporate information for millions of companies and officers worldwide.

26.6.3 Sources of CDOH Research Questions

Commercial determinants of health researchers need to recognize the complexity of the processes of election campaign donations, lobbying, and the reverse revolving door in order to avoid "straight-line thinking" of cause and effect in how laws, policies, and regulations come about; ask research questions within that complexity; and use equivalently complex designs, methodologies, and statistical techniques. For example, in assessing whether corporate campaign donations buy access to politicians, whether their behavior then changes, and if that translates into policy helpful to the corporation, researchers need to examine legislators' low-visibility reciprocal favors for donations (e.g., adding amendments in committee).[21] In addition to developing research questions based on previous empirical research[34] and theory,[35] ideas for meaningful policy research questions can come from advocacy organizations, serving policy roles in government or not-for-profit organizations, participating in political campaigns and party roles, observing policy hearings, participating in academic faculty governance, and from community research collaborators.

26.6.4 Dissemination of Policy Research Results

Commercial determinants of health policy researchers need to remember that factors other than health motivate policy and that facts alone are insufficient to bring about policy change. They must effectively communicate their methods and results to policymakers, advocates, and community members by making communication relevant to their interests and backgrounds.[36] Planning for communicating persuasively should occur at the beginning of the research, with consideration given to timing, context, circumstances, audience, and appropriate media. Policy briefings or a consensus statement from a credible panel of experts are commonly used to present results and policy recommendations.

26.7 CONCLUSION

In countries with democratically elected governments, lobbying, election campaign donations, and the reverse revolving door are the foundation of all other corporate tactics and should be priorities for quantitative and qualitative empirical CDOH policy research. Such CDOH research needs to be founded on existing social science theories, empirical research, methods, and data sources, and it needs to be conducted in interdisciplinary collaborative teams. Such research could significantly advance the CDOH field by contributing to policy reforms to liberate the ideals and practice of democratic governance from corporations' dominating power.[37]

REFERENCES

1. Wiist WH. Public health and the anticorporate movement: Rationale and recommendations. *Am J Public Health*. 2006; 96(8): 1370–1375.
2. Hartmann T. *Unequal Protection: The Rise of Corporate Dominance and the Theft of Human Rights*. Berrett-Koehler; 2002.
3. Brownell KD, Warner KE. The perils of ignoring history: Big Tobacco played dirty and millions died. How similar is Big Food? *Milbank Q*. 2009; 87(1): 259–294.
4. Wiist WH. The corporation: An overview of what it is, its tactics, and what public health can do. In: Wiist WH, ed. *The Bottom Line or Public Health: Tactics*

Corporations Use to Influence Health and Health Policy, and What We Can Do to Counter Them. Oxford University Press; 2010: 3–72.

5. Wiist WH. The corporate play book, health, and democracy: The snack food and beverage industry's tactics in context. In: Stuckler D, Siegel K, eds. *Sick Societies: Responding to the Global Challenge of Chronic Disease*. Oxford University Press; 2011: 204–216.

6. Beckert S, Rockman S. eds. *Slavery's Capitalism: A New History of American Economic Development*. University of Pennsylvania Press; 2016.

7. Stewart-Harawira M. *The New Imperial Order: Indigenous Responses to Globalization*. Zed; 2005.

8. Patel R, Moore JW. *A History of the World in Seven Cheap Things: A Guide to Capitalism, Nature, and the Future of the Planet*. University of California Press; 2017.

9. Wiist B. A framework for analyzing the corporation as a global governing agency. Paper presented at Simon Fraser University Corporations and Global Health Research Network, September 2013, Vancouver, Canada. 2013. Accessed April 15, 2021. https://www.academia.edu/45046063/A_Framework_for_Analyzing_the_Corporation_as_a_Global_Governing_Agency_public_health

10. Wiist WH. Citizens United, public health and democracy: The Supreme Court ruling, its implications, and proposed action. *Am J Public Health*. 2011; 101: 1172–1197.

11. Sheppard J. Justice at risk: An empirical analysis of campaign contributions and judicial decisions. American Constitution Society for Law and Policy. 2013. Accessed February 18, 2014. https://www.acslaw.org/analysis/reports/justice-at-risk

12. Puck J, Lawton T, Mohr A. The corporate political activity of MNCs: Taking stock and moving forward. *Manag Int Rev*. 2018; 58: 663–673.

13. Kalla JL, Broockman DE. Campaign contributions facilitate access to congressional officials: A randomized field experiment. *Am J Polit Sci*. 2016; 60(3): 545–558.

14. Wiist WH. Studying the influence of corporations on democratic processes. In: Lee K, Hawkins B, eds. *Researching Corporations and Global Health Governance: An Interdisciplinary Guide*. Rowman & Littlefield; 2017.

15. Stratmann T. Some talk: Money in politics. A (partial) review of the literature. *Public Choice*. 2005; 124: 135–156.

16. Harvey A. Is campaign spending a cause or an effect? Reexamining the empirical foundations of *Buckley v. Valeo* (1976). *Supreme Court Econ Rev*. 2019; 27: 67–110.

17. Witko C. Campaign contributions, access, and government contracting. *J Public Adm Res Theory*. 2011; 21(4): 761–778.

18. Roscoe DD, Jenkins S. A meta-analysis of campaign contributions' impact on roll call voting. *Soc Sci Q*. 2005; 86(1): 52–68.

19. Fellowes MC, Wolf PJ. Funding mechanisms and policy instruments: How business campaign contributions influence congressional votes. *Polit Res Q*. 2004; 57(2): 315–324.

20. Hall RL, Wayman FW. Buying time: Moneyed interests and the mobilization of bias in congressional committees. *Am Polit Sci Rev*. 1990; 84(3): 797–820.

21. McKay AM. Buying amendments? Lobbyists' campaign contributions and micro-legislation in the creation of the Affordable Care Act. *Legislative Stud Q*. 2020; 45(2): 327–360.

22. Witko C. Party government and variation in corporate influence on agency decision making: OSHA regulation, 1981–2006. *Soc Sci Q*. 2013; 94(4): 894–911.

23. Goldberga MH, Marlon JR, Wang X, van der Linden S, Leiserowitz A. Oil and gas companies invest in legislators that vote against the environment. *Proc Natl Acad Sci USA*. 2020; 117(10): 5111–5112.

24. Ard K, Garcia N, Kelly P. Another avenue of action: An examination of climate change countermovement industries' use of PAC donations and their relationship to congressional voting over time. *Environ Polit*. 2017; 26(6): 1107–1131.

25. Nichols J, McChesney RW. *Dollarocracy: How the Money-and-Media Election Complex Is Destroying America*. Nation Books; 2013.

26. Thomas HF, LaPira TM. How many lobbyists are in Washington? Shadow lobbying and the gray market for policy advocacy. *Int Groups Adv*. 2017; 6: 199–214.

27. Thurber JA. The contemporary presidency: Changing the way Washington works? Assessing President Obama's battle with lobbyists. *Presidential Stud Q*. 2011; 41(2): 358–374.

28. Drutman L. *The Business of America Is Lobbying: How Corporations Became Politicized and Politics Became More Corporate*. Oxford University Press; 2015.

29. Luechinger S, Moser C. The value of the revolving door: Political appointees and the stock market. *J Public Econ*. 2014; 119: 93–107.

30. Mellahi K, Frynas JG, Sun P, Siegel D. A review of the nonmarket strategy literature: Toward a multi-theoretical integration. *J Manag*. 2016; 42(1): 143–173.

31. Maani N, McKee M, Petticrew M, Galea S. Corporate practices and the health of populations: A research and translational agenda. *Lancet Public Health*. 2020; 5(2): e80–e81.

32. de Figueiredo JM, Richter BK. Advancing the empirical research on lobbying. *Annu Rev Polit Sci*. 2014; 17: 163–185.

33. Jost JT, Nam HH, Amodio DM, Van Bave JJ. Political neuroscience: The beginning of a beautiful friendship. *Adv Polit Psychol*. 2014; 35(Suppl 1): 3–42.

34. Lawton T, McGuire S, Rajwani T. Corporate political activity: a Literature review and research agenda. *Int J Manag Rev*. 2013; 15(1): 86–105.

35. Ciepley D. Beyond public and private: Toward a political theory of the corporation. *Am Polit Sci Rev*. 2013; 107(1): 139–158.

36. Moodie R. Where different worlds collide: Expanding the influence of research and researchers on policy. *J Public Health Policy*. 2009; 30: S33–S37.

37. Wood B, Baker P, Sacks G. Conceptualising the commercial determinants of health using a power lens: A review and synthesis of existing frameworks. *Int J Health Policy Manag*. 2021. doi:10.34172/ijhpm.2021.05

CHAPTER 27

The Influence of Commercial Industries on Public Discourse

SHONA HILTON

27.1 INTRODUCTION

This chapter investigates the influence that commercial industries have on public discourse about health and health policy. It first describes how commercial companies use the media to shape public and policymakers' opinion in favor of weak regulation aligned to their business interests. It explores how industries gain traction and legitimize their role in regulatory debates, especially through framing strategies. Next, the chapter outlines new empirical work that is advancing scholarship on how commercial companies influence public discourse. It identifies the need to build on this research by comparing different policy domains and industry sectors. Such comparative research could provide further explanation for variation in public discourses across harmful products and industries. The chapter concludes by suggesting that research in this domain could transform how the practices of corporate actors are publicly debated and help create a space for advocates and regulators to better influence and promote regulation to protect public health.

27.2 GAINING TRACTION AND LEGITIMACY IN HEALTH DEBATES

The media are one of the most powerful fora commercial actors have to influence public discourse (communications in the public domain). Such public discourses in the media are important because they determine the issues

Shona Hilton, *The Influence of Commercial Industries on Public Discourse* In: *The Commercial Determinants of Health.* Edited by: Nason Maani, Mark Petticrew, and Sandro Galea, Oxford University Press. © Oxford University Press 2023. DOI: 10.1093/oso/9780197578742.003.0027 and related information to which people are exposed.[1] The media reflect, reinforce, and shape common discourses about public health policy. Corporate actors are very aware of this, so they use the media to "gain traction" in such debates.[2] One way they do this is by supplying journalists with quotes and material for articles. This might include findings from industry-funded research, data from public opinion polls, and quotes in press releases. For instance, an analysis of stories in British daily newspapers showed that in many instances, media texts could be traced back verbatim to industry press releases.[3] Being directly quoted in the media in this way enables corporate actors to become part of the conversation, a "legitimate" stakeholder in the evolving debate, and, importantly, part of the solution.[4] An example of this in the fossil fuel industry refers to framing and advertorials in newspapers, linked to individual responsibility versus corporate liability.[5]

News coverage of health policies typically contains direct quotes from both commercial and other stakeholders.[6] Being quoted alongside representatives of academic, health, and government institutions may put commercial stakeholders on an equal footing in the eyes of audiences. This legitimacy is used to promote positive public and political perceptions of their activities and foster public support for regulations more in alignment with business interests.

As well as engaging directly and overtly in media content, corporations engage indirectly through sympathetic think tanks[7] or industry-sponsored organizations presenting themselves as grassroots movements.[8] For example, tobacco companies have funded a range of groups throughout the world intended to allow them to "speak as the smoker" in undermining evidence and resisting regulation[9]—for instance, Smokepeace in Sweden or Smokers' Rights Club in Denmark, which are often quoted in media reporting.[10] In these ways, commercial actors use both direct and indirect tactics in the media to influence and, at times, pollute public discourse to undermine or prevent health regulation that is perceived to impact on their profitability. Industry's conflicts of interest and ultimate responsibility to its shareholders are often missing in such debates, which works to industry's advantage.[11]

Twenty-four-hour broadcast and internet news mean tighter deadlines for journalists and increasing pressure to produce more material faster, often with fewer resources.[12] Thus, journalists often have less time to research issues in any depth, instead increasingly relying on externally produced stories and information.[13] These media pressures give commercial actors an opportunity to be an easy source of content, to construct themselves as legitimate partners, and to present arguments in debates, often with little journalistic scrutiny. It provides a public forum to present their own corporate-funded research using researchers sympathetic to corporate causes or products. In this unquestioning media climate, industry can attack legitimate scientific institutions and government agencies, presenting them as acting against market interests. Such tactics undermine the authenticity, integrity, and credibility of scientists and ultimately cast doubt over the strength of evidence in debates.[14] Importantly, these tactics allows corporate industries to lobby for less effective measures and voluntary codes while presenting themselves as a legitimate and responsible actor. In this way, corporations tactically achieve policy influence while emphasizing their corporate social responsibility credentials. An example of this is the ongoing sponsorship of *Washington Post* advertorials by Philip Morris International.[15,16]

27.3 FRAMING AND SETTING THE PARAMETERS OF THE DEBATE

In a contemporary and increasingly saturated information landscape, where people are bombarded daily with health information, highly skilled corporate actors need to direct public attention. They need to construct the issues and channel public attention to some elements while obscuring other elements, altering the public's perceptions of their relative importance.[17,18] In this way, they set the "parameters" of the debate through cherry-picking facts. Corporate actors often direct public attention to the fact that problems are complex and argue that uncertainty is inherent in scientific endeavor. This helps focus public attention on the challenges rather than the causes or solutions. It raises questions for the public on the status of established scientific knowledge, and, importantly, it encourages people to think that "nothing can be done until everything is done."[19] Such complexity narratives in public discourse are part of setting the parameters of the debate. It suggests that the problem is so complex and an insurmountable challenge that stalling regulation makes sense. In debates on sugar-sweetened beverage taxes to decrease the risk for obesity, causes were described as "far more complex" and the contribution of sugary drinks was downplayed.[20] Complexity arguments may also be created by offering facts that may be true but are irrelevant to the debate or by creating false dichotomies. This distracts public attention away from the real issues at hand and again leads us toward a sense that the challenge is insurmountable.

Another tactic that helps influence public opinion is to create consistent arguments over a period of time. Employing consistent messages in line with their business interests over time is important in cultivating and consolidating people's ideas on a debate and about viable policy options. This is central to Gerbner's cultivation theory of mass media processes and effects, which proposes that the more a person hears or sees a message, the more it might shape their social reality and worldview.[21] Indeed, by cultivating people's views over time in favor of a particular policy option, commercial industries engineer a societal "homogenization effect." This acts as a kind of mainstreaming of public discourse, priming people to accept policies that benefit commerce. Cultivating people's beliefs is important because the level of debate about policies or a particular public health issue does not always equate to any change in the severity of the problem. Taking the example of climate change, the refrain that technological advances will obviate the need for regulation is a common discourse linked to the notion that problems are best solved through the marketplace. Again, such narratives often channel public attention to less effective policies in line with corporate interests.

Another way commercial industry influences how the public thinks and informs its opinions about public health issues is *framing*. Rarely do people encounter messages about public health as a blank canvas. Corporate actors can use framing as a conduit to promote particular ways of thinking about an issue.[22] Within the broader media literature and study of political communications, there are various definitions of different framing methodologies.[23] Fundamentally, framing involves the generation of beliefs and ideas that provide a structure for thinking about an issue. Importantly, what makes it so powerful is that people are largely unaware of framing most of the time. This power in manipulating public views, voting patterns, and political strategies led framing to be described as a key "weapon of advocacy" and a potent tool to influence the public policy agenda.[24]

Scholars are becoming increasingly interested in examining how commercial actors frame and package ideas about public health policies. This may include how commercial actors construct meaning and open up or close down discursive debate in favor of certain policy options. It may identify which issues are prioritized or deprioritized in different aspects of policies and which issues are highlighted or omitted. And it may consider how specific aspects of frames are constructed to influence how people understand a policy.[6,25,26] An important construct in framing is what Entman describes as influential, salience-based conceptualization of framing.[18] He identifies four aspects of frames: They "define problems," "diagnose causes," "make moral judgements," and "suggest remedies."[18] In this way, framing has the capacity to characterize an issue as a political problem, befitting policy solutions.[24] Often, this requires commercial actors to contribute opinions on the definition of the problem as well as offering their own preferred policy solutions. Having a package of well-rehearsed arguments offers commercial actors a means to present their interpretation of the facts and problems, make moral judgments, and urge public support for potential solutions.

Generally, research examining public discourses shows that tobacco, alcohol, processed food, and soft drink corporate actors tend to promote frames that divert attention from harmful products.[27] Instead, commercial actors emphasize personal and parental responsibility, placing the focus on unhealthy lifestyles at an individual level. Such frames portray individuals as making less informed choices to smoke, consume alcohol, or consume unhealthy food and drinks. This focus suggests that government should have no role in curtailing individual freedoms to make choices, portraying them as anti-liberal.

Unsurprisingly, these frames often go hand-in-hand with arguments for supporting voluntary policies targeted at changing individual behavior such as education campaigns rather than regulatory systemic changes. Language is important in making these arguments persuasive, and in regulatory debates it is common to see or hear the use of pejorative terms in these frames such as "excessive," "over," or "unnecessary" regulation to promote distrust in the measures. In contrast, public health actors tend to frame debates very differently, drawing attention to systemic failures and the need for regulatory population-level intervention to protect citizens from dominant market interests. Researching commercial actors' intent and how they seek to influence policy debates through arguments is a valuable precursor to developing preventative strategies.[28] Indeed, advancing scholarship into the arguments used by commercial industries in public policy debates is important, and the rest of this chapter is dedicated to this by describing new empirical work that compares different policy domains and industry sectors.

27.4 ADVANCING SCHOLARSHIP INTO THE INFLUENCE OF COMMERCIAL ACTORS ON PUBLIC DISCOURSE

Many of the methods used to study corporate practices in health policy have focused on the content in documentary sources, such as internal documents, evidence submissions during policy development, annual reports, or court filings.[29] Studies have also combined data sources—media coverage, press releases, policy documents, and stakeholder interviews.[30,31] Triangulating multiple sources in this way helps identify public discourses in evolving policy debates, but it does not reveal the interplay between actors in the discourse network or how they argue for policy action across sectors of the unhealthy commodity industries.

Recent developments in this field include discourse network analysis, which stems from political sciences[32] and has recently been applied to public health polices across industry sectors.[26] Schmidt's commentary of this method highlights that this application is "likely to prove a particularly valuable tool for comparative research, allowing efficient, systematic, rigorous analysis to compare policy debates in the media internationally and across multiple unhealthy products."[33] Indeed, this work shows that commercial actors with shared interests coalesce around key arguments in media policy debates, suggesting they coordinate their communications to influence policy development.[26] This adds weight to the idea of a common industry "playbook."[19] In thinking about how commercial actors align messages in public discourses, it is useful to draw upon the wider policy literature. The Advocacy Coalition Framework posits that actors with shared ideological beliefs become entrenched in coalitions to influence policy design over time.[34] Changes in core policy preferences by political actors through consensus-seeking and alliance-building result in changes in the balance of coalitions and hence policy shifts. In relation to public discourse, Leifeld et al. suggest that it is the articulation of policy beliefs by interest groups in such discourse that reveals their policy preferences and encourages other stakeholders in the policy debate to support or reveal their opposition to them.[35] In this way, a discursive coalition forms and can be identified because actors influence each other through arguments and their position at "particular sites of discursive production."[35]

More detailed methods of investigating discursive networks are presented in several papers.[6,25,26] In short, discourse network analysis illuminates the discourse coalitions in a network through linking the quotations attributed to discursive frames in support of and in opposition to policies. This mapping of agreement or disagreement in discursive forums produces visual representations of actors that coalesce around particular assemblages of beliefs in a debate. This can be used to highlight and understand the complex interactions and alliances of stakeholders attempting to influence government policy. Its application to public health policy debates is new, but it has the potential to benefit commercial determinants of health research and advocacy as a rapid, cost-effective way to document content presented to the audience; make inferences about how that content may affect audiences' understandings; and synthesize strategies for improving the translation of public health evidence into public discourses and policies. Importantly, it offers new opportunities to better understand how different sectors of the unhealthy commodity industry strategically use the media and employ similar framing strategies to become effective coalitions of influence. As Smith et al. note, understanding coalitions, their relationships, and their interactions is necessary for elucidating advocacy strategies to counter industry and protect public health.[28]

Further research using discourse network analysis could be valuable in providing insights into changes in health debates over time and how actors converged on a policy solution—for instance, in frames that move away from individual-level problematization to frames supporting population-level solutions, as found in the news analysis of debates about regulating obesogenic environments.[36] Advancement could also be made into the relative prominence of different actors, including public health advocates and their arguments in public policy debates. This is particularly important given that interest groups presenting a united rather than separate front are more effective in having their preferred policy option adopted.[37] Discourse network research confirms this. It also confirms that by working together, public health advocates could be far more effective in countering the cumulative effects of corporate activity in public discourse.[26] For example, Hawkins and McCambridge suggest that a factor in the failure to implement minimum unit pricing for alcohol in England was that health advocates did not present as a coherent front with consistent arguments in the public policy debate.[38] Therefore, future research could usefully examine whether public health actors present a united front in debates to the public and policymakers through their use of arguments. This could direct advocacy efforts and help develop effective counterstrategies to industry coordination.

Further research into how different sectors of the unhealthy commodity industry are presented in public discourse may illuminate the current differences between the tobacco industry and alcohol, processed food, and soft drink corporations.[11] For example, Weishaar and colleagues found that media representations of alcohol, processed food, and soft drink companies overall seem to be predominantly positive compared to tobacco companies in public policy discourse.[27] This resonates with other research finding that alcohol and food companies were perceived as legitimate actors and policymaking partners in noncommunicable disease debates.[39]

27.5 CONCLUSION

Public health advocates have been proactive in developing a better understanding of both the harms and the influence of industries on health, social, and environmental issues. However, research that helps establish the role of public discourse in influencing strong government regulation of unhealthy product-producing industries is important. Heavily influenced by traditional market discourse, policymakers have been more receptive to industry calls for an unfettered marketplace and the rights of consumers to choose, often implementing weaker policy options that do not protect people. The investigation of commercial actors and their role in shaping public discourse is an under-researched area, despite the clear importance for population health, both nationally and globally. Adapted discourse network analysis offers scope to advance science into commercial determinants' influence on public health discourse. Such research could help transform how unhealthy commodities are presented in discourse, from being viewed as a harm to a few arising from a lack of individual responsibility to being more widely understood as a major, industry-driven risk factor. This could enable us to better counter industry influence so that the public and policymakers become more receptive to public health arguments supporting population-level regulation.

REFERENCES

1. McCombs M. A look at agenda-setting: Past, present and future. *Journal Stud.* 2005; 6(4): 543–557.
2. Leifeld P. *Policy Debates as Dynamic Networks: German Pension Politics and Privatization Discourse.* Campus Verlag; 2016.

3. Lewis J, Williams A, Franklin B. A compromised fourth estate? UK news journalism, public relations and news sources. *Journal Stud.* 2008; 9(1): 1–20.

4. Nixon L, Mejia P, Cheyne A, Wilking C, Dorfman L, Daynard R. "We're part of the solution": Evolution of the food and beverage industry's framing of obesity concerns between 2000 and 2012. *Am J Public Health.* 2015; 105(11): 2228–2236.

5. Supran G, Oreskes N. Rhetoric and frame analysis of ExxonMobil's climate change communications. *One Earth.* 2021; 4(5): 696–719.

6. Fergie G, Leifeld P, Hawkins B, Hilton S. Mapping discourse coalitions in the minimum unit pricing for alcohol debate: A discourse network analysis of UK newspaper coverage. *Addiction.* 2019; 114(4): 741–753.

7. McKee M, Stuckler D. Revisiting the corporate and commercial determinants of health. *Am J Public Health.* 2018; 108(9): 1167–1170.

8. Cho CH, Martens ML, Kim H, Rodrigue M. Astroturfing global warming: It isn't always greener on the other side of the fence. *J Bus Ethics.* 2011; 104(4): 571–587.

9. Smith EA, Malone RE. "We will speak as the smoker": The tobacco industry's smokers' rights groups. *Eur J Public Health.* 2007; 17(3): 306–313.

10. Apollonio DE, Bero LA. The creation of industry front groups: The tobacco industry and "get government off our back." *Am J Public Health.* 2007; 97(3): 419–427.

11. Casswell S. Vested interests in addiction research and policy. Why do we not see the corporate interests of the alcohol industry as clearly as we see those of the tobacco industry? *Addiction.* 2013; 108(4): 680–685.

12. Curran J. The future of journalism. *Journal Stud.* 2010; 11(4): 464–476.

13. Witschge T, Nygren G. Journalistic work: A profession under pressure? *J Media Bus Stud.* 2009; 6(1): 37–59.

14. Moodie AR. *What Public Health Practitioners Need to Know About Unhealthy Industry Tactics.* American Public Health Association; 2017.

15. Gilchrist M. Lost amid misinformation: Real people, real science, real progress. *The Washington Post.* May 25, 2021. https://www.washingtonpost.com/brand-studio/wp/2021/05/25/lost-amid-misinformation-real-people-real-science-real-progress/

16. PMI. Partner content. 2021. Accessed August 4, 2021.

17. Entman RM. Framing bias: Media in the distribution of power. *J Commun.* 2007; 57(1): 163–173.

18. Entman RM. Framing: Toward clarification of a fractured paradigm. *J Commun.* 1993; 43(4): 51–58.

19. Petticrew M, Katikireddi SV, Knai C, et al. "Nothing can be done until everything is done": The use of complexity arguments by food, beverage, alcohol and gambling industries. *J Epidemiol Community Health.* 2017; 71(11): 1078–1083.

20. Petticrew M, Katikireddi SV, Knai C, et al. "Nothing can be done until everything is done": The use of complexity arguments by food, beverage, alcohol and gambling industries. Supplementary file SF1. 2017. Accessed August 4, 2021. https://jech.bmj.com/content/71/11/1078#DC1

21. Gerbner G, Gross L. Living with television: The violence profile. In: *The Fear of Crime.* Routledge; 2017: 169–195.

22. Dorfman L, Wallack L, Woodruff K. More than a message: Framing public health advocacy to change corporate practices. *Health Educ Behav.* 2005; 32(3): 320–336.

23. Scheufele DA, Tewksbury D. Framing, agenda setting, and priming: The evolution of three media effects models. *J Commun.* 2007; 57(1): 9–20.

24. Hawkins B, Holden C. Framing the alcohol policy debate: Industry actors and the regulation of the UK beverage alcohol market. *Crit Policy Stud.* 2013; 7(1): 53–71.

25. Buckton CH, Fergie G, Leifeld P, Hilton S. A discourse network analysis of UK newspaper coverage of the "sugar tax" debate before and after the announcement of the soft drinks industry levy. *BMC Public Health*. 2019; 19(1): 1–14.

26. Hilton S, Buckton CH, Henrichsen T, Fergie G, Leifeld P. Policy congruence and advocacy strategies in the discourse networks of minimum unit pricing for alcohol and the soft drinks industry levy. *Addiction*. 2020; 115(12): 2303–2314.

27. Weishaar H, Dorfman L, Freudenberg N, et al. Why media representations of corporations matter for public health policy: A scoping review. *BMC Public Health*. 2016; 16(1): 1–11.

28. Smith K, Dorfman L, Freudenberg N, et al. Tobacco, alcohol, and processed food industries: Why do public health practitioners view them so differently? *Front Public Health*. 2016; 4: 64.

29. Maani N, Collin J, Friel S, et al. Bringing the commercial determinants of health out of the shadows: A review of how the commercial determinants are represented in conceptual frameworks. *Eur J Public Health*. 2020; 30(4): 660–664.

30. Katikireddi SV, Bond L, Hilton S. Changing policy framing as a deliberate strategy for public health advocacy: A qualitative policy case study of minimum unit pricing of alcohol. *Milbank Q*. 2014; 92(2): 250–283.

31. Katikireddi SV, Hilton S, Bonell C, Bond L. Understanding the development of minimum unit pricing of alcohol in Scotland: A qualitative study of the policy process. *PLoS One*. 2014; 9(3): e91185.

32. Leifeld P. Discourse Network Analyzer (DNA). 2018. Accessed July 27, 2018. https://github.com/leifeld/dna

33. Schmidt LA. Commentary on Fergie et al. (2019): A new tool for unpacking policy debates over unhealthy commodities. *Addiction*. 2019; 114(4): 754–755.

34. Cairney P. Policymaking in the UK: What is policy and how is it made? In: Policy *and* Policymaking *in the* UK. Palgrave; 2015: 1–22.

35. Leifeld P, Henrichsen T, Buckton C, Fergie G, Hilton S. Belief system alignment and cross-sectoral advocacy efforts in policy debates. *J Eur Public Policy*. 2021: 1–24.

36. Hilton S, Patterson C, Teyhan A. Escalating coverage of obesity in UK newspapers: The evolution and framing of the "obesity epidemic" from 1996 to 2010. *Obesity*. 2012; 20(8): 1688–1695.

37. Rasmussen A, Mäder LK, Reher S. With a little help from the people? The role of public opinion in advocacy success. *Comp Political Stud*. 2018; 51(2): 139–164.

38. Hawkins B, McCambridge J. Industry actors, think tanks, and alcohol policy in the United Kingdom. *Am J Public Health*. 2014; 104(8): 1363–1369.

39. Dorfman L, Cheyne A, Gottlieb MA, et al. Cigarettes become a dangerous product: Tobacco in the rearview mirror, 1952–1965. *Am J Public Health*. 2014; 104(1): 37–46.

CHAPTER 28

Commercial Determinants of Health in Low- and Middle-Income Countries

SALMA M. ABDALLA, LEONA OFEI, NASON MAANI, AND
SANDRO GALEA

28.1 INTRODUCTION

Commercial forces are playing an increasingly prominent role in low- and middle-income countries (LMICs) due to the rise of the local private sector and multinational corporations' (MNCs) investment, supply chains, and market penetration.[1,2] The growing presence of commercial actors in LMICs has had a short-term impact on behavior and consumption. During the past two decades, LMICs have recorded an increase in the rates of consumption of commodities such as soft drinks, processed foods, tobacco, and alcohol, with a faster pace than has occurred historically in high-income countries (HICs).[3] These changes are often part of a concerted effort by commercial entities to expand their base of operations—and client base—to LMICs. For example, whereas the global cultivation of tobacco decreased by 15.7% between 2012 and 2018, it increased by 3.4% in Africa.[4] There is also emerging evidence that the tobacco industry is strategizing to appeal to the growing young and middle-class population in Africa through techniques that diverge greatly from their activities in HICs. These include selling individual cigarettes, to increase their affordability particularly for children and young people, as well as providing free products and sponsoring youth programs.[5] Growing commercial actions in LMICs therefore hold portent for commercial determinants to have more impact on the health of populations in LMICs than ever before. This arises against a baseline of substantial disease burden in LMICs. LMICs

Salma M. Abdalla, Leona Ofei, Nason Maani, and Sandro Galea, *Commercial Determinants of Health in Low- and Middle-Income Countries* In: *The Commercial Determinants of Health.* Edited by: Nason Maani, Mark Petticrew, and Sandro Galea, Oxford University Press. © Oxford University Press 2023. DOI: 10.1093/oso/9780197578742.003.0028 account for a disproportionate percentage (77%) of global noncommunicable disease (NCD) deaths.[6]

Although during the past few years there has been growing recognition of the role the commercial determinants play in shaping the health of populations—with a particular focus on their role as important drivers of the burden of NCDs—that recognition is yet to fully extend to addressing commercial determinants of health (CDOH) in LMICs.[7-10] This chapter builds on existing CDOH research to highlight factors that can make LMICs particularly vulnerable to commercial forces in ways that impact on health. These factors include market globalization, which led to the expansion of MNCs into LMICs, and domestic conditions such as lack of strong regulatory enforcement mechanisms, taxation policies, and economic vulnerabilities. This work elaborates on these factors and provides examples of how they can exacerbate the impact of CDOH in LMICs.

28.2 GLOBALIZATION AND MULTINATIONAL CORPORATIONS

Growing market globalization during the past three decades has provided an array of opportunities for MNCs to invest in LMICs.[1] Between 1990 and 2006, foreign direct investment in LMICs increased 29-fold.[11] The scale of resources wielded by MNCs, and their political backing by governments in HICs where they and their shareholders are primarily based, often means that MNCs yield disproportionate power over governments and local producers in LMICs, dominating local markets and overwhelmingly shaping health through commercial decisions made thousands of miles away. Governments in HICs often use their own power—either through foreign aid or through trade agreement regulations—to pressure LMICs into commercial agreements that are favorable to MNCs. As a result, MNCs can become detrimental to the growth of local businesses in LMICs. MNCs often have greater access to monetary resources and technology to build their presence in a country than do local businesses.[1,12] MNCs also have greater brand recognition and the ability to offer less expensive products compared to local producers due to economies of scale. These conditions create difficulties for small and medium businesses to compete in LMICs markets. Moreover, MNCs may also take over local enterprises, eventually becoming monopolies.[1]

These practices mean that products generated by MNCs play an overwhelming role in shaping the health of LMIC populations. One example is the role the global food industry plays in shaping food systems and food choices in LMICs. For example, in 2013, three multi-national companies controlled 40% of the Coca-Cola market. These companies often have easy access to land in LMICs.[13] Between 2008 and 2009, land agreements between LMICs and foreign entities increased by almost 200%; these entities then used the land to grow products. These corporations use their considerable resources to produce processed food (e.g., soda and snacks), which results in both a dominant presence of these processed foods in the market and the reduced availability of land and water that can produce food of greater nutritional value for local communities.[13] MNCs may also create monopolies over local food and beverage supply systems. For example, in the early 2000s, Nestlé controlled the majority of collection stations of milk in the Shuangcheng District in China, which resulted in local farmers mostly selling to Nestlé and being compensated less than market rates.[13] Given that small farmers—particularly in rural areas in LMICs—already constitute a large percentage of people who experience hunger throughout the world, these corporate practices can exacerbate the poverty and hunger such small farmers face.[14]

There are a number of pathways through which MNCs can exert influence to maintain advantageous positions in LMICs. These include international trade agreements and regulations, bilateral and regional preferential trade agreements, structural adjustment requirements, and the use of litigation. We discuss each in turn.

28.2.1 International Trade Agreements and Regulations

The World Trade Organization (WTO) is the global authority on international trade agreements. The organization is tasked with limiting trade barriers such as tariffs, taxes, and other trade regulations and adjudicating relevant disputes. For example, the General Agreement on Tariffs and Trade (GATT) allows countries to put limits on trade for the purpose of health, but only if they can show that these trade limits are needed for public health purposes and that there are no other approaches to reduce their impact.[15] Another agreement, the Technical Barriers to Trade (TBT), aims to ensure that regulations and standards do not lead to unnecessary obstacles to trade.[16] The terms of these agreements can constrain the ability of LMICs to control the impact of commercial determinants on their population's health upon applying for WTO membership because many are not in a position of sufficient political or economic power to challenge trade agreements and decisions by WTO. For example, the United States disputed Vietnam's admission into the WTO by claiming that Vietnam's alcohol tax legislation was beneficial for local entities but not for foreign entities.

Furthermore, trade regulations can be used by MNCs to limit public health policy within LMICs, often with support from HICs. To illustrate this issue through the example of product packaging, evidence suggests that colored "traffic light" labels perform better in nudging people to make healthier food choices compared to monochrome labels.[17] In 2006, Thailand sought to place public health traffic light labels on snacks for children; several of these snacks were produced by MNCs based in the United States. The government of Thailand eventually settled for "monochrome" labels after the United States and other countries disputed the policy, arguing that it was not in line with TBT. In 2010, Thailand again sought to advance legislation with its Alcohol Beverage Control Act to improve warning messages on alcoholic products. These rules are considered "technical," and several countries such as Australia disputed whether the law is appropriate under the TBT.[18]

By way of another example, in the 1980s, U.S.-based tobacco corporations directed the U.S. Trade Representative to pressure four countries in Asia with trade penalties if they did not withdraw limitations for importing tobacco products (based on Section 301 from the 1974 Trade Act). This led to three countries (Japan, Taiwan, and South Korea) withdrawing their limitations and providing access to their markets. However, Thailand mounted a challenge that ultimately led to evaluating the disagreement under the GATT arbitration mechanism.[19] Thailand based its argument on the health exemption section of the GATT, highlighting that tobacco imports pose a public health risk because they would lead to more cigarette use. Thailand was required to provide proof that the market limitations placed on foreign tobacco corporations were needed to reduce smoking among its population and that this approach was the least limiting to achieve such goal. GATT evaluators did not rule in favor of Thailand, citing that the regulations by Thailand went against nondiscrimination requirements of the trade agreement and that Thailand could only enforce limitations that discriminated equally against local and foreign tobacco corporations.[19]

28.2.2 Bilateral and Regional Preferential Trade Agreements

Despite their limitations, multilateral trade agreements, as noted here, often allow for some recourse to address public health concerns. By contrast, bilateral and regional preferential trade agreements (PTAs) are less likely to have such protections. This leads to LMICs having even less ability to enforce public health guidelines under PTAs. By way of compelling example, in 2021, countries with free trade agreements with the United States had 63.4% greater soft drink consumption per capita compared to countries that did not have such agreements.[3]

A clear example of the role PTAs play in shaping how commercial forces enter LMICs and influence health is the North American Free Trade Agreement (NAFTA). The passage of the agreement in 1994 led to greater direct foreign investment and the rapid expansion of the sugary beverage and fast-food industry in Mexico. In 2019, Mexico had the highest consumption of soft drinks among the most populated countries in the world with 634 per capita consumption of 8-ounce servings.[20] Comparatively, despite experiencing high levels of economic growth, Venezuela, which was not part of NAFTA, maintained steady consumption rates of soft drinks during the 1990s and 2000s.[3]

Two corporations, Coca-Cola and PepsiCo, both primarily based in the United States, control 85% of the growing soda industry in Mexico.[21] This infiltration of processed food from U.S.-based corporations into Mexico contributed to poorer population health. When NAFTA was implemented in 1994, the prevalence of obesity among adults in Mexico was 17.9%, but by 2016 it had increased to 28.9%.[22] Mexico currently has the third highest obesity prevalence and the highest overweight prevalence among those 15 years or older among Organisation for Economic Co-operation and Development (OECD) countries.[23]

28.2.3 Structural Adjustment Requirements

In addition to trade agreements, the International Monetary Fund (IMF) can pressure LMICs to open their markets to MNCs through adding trade and market liberalization stipulations to loans. Such loans often come with requirements that LMIC governments reduce expenditure on certain public sectors, allow for greater trade and foreign direct investment, and support policies that encourage exports rather than support local markets.[24]

For example, in India, a bailout package by the IMF in the early 1990s contained a requirement that the Indian government undertake extensive market liberalization, which eventually led to changes in the local soft drink economy. Following this change, PepsiCo successfully penetrated the Indian market, followed by Coca-Cola. The price competition and marketing efforts by the two corporations led to significant shifts in the consumption of soft drinks among the Indian population. Between 1998 and 2012, the consumption of soft drinks in India rose from 1.2 to 4.4 million liters.[24]

28.2.4 Use of Litigation

Building on the existence of multilateral, regional, and bilateral trade agreements and the lack of government resources in LMICs, MNCs are often able to use their expansive resources to block or delay government actions to address particular corporate practices in LMICs. For example, in Sri Lanka, the government introduced a policy for health cautionary messages to appear on the majority (80%) of tobacco packaging. Ceylon Tobacco Company (CTC), a branch of the British American Tobacco (BAT) company, brought lawsuits against the government for that policy. The Sri Lankan government subsequently reduced warning labels to 60% of packaging. However, the case proceeded, eventually reaching the Supreme Court in Sri Lanka, which delayed the enactment of the policy but ultimately determined that the Ministry of Health could implement a policy with a 50–60% packaging requirement. Tobacco companies were expected to begin implementation of the policy in 2014, but the CTC applied for a delay to be allowed to sell existing products. The delay was approved and implementation was extended to 2015. In Nigeria, the tobacco industry—which was dominated by branches of international corporations such as BAT and the International Tobacco Company—lobbied to impede the country's efforts to implement tobacco control measures through a decree in 1990, during the re-evaluation of the decree in 1995, and Nigeria's 2015 Tobacco Control Act.

28.3 DOMESTIC FACTORS

In addition to the aforementioned global forces, several other factors may facilitate the role that commercial forces play in shaping the sale and consumption patterns of harmful products and, by extension, the health of populations in LMICs. Central among these are the regulatory environments, taxation policies, and the realities of the economic trade-offs embedded in the government policies toward private actors.

28.3.1 Regulatory Environments

The development and enforcement of regulations are central to good governance and achieving economic and social policy objectives. There is ample evidence that most governments experience regulatory failure—through over- or under-regulation and through poor design and implementation of regulations—that undermines policies and increases the costs and risk of commercial activities. LMICs generally perform worse than HICs in their regulatory governance approaches.[25] Moreover, regulations in LMICs may not be enforced due to resource constraints.[26]

The lack of strong regulatory mechanisms in LMICs makes them more likely to implement guidance by international organizations, which may put them at a disadvantage if that guidance is influenced by MNCs. For example, WHO consultations on NCDs between 2015 and 2018 included representatives from the global food industry in the form of business associations. These groups were against statutory proposals that included taxation, marketing limitations, and mandatory labeling, and they argued instead for voluntary proposals that focused on education or self-regulation.[27] This is despite the mounting evidence that mandatory population-level measures such as taxation and limiting marketing have a positive impact on reducing the consumption of harmful products.[28-30]

28.3.2 Taxation Policies

Overall, LMICs have lower taxation rates compared to HICs. This can be due to the informal nature of LMIC markets; reliance on natural resources and foreign aid; and weaker tax regulations and administrative barriers, which create an environment that is less likely to support progressive taxation.[31,32] LMICs are therefore particularly lucrative to corporations and potentially more vulnerable to a disproportionate impact of commercial forces on the health of populations. For example, mining corporations, which contribute to the global burden of injury, operate heavily in LMICs. If African countries taxed mining companies at similar levels to those in Australia between 2003 and 2008, these countries would have generated an additional $70 billion in tax revenue for budgets.[31] Furthermore, limited regulation can lead to inability to introduce or enforce excise taxes on harmful products to either discourage the consumption of these products or use the tax revenue to improve their health systems.

28.3.3 Economic Reality and Trade-Offs

The economic reality in many LMICs contributes to the complexity of the role commercial forces play in shaping the health of population in LMICs. In theory, economic growth should lead to better health outcomes.[33] As such, for many LMICs, the rise of the engagement of the private sector can also lead to improved health outcomes. This creates the need to balance the potential positive impact of commercial forces with the negative impact of commercial forces on population health.

Moreover, the same economic conditions in some LMICs can both contribute to and exacerbate the role of a range of global and domestic factors that led to the increasing influence of commercial entities in LMICs. As demonstrated in this chapter, the power imbalances MNCs exert on LMICs are largely driven by the global pressures LMICs face in seeking monetary support from HICs and other international actors. Resource scarcity in LMICs shapes the limits of regulatory and taxation policies in LMICs. There is a need for economic development, and potentially social development by extension, that comes from the increasing presence of foreign aid and commercial forces in LMICs. This creates a substantial obstacle to LMIC efforts to grapple with the influence of commercial forces, generate positive social good, promote health, and limit harm to health.

28.4 CONCLUSION

Several factors, both global and domestic, make LMICs vulnerable to the increasing influence of commercial forces on their population health.

Ultimately, addressing the CDOH cannot occur in isolation of the global structure that creates power imbalances and the economic realities in LMICs. This highlights the need to invest in locally produced CDOH research to address the unique and increasing influence of commercial forces in LMICs and also to guide how commercial development in LMICs can optimize the benefits to the health of the population that originate from economy prosperity, while limiting the public health harms from corporate practices.

REFERENCES

1. Masroor N, Asim M. SMEs in the contemporary era of global competition. *Proc Comput Sci.* 2019; 158: 632–641. doi:10.1016/j.procs.2019.09.097
2. Tanchua J, Shand J. Emerging markets may offer the most potential for the world's largest consumer-focused companies. S&P Global. August 3, 2016. Accessed May 14, 2021. https://www.spglobal.com/en/research-insights/artic les/emerging-markets-may-offer-the-most-potential-for-the-worlds-largest-consumer-focused-companies
3. Stuckler D, McKee M, Ebrahim S, Basu S. Manufacturing epidemics: The role of global producers in increased consumption of unhealthy commodities including processed foods, alcohol, and tobacco. *PLoS Med.* 2012; 9(6): 10. doi:10.1371/journal.pmed.1001235
4. Blum A, Eke R. Tobacco control: All research, no action. *Lancet.* 2021; 397(10292): 2310–2311. doi:10.1016/S0140-6736(21)01193-4
5. Gilmore AB, Fooks G, Drope J, Bialous SA, Jackson RR. Exposing and addressing tobacco industry conduct in low-income and middle-income countries. *Lancet.* 2015; 385(9972): 1029–1043. doi:10.1016/S0140-6736(15)60312-9
6. World Health Organization. Noncommunicable diseases. April 13, 2021. Accessed June 21, 2021. https://www.who.int/news-room/fact-sheets/detail/noncommu nicable-diseases
7. Maani N, McKee M, Petticrew M, Galea S. Corporate practices and the health of populations: A research and translational agenda. *Lancet Public Health.* 2020; 5(2): e80–e81. doi:10.1016/S2468-2667(19)30270-1
8. Kickbusch I, Allen L, Franz C. The commercial determinants of health. *Lancet Glob Health.* 2016; 4(12): e895–e896. doi:10.1016/S2214-109X(16)30217-0
9. Chaloupka FJ, Powell LM, Warner KE. The use of excise taxes to reduce tobacco, alcohol, and sugary beverage consumption. *Annu Rev Public Health.* 2019; 40: 187–201. https://pubmed.ncbi.nlm.nih.gov/30601721
10. World Health Organization. Noncommunicable diseases. April 13, 2021. Accessed June 14, 2021. https://www.who.int/news-room/fact-sheets/detail/noncommu nicable-diseases
11. UNCTAD. Transnational corporations and the infrastructure challenge. *World Investment Report.* 2008. Accessed May 14, 2021. https://worldinvestmentrep ort.unctad.org/wir2008/part-2-transnational-corporations-and-the-infrastruct ure-challenge
12. Oshionebo E. Corporations and nations: Power imbalance in the extractive sector. *Am J Econ Sociol.* 2018; 77(2): 419–446. doi:10.1111/ajes.12209

13. Oxfam. Behind the brands: Food justice and the "Big 10" food and beverage companies. February 26, 2013. Accessed June 3, 2021. https://policy-practice.oxfam.org/resources/behind-the-brands-food-justice-and-the-big-10-food-and-beverage-companies-270393

14. Action Against Hunger. World hunger: Key facts and statistics 2021. 2021. Accessed June 3, 2021. https://www.actionagainsthunger.org/world-hunger-facts-statistics

15. Baker P, Kay A, Walls H. Trade and investment liberalization and Asia's noncommunicable disease epidemic: A synthesis of data and existing literature. *Global Health*. 2014; 10(1): 66. doi:10.1186/s12992-014-0066-8

16. World Trade Organization. Technical barriers to trade. n.d. Accessed June 14, 2021. https://www.wto.org/english/tratop_e/tbt_e/tbt_e.htm

17. Borgmeier I, Westenhoefer J. Impact of different food label formats on healthiness evaluation and food choice of consumers: A randomized-controlled study. *BMC Public Health*. 2009; 9(1): 1–12. doi:10.1186/1471-2458-9-184

18. Friel S, Hattersley L, Townsend R. Trade policy and public health. *Annu Rev Public Health*. 2015; 36: 325–344. doi:10.1146/annurev-publhealth-031914-122739

19. MacKenzie R, Collin J. "Trade policy, not morals or health policy": The US Trade Representative, tobacco companies and market liberalization in Thailand. *Glob Soc Policy*. 2012; 12(2): 149–172. doi:10.1177/1468018112443686

20. Statista. Per capita consumption of carbonated soft drinks in 2019 in the ten most populated countries worldwide. 2020. Accessed June 1, 2021. https://www.statista.com/statistics/505794/cds-per-capita-consumption-in-worlds-top-ten-population-countries

21. Gómez EJ. Coca-Cola's political and policy influence in Mexico: Understanding the role of institutions, interests and divided society. *Health Policy Plan*. 2019; 34(7): 520–528. doi:10.1093/heapol/czz063

22. Our World in Data. Obesity. 2017. Accessed June 1, 2021. https://ourworldindata.org/obesity

23. Organisation for Economic Co-operation and Development. Obesity update. 2017. Accessed June 1, 2021. https://www.oecd.org/health/obesity-update.htm

24. Baker P, Kay A, Walls H. Trade and investment liberalization and Asia's noncommunicable disease epidemic: A synthesis of data and existing literature. *Global Health*. 2014; 10(1): 1–20. doi:10.1186/s12992-014-0066-8

25. The World Bank. Global Indicators of Regulatory Governance key findings. n.d. Accessed May 14, 2021. https://rulemaking.worldbank.org/en/key-findings#4

26. Nordhagen S. Improving food safety: An emerging imperative in low-income countries. Global Alliance for Improved Nutrition. June 7, 2020. Accessed May 14, 2021. https://www.gainhealth.org/media/news/improving-food-safety-emerging-imperative-low-income-countries

27. Lauber K, Ralston R, Mialon M, Carriedo A, Gilmore AB. Non-communicable disease governance in the era of the sustainable development goals: A qualitative analysis of food industry framing in WHO consultations. *Global Health*. 2020; 16(1): 1–15. doi:10.1186/s12992-020-00611-1

28. Mytton OT, Boyland E, Adams J, et al. The potential health impact of restricting less-healthy food and beverage advertising on UK television between 05.30 and 21.00 hours: A modelling study. *PLoS Med*. 2020; 17(10): e1003212. doi:10.1371/journal.pmed.1003212

29. Miracolo A, Sophiea M, Mills M, Kanavos P. Sin taxes and their effect on consumption, revenue generation and health improvement: A systematic literature

review in Latin America. *Health Policy Plan*. 2021; 36(5): 790–810. doi:10.1093/heapol/czaa168

30. Chaloupka FJ, Powell LM, Warner KE. The use of excise taxes to reduce tobacco, alcohol, and sugary beverage consumption. *Annu Rev Public Health*. 2019; 40: 187–201.

31. Mills L. *Barriers to Increasing Tax Revenue in Developing Countries*. UK Department for International Development; 2017.

32. Besley T, Persson T. Why do developing countries tax so little? *J Econ Perspect*. 2014; 28: 99–120. doi:10.1257/jep.28.4.99

33. Lange S, Vollmer S. The effect of economic development on population health: A review of the empirical evidence. *Br Med Bull*. 2017; 121(1): 47–60. doi:10.1093/bmb/ldw052

A Way Forward

CHAPTER 29
The Question of Industry Partnerships

PETER J. ADAMS

29.1 INTRODUCTION

In March 1998, the United Nations (UN) set up its Office for Partnerships as a "global gateway for catalyzing and building partnership initiatives between public and private sector stakeholders."[1] The scheme that evolved, its Fund for International Partnership, has resourced a wide range of public good projects.[2] Although receiving some criticism for enabling corporate interests to over-take democratic governance,[3,4] interest in public–private partnerships (PPPs) has continued to flourish and has resulted in a range of productive partner-ships in areas as diverse as women's health, child health, and infectious dis-eases.[5-7] Following from this spirit of cooperation, in 2015 the UN together with the World Health Organization (WHO) adopted "Partnerships for the Goals" as Goal 17 of their Sustainable Development Goals. This goal sought to "revitalize" global partnerships by bringing together a range of non-state ac-tors, including "private sector entities" and "businesses," into PPP enterprises at both global and local levels.[8] Over the next 3 years, such partnerships had resulted in projects worth $1.46 billion, aimed at tackling major global health challenges such as measles and rubella, malaria, and reproductive health.[9]

This chapter examines whether this spirit of industry partnerships can ef-fectively and wisely be extended to partnerships with unhealthy commodity industries, such as alcohol, ultra-processed food, or fossil fuels. There are strong reasons to exercise caution. A unifying characteristic of unhealthy commodities is the presence of profit-driven corporations whose success is reliant on consumptions linked to a range of health, social, psychological, and financial harms.[10,11] What on the surface might appear as sensible co-operative ventures—such as improved product labeling or safer consuming

Peter J. Adams, *The Question of Industry Partnerships* In: *The Commercial Determinants of Health.*
Edited by: Nason Maani, Mark Petticrew, and Sandro Galea, Oxford University Press.
© Oxford University Press 2023. DOI: 10.1093/oso/9780197578742.003.0029

environments—at a deeper level serve to lock those involved in with health initiatives of dubious effectiveness and provide a platform for corporations to position themselves as positive agents of change. By this route, partnerships can be viewed as a channel for private interests to exert stronger influence in the public sphere and, thereby, providing a vehicle for corporations to further their interests in diverting, confusing, and stalling healthy public policy.[12,13]

29.2 MODELS OF ASSOCIATION

To explore the assumptions underpinning such collaborations, the following groups the various parties into three broad sectors.[14] First, the *government sector* refers to the complex set of relationships and processes involving politicians, legislative bodies, government departments and their officials, regulatory bodies, and quasi-government organizations, each of which works collaboratively through policy, regulation, and project streams to set the scene for how populations engage with unhealthy commodities. Outside of the government sector, the *health sector* combines the energies of a broad range of community and service organizations supported by input from local bodies, researchers and advocates, along with a broad array of nongovernment and civil society organizations, all seeking ways to minimize the harms to health generated by unhealthy commodities. The third sector consists of the *unhealthy commodity industries* and is made up of the complex of companies and business systems—some collaborative, some competitive—that integrate the efforts of manufacturers, wholesalers, retailers, and marketers to produce, distribute, market, and sell these commodities to maximize profits for their owners. Also as part of this complex are the various forms of associations, front groups, and lobbying bodies that advance industry interests in the political environment.[15,16]

These three sectors can be seen as engaging in partnerships in a variety of ways. The first model worth considering, the three-way *equal association model*, assumes each sector has an equal voice, is equally resourced, and has an equal capacity to contribute and to influence how events unfold. For example, in an initiative in bars aimed at more responsible hosting, industry might provide access to venues and staff, government provides some development funding, and the health sector provides professional support and expertise. Figure 29.1 provides a simple representation of this arrangement.

This model faces a range of significant pitfalls and challenges. The most worrying concerns the high likelihood of differences in power between the sectors. Without a guarantee of sufficient power, any weaker party can be dominated and perhaps find themselves absorbed by the interests of the dominant players. Contrary to claims of equality, the power relationships in this arrangement tend to tip naturally away from health sector interests. Another challenge is the presence of explicit and implicit relationships

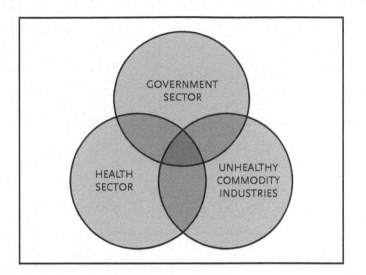

Figure 29.1 Equal association model.
Adapted from Adams et al.[14]

between government and industry actors.[17] For example, actors within the food and beverage industry are likely to have built up ongoing relationships with government actors for reasons that stem from their importance to the economy, their contributions to taxation, and their investment in relationship building.[18,19] Health sector representatives, often hand-picked for their moderate views by government actors, find themselves buying into talk of "cooperation" and "collaboration" soon to discover their own priorities sidelined and themselves wedded to strategies that they only partially endorse.[20]

An alternative model for engagement, the *managed association model*, has the government sector assuming responsibility for managing a limited and highly constrained level of direct involvement between health and industry sectors (Figure 29.2).

Examples of joint activities include research on substitute products (e.g., snus), venue modifications (e.g., socialized gambling), compulsory standards (e.g., food advertising codes), and environmental controls (e.g., air pollution standards). The model's success relies heavily on the active and assertive involvement of key government agencies in carefully monitoring and mandating all contact and joint activities. Any sign of compromised funding arrangements, industry ambivalence, or loss of health sector independence would require prompt intervention to review whether to terminate activities or renegotiate understandings. In the case of unhealthy commodity industries, it is difficult to envisage governments achieving sufficient clarity because of their own interests and involvements with industry activities, and this would risk sliding back into the power imbalances of the equal association model.

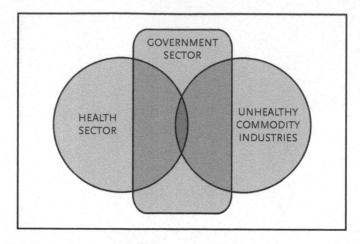

Figure 29.2 Managed association model.
Adapted from Adams et al.[14]

The third alternative arrangement, the *non-association model*, recognizes that government sector agencies will need to maintain some ongoing relationships with the industry sector for purposes such as monitoring standards, regulation compliance, and harm minimization. However, it also acknowledges that health sector engagement with industry comes with too many negative consequences and that any contribution of the health sector to improving consumption environments must be managed through the government sector in ways that avoid direct exposure. In this way, and as depicted in Figure 29.3, the government's role becomes one of relating to both sectors while at the same time accepting, and perhaps supporting, health sector interests in maintaining their separation.

The strongest and most consistent example of this model, at least up until the advent of e-cigarettes, has been the health sector stance of non-association with tobacco companies.[21,22] The stance has the advantages of clarity and

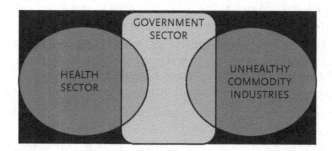

Figure 29.3 Non-association model.
Adapted from Adams et al.[14]

preserving health sector integrity; however, it assumes that the government sector will be strong and independent enough to maintain this separation. As with the managed association model, government interests and involvements with the products make this difficult to achieve, particularly with corporates promoting the perceived social benefits of their products to the public, as happens with alcohol and unhealthy food and beverages.

29.3 CATEGORIES OF CONSUMPTION

In the United Kingdom, one example of a high-profile PPP, the Public Health Responsibility Deal, was launched in 2011 as a system of PPPs targeting health improvements with alcohol, food, physical activity, and workplace networks.[23] By May 2017, 776 organizations were reported to have pledged their contributions to partnership initiatives.[24] However, by this time, a range of public health concerns had already been raised about the value of this network of deals. Some criticized the arrangements as prioritizing private interests over public good.[25,26] Others highlighted the way these deals had led to conflict and fragmentation in the health sector. For example, Hawkins and McCambridge interviewed 26 policy actors whose accounts detailed how the Responsibility Deal had reshaped the policy terrain in ways that "led to both disagreements and divisions within the public health sector and marginalized these bodies from policy debates."[27(p11)] Another group noted how adopting partnership arrangements with different consumptions—for example, alcohol compared to food—involves a different set of risks. Indeed, leaders in the alcohol field expressed concern from the outset.[28,29]

The idea that different commodities entail different risks highlights whether partnership approaches with one type of consumption require different terms of engagement and different models of association compared to those with other consumptions. What might be appropriate for fossil fuels may not be as appropriate for tobacco or gambling. In other words, the risk of engaging in conflicted or ineffective partnership varies according to a range of factors, including the nature of the products. To assist with this discussion, I propose dividing unhealthy commodities according to three broad categories as listed in Table 29.1.

Category A (addictive) consumptions need to be treated differently than other unhealthy commodities primarily because addicted consumers differ from non-addicted consumers in several important ways. First, addicted consumers consume far more than non-addicted consumers. Not that addicted consumers are necessarily any more numerous than non-addicted consumers, but their excess consumption means they spend considerably more and are, therefore, responsible for a larger proportion of the profits. For example, a significant proportion of profits from tobacco and alcohol is derived directly

Table 29.1 TYPES OF UNHEALTHY CONSUMPTION

Category	Type of Consumption	Description of Commodity	Examples
A	Addictive	Products with the potential for addiction-driven consumption	Tobacco, alcohol, gambling, legalized cannabis, prescribed opiates
B	Behaviorally challenging	Products that are likely to lead to impacts on well-being	Unhealthy food, pornography, cosmetic surgery, retirement villages
C	Contextually damaging	Products impacting on environment in ways that affect health	Fossil fuels, nuclear power, ocean harvesting, petroleum vehicles

from those consuming addictively. Second, this add-on amount of money provides a strong incentive for producers and retailers to do their utmost in both maintaining addictive consumption and guarding against legislative measures that might curb such consumption.[30] Third, addiction surplus provides an accessible and convenient financial base to resource initiatives aimed at diverting healthy public policy by means of a range of well-documented strategies, such as downloading responsibility for harm onto consumers and manipulations of the knowledge base.[31,32] Together, these three aspects combine in positioning public sector interests in diametrically opposed ways to corporate interests.

Category B (behaviorally challenging) consumptions, such as unhealthy food and pornography, miss out on the add-on effects of addiction surplus, and this effectively reduces the incentives that place industry at odds with public health. Kraak et al. argue that when it comes to partnerships with food industries in addressing issues of global malnutrition, as long as commercial interests, conflicts of interest, and effectiveness issues are well managed, then positive initiatives can take place.[33] Similarly, Rouvière and Royer, although cautious about partnerships with the food industry, argue they can be productive, and they developed a framework for managing "incentive mechanisms" to enable partnerships more chances of success.[34] However, others in the field note the extent that unhealthy food and beverage corporations are involved in the promotion and distribution of their products, their investments in influencing policymakers and scientists, and how attachment to profits makes it virtually impossible to conceive of engaging in genuine partnerships for minimizing harm.[35-38]

Category C (contextually damaging), such as fossil fuels and nuclear power, focuses less on consumption by specific individuals and more on consumptions by groups and collectives of people. Although they miss out on the dynamics of addiction surplus, they are exposed to the power play of large multinationals that, unsurprisingly, leads to a similar use of influence strategies common with consumption categories A and B.[39] Accordingly, health sector and civil society organizations that engage in these arrangements can find their goals eclipsed by corporate interests.[40] Mert has highlighted how multinational alliances have encouraged the privatization of global governance and that this has enabled corporations to effectively dominate sustainability partnerships.[41,42] Nonetheless, the mounting urgency regarding global warming and other environmental threats, in addition to the high costs involved in preventing degradation, makes industry partnerships involving large injections of funding highly attractive. This has prompted work exploring the conditions under which multilateral partnerships might prove effective.[43,44] For example, Bäckstrand has evaluated different frameworks for climate partnerships and argues that multilateral PPPs with clear goals, independent monitoring, and high standards of accountability show signs of making a difference.[45]

29.4 ISSUES OF EFFECTIVENESS AND GOVERNANCE

Another issue for the UK Responsibility Deal concerned questions regarding whether the large amounts of money invested in partnership projects resulted in efficient and effective interventions.[46] In an attempt to address these questions, Knai et al. used a systems approach to analyze findings from evaluations of Responsibility Deal projects and concluded that they were largely driven by the interests of partners themselves, "enabling the wider business systems within which RD [Responsibility Deal] was operating to remain resistant to change."[24(p12)] Their findings are consistent with other literature on the effectiveness of PPPs in health. In a systematic review, Torchia et al. identified 46 quality studies, most of which pointed to issues with claims of effectiveness and efficiency, as well as raising concerns that the primary driver for the projects was public attention rather than health goals.[47]

These studies highlight an emerging awareness in public health that health is largely shaped by upstream forces, such as the distribution of power and wealth, and influenced by changes at the level of systems and environments— such as price and availability interventions—and less so by downstream and individualized approaches—such as awareness and behavioral interventions. The voluntary nature of health PPPs enables a significant degree of latitude in the choice of intervention, particularly when government sector agencies take a minor role.[48,49] In these circumstances, corporations will, understandably, seek to engage with approaches that have minimal impacts on profits while at the same time appearing to make a difference. What follows is a tendency for partnerships to focus less on reducing upstream impacts and more on downstream drivers. This has led some commentators to view industry-led health initiatives as taking more the forms of self-promotion rather than genuine and effective attempts to minimize harm.[50,51] For example, Babor et al. rated the quality of 3,551 alcohol industry corporate social responsibility initiatives throughout the world, most of which involved partnerships with government or health sector entities.[52] They found the majority (97%) lacked evidence of effectiveness, and 11% had the potential of doing harm. They concluded that these initiatives functioned more in terms of brand marketing and in managing risks from public health policies.[52]

A further challenge for joint initiatives is clarity over who owns and governs the partnerships that evolve. Ideally, governance should be shared and should reflect the level of contribution of the parties to the project, but clarity over governance is difficult to achieve when vested interests are minimized, concealed, or ignored. Honest and fulsome declarations of conflicts of interest are required to ensure levels of trust required in building sustainable partnerships. However, despite the attractiveness of cooperative arrangements, three aspects can get in the way. First, vested interests can occur at varying levels that include individual, organizational, and systemic conflicts. Declaring conflicts at one level may fail to address conflicts at another level. For instance, in Aotearoa, New Zealand, government guidelines on managing conflicts of interest focus primarily on individual conflicts, such as personal ownership of shares in a relevant company. This means a food or alcohol industry representative can claim to have no conflict despite working for a highly conflicted organization. Second, even in situations in which conflicts are openly declared, more is required before governance risks are addressed; a declaration of vested interest is simply insufficient. What is needed are robust procedures for responding to declared conflicts aimed at ensuring agendas are open and above board. Third, an outstanding challenge is finding solid enough points of accountability in governments for them to adequately monitor and manage conflicts of interest. This is most obvious in the blurring between public and private with state-owned category A consumptions, such as gambling in Nordic countries and tobacco in China.[53,54]

29.5 A HEALTH WARNING

This brief overview of partnership arrangements with unhealthy commodity industries has unearthed more reasons to be cautious than optimistic. Although partnerships have proved productive in other areas of health, the influence and relationship-building potential of unhealthy commodity industries will continue to overshadow efforts in the health sector. Table 29.2 presents my reading of what the literature on partnerships is suggesting.

With the equal association model, for all three consumption categories, the assumption of equality generates an unsafe space for partnership relationships in addressing harms to health. When heavy consumption sits at the center of profits, industry purposes place them at loggerheads with health and well-being purposes. With the managed association model, an independent body, usually a government agency, needs to play an assertive role in monitoring and managing engagement between parties. This is challenging when the independence of such bodies is likely to be eroded by their own interests in the commodities. With the non-association model, industry and health sector actors are kept apart while both contributing to government-led initiatives. This model, arguably, holds promise for consumption categories B and C, but the integrity of initiatives will continue to face challenges in terms of goal-setting, the monitoring of conflicts of interest, and independent accountability.

It is tempting to join in with the spirit of cooperation that underpins the UN and the WHO drive for health PPPs, but in the case of unhealthy commodities, this spirit needs to be tempered by adopting a precautionary approach. In principle, partnerships with unhealthy commodity industries might seem possible as long as the terms of engagement are well defined and implemented. In practice, the history of corporate power strategies, conflicts of interest, and poor accountability make it more likely for partnership initiatives to result in token and ineffective outcomes.

Table 29.2 SUMMARY OF PROBABLE RISK ACROSS ASSOCIATION MODELS AND TYPES OF CONSUMPTION

Category	Equal Association	Managed Association	Non-Association
A (addictive)	Too risky: purposes not aligned	Too risky: Government likely to be conflicted by own interests in commodities	Very high risk: Requires strong, clear, and independent management
B (behavioral)	Too risky: purposes not aligned	Very high risk: Requires strong, clear, and independent management	High risk: Industry influence strategies likely to derail government independence
C (contextual)	Too risky: purposes not aligned	High risk: Requires constant and independent monitoring of conflicts of interest	Moderate risk: Requires high-level monitoring of conflicts of interest

REFERENCES

1. United Nations Office for Partnerships. What we do. 2021. Accessed April 12, 2021. https://www.un.org/partnerships/content/what-we-do-1
2. United Nations Joint Inspection Unit. *The United Nations system: Private sector partnerships arrangements in the context of the 2030 agenda for sustainable development*. United Nations; 2017. https://www.unjiu.org/sites/www.unjiu.org/files/jiu_rep_2017_8_english_1.pdf
3. Bäckstrand K. Are partnerships for sustainable development democratic and legitimate? In: Pattberg P, Biermann F, Chan S, et al., eds. *Public–Private Partnerships for Sustainable Development*. Elgar; 2012: 165.
4. Utting P, Zammit A. United Nations–business partnerships: Good intentions and contradictory agendas. *J Bus Ethics*. 2009; 90: 39–56.
5. Buse K. Governing public–private infectious disease partnerships. *Brown J World Affairs*. 2004; 10(2): 225–242.
6. Lynch T. *The Future of Health, Wellbeing and Physical Education*. Palgrave Macmillan; 2016.
7. Timmermann M, Kruesmann M. *Partnerships for Women's Health: Striving for Best Practice Within the UN Global Compact*. United Nations University Press; 2009.
8. SDG Tracker. Revitalize the global partnership for sustainable development. 2021. Accessed May 10, 2021. https://sdg-tracker.org/global-partnerships
9. United Nations Office for Partnerships. Report of the Secretary-General to UN General Assembly on UN Office for Partnerships. 2019. Accessed May 10, 2021. https://undocs.org/pdf?symbol=en/A/74/266
10. Adams P. *Moral Jeopardy: The Risks of Accepting Money from Tobacco, Alcohol and Gambling Industries*. Cambridge University Press; 2016.
11. Moodie A. What public health practitioners need to know about unhealthy industry tactics. *Am J Public Health*. 2017; 107(7): 1047–1049.
12. McCambridge J, Mialon M, Hawkins B. Alcohol industry involvement in policymaking: A systematic review. *Addiction*. 2018; 113: 1571–1584.
13. Ruckert A, Labonté R. Public–private partnerships (PPPs) in global health: The good, the bad and the ugly. *Third World Q*. 2014; 35(9): 1598–1614.
14. Adams P, Buetow S, Rossen F. Poisonous partnerships: Health sector buy-in to arrangements with government and addictive consumption industries. *Addiction*. 2010; 105: 585–590.
15. Babor T, Robaina K. Public health, academic medicine, and the alcohol industry's corporate social responsibility activities. *Am J Public Health*. 2013; 103(2): 206–214.
16. Petticrew M, Maani Hessari N, Knai C, et al. The strategies of alcohol industry SAPROs: Inaccurate information, misleading language and the use of confounders to downplay and misrepresent the risk of cancer. *Drug Alcohol Rev*. 2018; 37(3): 313–315.
17. Hawkins B, Holden C. "Water dripping on stone?" Industry lobbying and UK alcohol policy. *Policy Polit*. 2014; 42(1): 55–70.
18. Gornall J. Sugar: Spinning a web of influence. *Br Med J*. 2015; 350: h231.
19. Miller D, Harkins C. Corporate strategy, corporate capture: Food and alcohol industry lobbying and public health. *Crit Soc Policy*. 2010; 30(4): 564–589.
20. Petticrew M, McKee M, Marteau T. Partnerships with the alcohol industry at the expense of public health. *Lancet*. 2018; 392(10152): 992–993.

21. Chapman S. *Public Health Advocacy and Tobacco Control: Making Smoking History*. Blackwell; 2007.

22. World Health Organization. Tobacco industry interference with tobacco control. 2008. Accessed May 20, 2021. https://escholarship.org/uc/item/98w687x5

23. Durand M, Petticrew M, Goulding L, et al. An evaluation of the Public Health Responsibility Deal: Informants' experiences and views of the development, implementation and achievements of a pledge-based, public–private partnership to improve population health in England. *Health Policy*. 2015; 119(11): 1506–1514.

24. Knai C, Petticrew M, Douglas N, et al. The Public Health Responsibility Deal: Using a systems-level analysis to understand the lack of impact on alcohol, food, physical activity, and workplace health sub-systems. *Int J Environ Res Public Health*. 2018; 15(12): 2895.

25. Brown K. The Public Health Responsibility Deal: Why alcohol industry partnerships are bad for health? *Addiction*. 2015; 110(8): 1227–1228.

26. Panjwani C, Caraher M. The Public Health Responsibility Deal: Brokering a deal for public health, but on whose terms? *Health Policy*. 2014; 114(2): 163–173.

27. Hawkins B, McCambridge J. Public–private partnerships and the politics of alcohol policy in England: The Coalition Government's Public Health "Responsibility Deal." *BMC Public Health*. 2019; 19(1): 1477.

28. Bonner A, Gilmore I. The UK Responsibility Deal and its implications for effective alcohol policy in the UK and internationally. *Addiction*. 2012; 107(12): 2063–2065.

29. Gilmore A, Savell E, Collin J. Public health, corporations and the New Responsibility Deal: Promoting partnerships with vectors of disease? *J Public Health*. 2011; 33(1): 2–4.

30. Adams P, Livingstone C. Addiction surplus: The add-on margin that makes addictive consumptions difficult to contain. *Int J Drug Policy*. 2015; 26(1): 107–111.

31. Adams P. Commercialization: The role of unhealthy commodity industries. In: Chamberlain K, Lyons A, eds. *Routledge International Handbook of Critical Issues in Health and Illness*. Routledge; 2022: 312–327.

32. White J, Bero L. Corporate manipulation of research: Strategies are similar across five industries. *Stan Law Pol Rev*. 2010; 21: 105–133.

33. Kraak V, Harrigan P, Lawrence M, et al. Balancing the benefits and risks of public–private partnerships to address the global double burden of malnutrition. *Public Health Nutr*. 2012; 15(3): 503–517.

34. Rouvière E, Royer A. Public private partnerships in food industries: A road to success? *Food Policy*. 2017; 69: 135–144.

35. Freedhoff Y, Hébert P. Partnerships between health organizations and the food industry risk derailing public health nutrition. *Can Med Assoc J*. 2011; 183(3): 291–292.

36. James J. "Third-party" threats to research integrity of public–private partnerships. *Addiction*. 2002; 97(10): 1251–2355.

37. Ludwig D, Nestle M. Can the food industry play a constructive role in the obesity epidemic? *JAMA*. 2008; 300(15): 1808–1811.

38. Mialon M, Swinburn B, Wate J, et al. Analysis of the corporate political activity of major food industry actors in Fiji. *Global Health*. 2016; 12(1): 18–32.

39. Supran G, Oreskes, N. Rhetoric and frame analysis of ExxonMobil's climate change communications. *One Earth*. 2021; 4: 1–24.

40. Ählström J, Sjöström E. CSOs and business partnerships: Strategies for interaction. *Bus Strateg Environ*. 2005; 14(4): 230–240.

41. Mert A. Partnerships and the privatisation of environmental governance of nature and other inevitabilities. *Environ Value*. 2012; 21(4): 475–498.
42. Mert A. *Environmental Governance Through Partnerships: A Discourse Theoretical Study*. Elgar; 2015.
43. Abbott K. Orchestrating experimentation in non-state environmental commitments. *Environ Polit*. 2017; 26(4): 738–763.
44. Chan S, van Asselt H, Hale T, et al. Reinvigorating international climate policy: A comprehensive framework for effective nonstate action. *Glob Policy*. 2015; 6(4): 466–473.
45. Bäckstrand K. Accountability of networked climate governance: The rise of transnational climate partnerships. *Global Environ Polit*. 2008; 8(3): 74–102.
46. Laverty A, Kypridemos C, Seferidi P, et al. Quantifying the impact of the Public Health Responsibility Deal on salt intake, cardiovascular disease and gastric cancer burdens. *J Epidemiol Community Health*. 2019; 73(9): 881–887.
47. Torchia M, Calabrò A, Morner M. Public–private partnerships in the health care sector: A systematic review of the literature. *Public Manag Rev*. 2015; 17(2): 236–261.
48. Jahiel R. Corporate-induced diseases, upstream epidemiologic surveillance, and urban health. *J Urban Health*. 2008; 45(4): 517–530.
49. Marmot M. Social determinants of health inequalities. *Lancet*. 2005; 365(9464): 1099–1104.
50. Cai Y, Jo H, Pan C. Doing well while doing bad? CSR in controversial industry sectors. *J Bus Ethics*. 2012; 108(4): 467–480.
51. Yoon S. Lam T. The illusion of righteousness: Corporate social responsibility practices of the alcohol industry. *BMC Public Health*. 2013; 13: 630.
52. Babor T, Robaina K, Brown K, et al. Is the alcohol industry doing well by "doing good"? Findings from a content analysis of the alcohol industry's actions to reduce harmful drinking. *BMJ Open*. 2018; 8(10): e024325.
53. Nikkinen J. Is there a need for personal gambling licences? *Nord Stud Alcohol Drugs*. 2019; 36(2): 108–124.
54. Malone R. China's chances, China's choices in global tobacco control. *Tob Control*. 2010; 19(1): 1–2.

CHAPTER 30

Understanding and Managing Corporate Conflicts of Interest

KATHERINE CULLERTON AND MARTIN WHITE

30.1 WHAT IS A CONFLICT OF INTEREST?

The primary purpose of commercial enterprises is to make or maximize profits and often to grow the company in question. Although companies may increasingly claim to have subsidiary aims, such as responsibilities for human or planetary health and well-being, their primary goal is for the most part poorly aligned with such prosocial goals. Indeed, a major systemic failure of the post-Industrial Revolution era is the huge external costs of commercial enterprises, which range from poor human health to environmental degradation.[1] The goals of commerce are thus often poorly aligned with the goals of public policies designed to improve health and well-being and also with those of health research. This fundamental misalignment leads to the potential for conflicts of interest. These conflicts of interest can undermine the credibility of health policy or research and professionals who pursue them. They can also result in the erosion of public trust in health policymaking and research.

A conflict of interest can be defined as "a set of conditions in which professional judgment concerning a primary interest (such as a patient's welfare or the validity of research) tends to be unduly influenced by a secondary interest (such as financial gain)."[2] The transfer of money between parties clearly leads to indebtedness (see Chapter 23), but this is not the only such transaction that can create the conditions that lead to a conflict of interest. Secondary interests therefore need to be widely defined, including intellectual conflicts. Importantly, although intellectual conflicts of interest do exist, we recognize that they are of lower ethical priority than conflicts of interest flowing from

Katherine Cullerton and Martin White, *Understanding and Managing Corporate Conflicts of Interest* In: *The Commercial Determinants of Health.* Edited by: Nason Maani, Mark Petticrew, and Sandro Galea, Oxford University Press.
© Oxford University Press 2023. DOI: 10.1093/oso/9780197578742.003.0030

Table 30.1 EXAMPLES OF CONFLICTS OF INTEREST INVOLVING COMMERCIAL
ORGANIZATIONS

Conflicted Party	Primary Interest	Examples of Secondary Interests That Would Likely Conflict
Health policymaker	Developing policy on alcohol regulation	Non-executive directorship of a beer company
		Receipt of funds from a spirits company to support political campaigning
		Board membership of a charitable foundation funded by the alcohol industry
Health researcher	Research on sugar-sweetened beverage taxes	Receipt of research funding from a sugar producer
		Holding shares in a sugar-sweetened beverage company
		Presenting work at a symposium sponsored by a sugary beverage or trade organization

relationships between the health sector and commercial industry character-ized by financial exchange.[3] Of relevance to this book, primary interests can include policymaking that is relevant to human health, health care and public health services, and health research. Some concrete examples are given in Table 30.1. We have limited these to conflicts involving commercial organi-zations, given the focus of this book; however, conflicts of interest can occur in relation to other entities, including public bodies and the charitable sector. All interactions between two parties result in an exchange—and this does not necessarily need to be a financial one for it to create the conditions of suscep-tibility to conflicts of interest. However, it is widely regarded that financial conflicts of interest are the most significant problem involving harmful com-modity industries.[3]

30.2 WHO IS SUSCEPTIBLE TO CONFLICTS OF INTEREST?

In relation to the commercial determinants of health, those susceptible to conflicts of interest include anyone involved in health-related policymaking or health-related research at any organizational level. Susceptibility is also a function of awareness. In our research on interactions between researchers and the food industry, we identified widely varying levels of awareness of the problem of conflicts of interest.[4] Many researchers in nutrition, for example, do not recognize that receiving money from industry may influence their scientific judgment or interpretation of research findings. This blindness to the problem appears to be borne out of long-standing, historical normalization of funding policies and practices by universities, scientific associations, and researchers themselves. There are, of course, contextual explanations for this. Historically, public (governmental) research funding has not been as generous as it is now in many high-income countries, and in many low-resource settings, industry funding may still represent one of the only readily available sources of research funding. In many countries, governments also actively encourage industry involvement in publicly funded research, often without clear guidance on managing potential conflicts of interest. For example, in the United Kingdom, the Medical Research Council strongly encourages researchers to work with industry. The terms of such relationships are guided by a charter.[5] However, this only makes one mention of conflicts of interest: "Potential conflicts of interest, at corporate and individual levels, will be declared and managed."[5(p2)] Guidance on such declaration and management is not given, and it is recognized that declaring interests alone does not necessarily mitigate conflicts of interest.[3,6]

Among policymakers, especially but not exclusively politicians, relationships with the commercial world are commonplace. In most administrations, whether local or national, the economy is the highest priority, and so politicians seek to enhance commerce. Although this may often seem to be at the expense of human and planetary health and well-being because of the large and direct external costs of commerce, there is also a strong and direct relationship between overall wealth and health in all nations. Unfortunately, these trade-offs are often poorly recognized and quantified, so it remains difficult to be clear about the relative benefits of prioritizing the economy versus health. Nevertheless, this general favoring of commerce over health does create the conditions of susceptibility to conflicts of interest.[7]

30.3 WHEN ARE CONFLICTS OF INTEREST A PROBLEM?

In some circumstances, some conflicts of interest are considered "worse" (of higher ethical priority) than others.[3] Goldberg has argued that financial conflicts of interest are more serious than intellectual conflicts.[3] But are there degrees of either type? One nongovernmental health organization has a policy on financial relationships that considers risk on the basis of the *amount* of money involved in a transaction, an approach that is not uncommon.[8] Defining interests as greater or lesser risks suggests that some things are less worth worrying about—that the level of some conflicts may not unduly influence professional judgment. But indebtedness is surely created by the interaction itself, rather than its scale. Arguably a stronger approach is a more neutral appraisal of interests across a number of categories, such as that adopted by the International Committee of Medical Journal Editors, which asks authors to specify interests as (a) funding received for the research itself; (b) financial relationships (including receipt of materials or services in kind) outside the research under consideration that might be perceived to influence, or that give the appearance of potentially influencing, the research; (c) interests in intellectual property related to the research; and (d) other relationships or activities that could be perceive to have influenced or that give the appearance of potentially influencing the research—which might include personal or working relationships, involvement in company activities, etc.[9] The intention of such a declaration is to surface any issues that may result in a conflict of interest. However, no judgment is made about the actual influence such issues may have had—the purpose is simply to achieve transparency, on which we say more below. However, the declaration relates only to "the time frame for this reporting . . . the work itself, from the initial conception and planning to the present."[9] Thus, if any of the above conflicts existed the day before or the day after the research took place, then there is no obligation to declare them—yet, in our view, the conflict very likely still exists. Again, this is an issue on which there seems to be little consensus. Moreover, it is recognized that disclosure alone does not mitigate conflicts of interest, and it may even increase the effects of bias.[10] Several studies have demonstrated that disclosure intensifies behavior of partiality flowing from conflicts of interest.[6,11] However, it would also be wrong to assume that a researcher or policymaker who once had a relationship with a commercial entity is forever indebted to it. Indeed, the opposite may be true.

A key question that has arisen in relation to interactions between researchers and commercial entities is, what defines a commercial entity that is of concern with regard to population health? As previous chapters have identified, commercial companies are of concern when their products, services, or other activities are damaging to health. For some, this is straightforward—for example, tobacco and alcohol companies, gambling companies, and armament manufacturers. However, there are others for which it is less clear-cut, and this is generally because the company has a mixed portfolio of products or services—some good and some bad for health—or because it engages in other activities associated with risk to health, such as causing pollution, tax avoidance, or political activities. For example, approximately 80% of UK households do all their main food shopping at a supermarket for reasons of convenience and value for money. Supermarkets have contributed importantly to improving food supply and safety during approximately the past 60 years, including a substantial widening of the availability of healthy, fresh produce. Yet, they also market a wide range of unhealthy products, including ultra-processed foods, alcohol, and tobacco. The same applies to the vast array of smaller convenience stores. This makes the question of whether researchers should interact with such companies in the interests of better understanding and transforming commercial food systems a challenging one.

Personal behaviors among researchers and policymakers have also been suggested to represent potential conflicts of interest.[12] For example, at a recent international conference on the science and politics of food, speakers were encouraged to declare whether they had any personal dietary preferences (e.g., vegan).[13] There is no consensus on the issue of personal behaviors and other intellectual interests, although some have argued that nonfinancial interests should be managed differently to ensure accountability—for example, by applying the principles of fair representation of differing interests and the application of reflexivity.[14,15]

So far, we have considered the challenges of conflicts of interests that arise from the activities of individual researchers. However, conflicts of interest can also occur at the institutional level (e.g., in universities), when an organization has financial ties that conflict with its vision and mission. Institutional conflicts of interest can also damage public trust in and the credibility of public sector officials or agencies (including research institutions) and undermine the quality of outcomes and services they deliver. Relationships between academic institutions and commercial entities are increasingly encouraged by governments, and this normalizes the involvement of commerce in science, despite its risks to scientific integrity. Commercial partnerships also reinforce the framing of public health problems and their solutions in ways that are least threatening to the interests of corporations.[16]

30.4 WHAT PROBLEMS DO CONFLICTS OF INTEREST CAUSE?

Whether or not we can identify and classify potential conflicts of interest, or grade them according to their implications for policy or research, it is clear from empirical evidence that such conflicts can affect judgments. For example, in an evidence synthesis on the association between sugar-sweetened beverage consumption and weight gain or obesity, systematic reviews that declared financial interest with relevant companies were five times more likely to present a conclusion of no positive association compared to those without them (relative risk: 5.0; 95% confidence interval: 1.3–19.3).[17] Many such studies have been conducted in relation to industry funding across many fields of medicine, health care, and public health with similar conclusions (e.g., medical and surgical trials,[18] pharmaceutical research,[19] and physician prescribing practices[20]).

A conflict of interest, of whatever sort, with a commercial entity can lead to a sense of indebtedness that is not always explicitly recognized by its owner.

Such indebtedness leads to bias in decision-making. This may be subtle and difficult to recognize. Such biases lead to favoring commercial entities in a variety of ways, which may include interpretation of research results that favor a company's products, corporate image, brand, or services; preferential access to policymaking forums; and direct influence over policymakers (e.g., in relation to regulatory policies that might be unfavorable to the company). Conflicts of interest can also lead to reputational damage among all parties concerned. However, the implications and sanctions for those in the public sector can be serious, whereas the actions that lead to conflicts of interest are calculated and deliberate on the part of commercial entities and thus of limited reputational consequence.

Decisions regarding whether a relationship represents a conflict of interest and the level of reputational risk that is acceptable remain a matter of judgment for individuals and their employers, and there is as yet little consensus. In addition to the growth of interest in research on the commercial determinants of health, there has been a growing interest in developing ways to manage such conflicts of interest. This forms the subject of the remainder of this chapter.

30.5 WHAT PRINCIPLES SHOULD UNDERLIE THE MANAGEMENT OF CONFLICTS OF INTEREST?

Our own experience is limited to interactions between researchers and industry, which we use as a case study here. We believe that this encapsulates key principles that can be applied in multiple contexts. To date, limited empirical work has been conducted on what constitutes acceptable interactions between population health researchers or practitioners and the commercial sector, and consensus is urgently needed. In 2015, we commenced a program of work aimed at gaining a deeper insight into the issue.[21] We anticipate that in due course, this should provide the basis for developing internationally agreed guidance for population health researchers.

In a systematic scoping review, we identified the principles and strategies that currently exist to prevent and manage conflicts of interest for population health researchers.[22] We focused our enquiry on the field of diet and nutrition. However, we realized that for these principles to be acceptable and useful, consensus was needed to identify which ones were acceptable for the majority of population health researchers. This would help clarify the conditions under which it may be acceptable to interact with the food industry as well as identify when this interaction should not occur. To gain insight into this, we examined which of the strategies found in our scoping review were supported by the population health research community as well as population health stakeholders.[4] We found that the principles which attracted the highest levels of agreement were those derived from widely accepted research governance frameworks and involved limited values-based decision-making, such as the following:

- Have a clearly identified system to identify and assess interests of potential partners.
- Ensure research governance practices are in place before work commences.
- Establish upfront control and ownership of data.
- Have a clearly identified system to identify and manage conflict of interests and clearly stated exit mechanisms.
- Ensure researchers retain full rights to publish all results.

We also found broad agreement on more aspirational principles, with researchers and stakeholders agreeing that the organizational values and overarching goals of the partners should be compatible and that whether the partnership maximizes benefit to society should be considered.

The most contentious statements, in terms of both agreement levels and emotive comments from participants, were concerned with which elements of the commercial sector it is acceptable for population health researchers to interact. Most researchers and stakeholders believed it was appropriate for population health researchers to accept funding from commercial organizations in general. However, the level of agreement decreased significantly when statements specified accepting funding from the food industry and, in particular, processed food and beverage companies. This is unsurprising because many view the primary goal of population health researchers (to discover new knowledge to improve the health of the population) as being poorly aligned with the primary goal of most processed food and beverage companies (to generate profit).[23–25] Furthermore, recommendations from population health researchers frequently encourage government actions that are contrary to the preferences of the commercial sector.

30.6 HOW SHOULD CONFLICTS OF INTEREST BE MANAGED?

Through our consensus-building work, we recognized that most researchers sought a practical decision-making tool that would both provide clarity and increase their agency to assess potential opportunities or risks associated with interacting with industry, as well as manage such relationships. We set out to design such a toolkit based on our research.

30.6.1 Assessing Risks

Central to our research findings has been the importance of assessing the potential risk of interacting with the food industry *prior* to any formal interaction. Risk assessments are inherently difficult because people tend to be overconfident about their ability to independently assess risk and the range of outcomes that may occur,[26] and so we recommend this always be undertaken by one or more independent professional colleagues. The risk assessment should assess the risk profile of the organization and the type of interaction proposed with the organization. Only if both of these categories of risk are considered low would we recommend proceeding to a "risk–benefit analysis." Importantly, the type of interaction a researcher or research institution has with a commercial organization may change over time. Therefore, it is important to re-evaluate risk regularly and at every stage of the research.

30.6.2 Negotiating Interaction

If the risk of interaction is low and the benefit to society is high, then one may decide to proceed with an interaction. However, research governance and integrity requirements need to be established before a formal interaction can take place. This is likely to require negotiation of a number of terms, which might include the following:

- Agreement with the commercial organization that it should not be involved in study design and analyzing and/or interpreting scientific findings due to the potential for conflicts of interest
- Establishing upfront control and ownership of the research data
- Considering whether it is possible to have oversight of the research by a party independent of the researchers, irrespective of the funding source
- Consideration of whether the commercial partner should be allowed to co-brand research project materials (e.g., use its logo)

30.6.3 Research Governance

If negotiations have proceeded satisfactorily and all parties are satisfied that the risks of conflict of interest are low, then it should be possible to commence interaction with the commercial organization formally. This will require researchers to adhere to the usual standards of research conduct—for example, using the standards set by the EQUATOR Network (a network aimed at enhancing the quality and transparency of health research).[27] But, we also encourage researchers to go above and beyond these standards and consider further governance standards, such as the following:

• Publicly reporting funding arrangements, governance structures, research frameworks, and findings
• Using established mechanisms to continuously monitor for conflicts of interest among the research team
• Providing a comprehensive declaration of interests near the start of any research presentation when the research has involved interactions with industry, and ensuring such a declaration is provided in full with all publications arising from the research (including press releases)

30.7 BY WHOM SHOULD CONFLICTS OF INTEREST BE MANAGED?

Ideally, we believe the risk assessment process outlined above should be undertaken by an independent body—perhaps an ethics committee. The negotiating interaction stage can be undertaken by the research team, although it may also require legal advice from one's institution. The research governance process can by undertaken by the research team, often with support from an institutional research governance team. We consider it good practice to seek independent oversight of one's research (in terms of both the science and governance arrangements, including commercial interactions) by an independent advisory committee, irrespective of the funding source.

The approach described above has been developed for researchers, specifically in relation to the food industry, but the principles on which it is based are generic and could be adapted for all research areas. An international group of research funders, led by the Canadian Institutes of Health Research, has shown interest in this approach, although a planned consensus building workshop in 2020 was postponed due to the coronavirus pandemic.

Guidance regarding acceptable interactions and conflicts of interest involving the commercial sector has also been developed for nongovernment organizations[28] and for policymakers.[29-31] Most widely adopted among these is the World Health Organization (WHO) Framework Convention on Tobacco Control, adopted by 168 countries.[31] Although this covers a much broader range of activities, Article 5.3 exists to protect health policy from the "commercial and vested interests of the tobacco industry."[31(p14)] However, it does not state how this should be achieved, and it provides no clear framework for the avoidance of conflicts of interest. Similar criticisms have been leveled at other frameworks,[32] such as WHO's Framework of Engagement with Non-State Actors.[30]

30.8 FUTURE DEVELOPMENTS

Our studies in this field have revealed differing views on the complex issues of preventing and managing conflicts of interest, and it was clear that experience of these issues varied across different nations and cultures. We need to better understand the experience of these issues and the ways they are handled in low- and middle-income countries in particular. This understanding will help assess the barriers to implementing guidelines in the future. We also believe there is much to be gained from discerning the similarities and differences between our findings and those of other research fields, such as biomedical and pharmaceutical research, in which industry research collaborations are widespread and the goals of industry and research are often more closely aligned.

REFERENCES

1. White M, Aguirre E, Finegood DT, Holmes C, Sacks G, Smith R. What role should the commercial food system play in promoting health through better diet? *BMJ.* 2020; 368: m545. doi:10.1136/bmj.m545
2. Thompson DF. Understanding financial conflicts of interest. *N Engl J Med.* 1993; 329(8): 573–576. doi:10.1056/nejm199308193290812
3. Goldberg DS. Financial conflicts of interest are of higher ethical priority than "intellectual" conflicts of interest. *J Bioeth Inq.* 2020; 17(2): 217–227. doi:10.1007/s11673-020-09989-4
4. Cullerton K, Adams J, Francis O, Forouhi N, White M. Building consensus on interactions between population health researchers and the food industry: Two-stage, online, international Delphi study and stakeholder survey. *PLoS One.* 2019; 14(8): e0221250. https://doi.org/10.1371/journal.pone.0221250
5. Medical Research Council. *The Medical Research Council Industry Charter.* 2017.
6. Loewenstein G, Sah S, Cain DM. The unintended consequences of conflict of interest disclosure. *JAMA.* 2012; 307(7): 669–670. doi:10.1001/jama.2012.154
7. Cullerton K, Donnet T, Lee A, Gallegos D. Playing the policy game: A review of the barriers to and enablers of nutrition policy change. *Public Health Nutr.* 2016; 19(14): 2643–2653. doi:10.1017/s1368980016000677
8. World Obesity Federation. World Obesity's financial relationship policy 2015. http://s3-eu-west-1.amazonaws.com/wof-files/WOF_Financial_Relationship_Policy_June2015.pdf
9. International Committee of Medical Journal Editors. Disclosure of financial and non-financial relationships and activities, and conflicts of interest. 2022. http://www.icmje.org/recommendations/browse/roles-and-responsibilities/author-responsibilities--conflicts-of-interest.html
10. Goldberg DS. The shadows of sunlight: Why disclosure should not be a priority in addressing conflicts of interest. *Public Health Ethics.* 2018; 12(2): 202–212. doi:10.1093/phe/phy016
11. Cain DM, Loewenstein G, Moore DA. When sunlight fails to disinfect: Understanding the perverse effects of disclosing conflicts of interest. *J Consume Res.* 2010; 37(5): 836–857. doi:10.1086/656252

12. Ioannidis JPA, Trepanowski JF. Disclosures in nutrition research: Why it is different. *JAMA*. 2018; 319(6): 547–548. doi:10.1001/jama.2017.18571
13. The BMJ and Swiss Re. Food for thought: The science and politics of nutrition conference. n.d. https://www.bmj.com/food-for-thought
14. Bero LA, Grundy Q. Why having a (nonfinancial) interest is not a conflict of interest. *PLoS Biol*. 2016; 14(12): e2001221. doi:10.1371/journal.pbio.2001221
15. Bero L, Grundy Q. Conflicts of interest in nutrition research. *JAMA*. 2018; 320(1): 93–94. doi:10.1001/jama.2018.5662
16. Marks JH. Toward a systemic ethics of public–private partnerships related to food and health. *Kennedy Inst Ethics J*. 2014; 24(3): 267–299. doi:10.1353/ken.2014.0022
17. Bes-Rastrollo M, Schulze MB, Ruiz-Canela M, Martinez-Gonzalez MA. Financial conflicts of interest and reporting bias regarding the association between sugar-sweetened beverages and weight gain: A systematic review of systematic reviews. *PLoS Med*. 2014; 10(12): e1001578. doi:10.1371/journal.pmed.1001578
18. Bhandari M, Busse JW, Jackowski D, et al. Association between industry funding and statistically significant pro-industry findings in medical and surgical randomized trials. *Can Med Assoc J*. 2004; 170(4): 477–480.
19. Sismondo S. How pharmaceutical industry funding affects trial outcomes: Causal structures and responses. *Social Sci Med*. 2008; 66(9): 1909–1914. https://doi.org/10.1016/j.socscimed.2008.01.010
20. Yeh JS, Franklin JM, Avorn J, Landon J, Kesselheim AS. Association of industry payments to physicians with the prescribing of brand-name statins in Massachusetts. *JAMA Intern Med*. 2016; 176(6): 763–768. doi:10.1001/jamainternmed.2016.1709
21. Centre for Diet & Activity Research. Dietary public health research and the food industry. University of Cambridge. n.d. Accessed June 20, 2021. https://www.cedar.iph.cam.ac.uk/research/dietary-public-health/food-systems-public-health/diet-research-food-industry-project
22. Cullerton K, Adams J, Forouhi N, Francis O, White M. What principles should guide interactions between population health researchers and the food industry? Systematic scoping review of peer-reviewed and grey literature. *Obes Rev*. 2019; 20(8): 1073–1084. doi:10.1111/obr.12851
23. Aveyard P, Yach D, Gilmore AB, Capewell S. Should we welcome food industry funding of public health research? *BMJ*. 2016; 353: i2161. doi:10.1136/bmj.i2161
24. Collin J, Hill SE, Kandlik Eltanani M, Plotnikova E, Ralston R, Smith KE. Can public health reconcile profits and pandemics? An analysis of attitudes to commercial sector engagement in health policy and research. *PLoS One*. 2017; 12(9): e0182612. doi:10.1371/journal.pone.0182612
25. Nestle M. Food company sponsorship of nutrition research and professional activities: A conflict of interest? *Public Health Nutr*. 2001; 4(5): 1015–1022. doi:10.1079/phn2001253
26. Fabricius G, Büttgen M. Project managers' overconfidence: How is risk reflected in anticipated project success? *Bus Res*. 2015; 8(2): 239–263. doi:10.1007/s40685-015-0022-3
27. EQUATOR network. Enhancing the QUAlity and Transparency Of health Research. n.d. https://www.equator-network.org

28. Kraak VI, Story M. Guiding principles and a decision-making framework for stake-holders pursuing healthy food environments. *Health Aff*. 2015; 34(11): 1972–1978. doi:10.1377/hlthaff.2015.0635

29. World Health Organization. Addressing and managing conflicts of interest in the planning and delivery of nutrition programmes at country level: Report of a technical consultation convened in Geneva, Switzerland, on 8–9 October 2015. 2016. https://apps.who.int/iris/bitstream/handle/10665/206554/9789241510530_eng.pdf

30. World Health Organization. Framework of engagement with non-state actors. 2016. https://apps.who.int/gb/ebwha/pdf_files/wha69/a69_r10-en.pdf

31. Conference of the Parties to the WHO FCTC. WHO Framework Convention on Tobacco Control. 2003. https://apps.who.int/iris/bitstream/handle/10665/42811/9241591013.pdf

32. Buse K, Hawkes S. Sitting on the FENSA: WHO engagement with industry. *Lancet*. 2016; 388(10043): 446–447. https://doi.org/10.1016/S0140-6736(16)31141-2

CHAPTER 31

Teaching the Commercial Determinants of Health

NICHOLAS FREUDENBERG AND ERIC CROSBIE

31.1 BACKGROUND

Public health and health care professionals, researchers, lawyers, journalists, policymakers, regulators, and activists will inevitably find themselves in situations in which they encounter and must engage with the actions and health consequences of commercial actors. Consider the local health official who must decide whether and how to regulate the promotion of unhealthy food, alcohol, or tobacco; the legislator who wants to reduce carbon emissions from fossil fuels; the labor activist seeking to protect members from unsafe working conditions; or the researcher who wants to elucidate the pathways by which corporate investment decisions shape patterns of health and disease. To make informed decisions that protect public health, each of these actors will need conceptual and practical skills to gather, analyze, and interpret the available evidence.

In this chapter, we describe the rationale, challenges, and opportunities of teaching a variety of audiences about the commercial determinants of health (CDOH) in ways that enable them to make informed decisions that protect public health. We draw from a wide base of research, scholarship, and practical experience and seek to synthesize this evidence into practical suggestions for those teaching inside and outside of academia.

A common starting point for the design of educational programs for professional preparation is to identify the competencies—defined as what students should be able to do by the time they graduate—needed for competent, ethical professional practice. To develop the educational field of CDOH will

Nicholas Freudenberg and Eric Crosbie, *Teaching the Commercial Determinants of Health* In: *The Commercial Determinants of Health*. Edited by: Nason Maani, Mark Petticrew, and Sandro Galea, Oxford University Press.
© Oxford University Press 2023. DOI: 10.1093/oso/9780197578742.003.0031

require preparation of a cadre of researchers, practitioners, and advocates who can apply this framework to practice, research, and policy advocacy.

31.2 COMPETENCIES/SKILLS

Effective teaching of CDOH will require identifying clear competencies that serve as goals for teaching. Our primary focus in this chapter is on teaching students in graduate schools of public health, the foundation of the public health workforce in the United States and many other nations. However, because many other disciplines contribute to the public health workforce and those working in other settings and with other levels of formal education also contribute to the task of addressing CDOH, we briefly consider some of the issues confronting teaching about CDOH to these other key players.

Based on our experience teaching CDOH and our scan of the relevant literature, we propose that graduates of schools of public health should be able to do the following:

1. Define CDOH and discuss the history of the framework and evolving conceptions of its meaning, importance, and its relationship to other determinants (e.g., biological and behavioral) and public health frameworks such as the social determinants of health (SDOH)
2. Apply CDOH frameworks to the analysis of public health practice, research, and policy analysis in order to develop research studies and interventions that contribute to effective strategies for minimizing the harms and maximizing the benefits of CDOH
3. Assess marketing practices and corporate political activity among major health harming industries such as tobacco, alcohol, food and beverage, pharmaceuticals, gaming, social media, fossil fuels, and others
4. Identify key sources of evidence and data on the distribution, impact, and pathways by which commercial factors influence health and assess the strengths and limitations of these sources
5. Assess the strengths and weakness of various supply-side and demand-side government policy solutions and intergovernmental agreements to reduce the harmful consequences of CDOH
6. Assess the various strategies, tactics, counter-marketing, and campaigns by advocacy groups and coalitions to address the harms of CDOH and help reduce noncommunicable diseases (NCDs) and other adverse outcomes, including infectious diseases
7. Evaluate the impact of strategies designed to reduce the harms and enhance the benefits of CDOH and communicate the findings clearly to various constituencies

8. Make the case for public health practice and research that address CDOH as fundamental determinants of health and health equity

In our view, each academic institution and department will need to tailor these broad competencies to meet the specific needs of their students and identify the specific criteria they will use to assess whether learners have met each competency.

31.3 WHAT TO TEACH

Those who teach must ask both what to teach and how to teach. To acquire the skills and competencies needed to address CDOH, students will need to grasp several key concepts, frameworks, and theoretical approaches. Table 31.1 defines a few key concepts that have emerged in the recent literature—concepts that both faculty and students should grasp. By encouraging reading, critical analysis, and application of these concepts inside and outside the classroom, faculty can help students use them as they enter professional practice.

Although the use of the term CDOH began in the second decade of this century, its foundations lie in more than two centuries of interactions between markets, governments, and people.[5] (Tracing these origins can help students develop a historical perspective and link the concept to other disciplines, including political economy, history, business, law, medicine, and sociology.)

A more recent intellectual ancestor of the CDOH concept is the SDOH framework.[13] By expanding the 20th-century focus of public health research and action from biomedical and behavioral causes and interventions to the inclusion of deeper social, economic, and political forces that SDOH theorists called the "causes of the causes," this school of thought opened the door for investigation of a wide array of market actor influences on health. Are CDOH a subset of SDOH or themselves a cause (i.e., drivers) of other social influences? Although there is no academic consensus on this question, students should be familiar with this debate and encouraged to examine the implications for prevention and public health improvement of how the CDOH/SDOH nexus is framed.[14]

Several public health methodologies and approaches can be useful to public health professionals who seek to apply the CDOH concept to their practice and research. Early research on the tobacco industry used archival research on internal industry documents to understand commercial industries as vectors of disease that help transmit NCDs by producing and marketing unhealthy products and influencing science and public policy to protect their profits. The University of California, San Francisco's Industry Documents Library contains more than 80 million previously secret tobacco internal industry documents. In the 2010s, this collection expanded to include internal documents from

Table 31.1 KEY CONCEPTS IN CDOH

Term	Definitions and References
Capitalism	An economic and political system in which the quest for profit motivates business activities, and corporate, cultural, political, and ideological practices shape a system of accumulation.[1] In the 21st century, a variety of heterogeneous varieties of capitalism are in operation.[2]
Commercial determinants of health	"Actors that influence health which stem from the profit motive."[3] "Strategies and approaches used by the private sector to promote products and choices that are detrimental to health."[4] "The social, political and economic structures, norms, rules, and practices by which business activities designed to generate profits and increase market share influence patterns of health, disease, injury, disability, and death within and across populations."[5]
Commodification	Transformation of goods and services to commodities (material or product that can be sold).[6]
Corporate accountability	The degree to which a company is accountable to the public for its performance in nonfinancial areas, such as social responsibility and sustainability.[7]
Corporate social responsibility	Self-regulating business model that has the goal of helping a corporation be socially accountable to itself, its shareholders, and the public.
Corporation	Legal entity that is separate from its owners, owned by shareholders who elect a board of directors.
Externalities	Cost or benefit incurred or received by a third party that lacks control over these positive or negative externalities.[8] Health and environmental effects of corporate practices can be considered externalities.
Globalization	"Multidimensional set of *social processes* that create, multiply, stretch, and intensify worldwide social *interdependencies and exchanges* while at the same time fostering in people a growing awareness of deepening connections between the local and the distant."[9]
Marketing	Marketing is a *process* that involves design, creation, research, and data mining about how to best align the idea of a product or service with the *target audience*.[10] Marketing helps define the product even more than the actual product does. Advertising is one component of the marketing process.
Public–private partnerships	Partnerships among public or nonprofit entities such as health departments, universities, or civil society groups and for-profit businesses designed to achieve research, practice, or other public health goals.[11]
Trade liberalization	Reducing or eliminating barriers to trade, including tariff barriers (taxes on imported goods and services)s and non-tariff barriers (e.g., quotas and subsidies).[12]

CDOH, commercial determinants of health.

food, chemical, drug, and fossil fuel industries.[15] Research using the archival library has already led to more than 1,000 research publications. Other such archives have recently been established.[16]

A second approach, systems thinking, is defined by Arnold and Wade as "a set of synergistic analytic skills used to improve the capability of identifying and understanding systems, predicting their behaviors, and devising modifications to them in order to produce desired effects."[17] Knai et al. (see also Chapter 2, this volume) note that systems thinking enables CDOH researchers to embed their work

> in the wider political, economic, institutional, and cultural systems; reveal the underlying characteristics and relationships of systems; and show how they interrelate to produce outcomes. . . . It also enables moving away from "factors thinking" (listing factors that may influence a result) and "intervention thinking" (which recommends solutions based on isolated, discrete interventions) toward "operational thinking" (understanding how interventions work in combination and interact with their context).[18]

Systems thinking provides a foundation for systems science and modeling approaches that can help CDOH practitioners and researchers identify pathways by which commercial influences shape health and promising opportunities for intervention.[19]

Implementation science, a third approach, studies the use of strategies to adapt and use evidence-based targeted interventions to initiate and sustain improvements to population health.[20] The rich variety of natural and planned efforts to modify commercial influences on health provides an ideal opportunity to apply implementation science to understand more and less effective strategies to minimize harmful CDOH and to guide the process of implementation in diverse settings. The growing interest in "practice-based evidence" as a source for policy guidance builds on the methods of implementation science.[21] For example, the decision to expand bans on trans fats in commercial food after the New York City Department of Health showed that such a ban led to decreases in consumption of this addiction, reductions in associated cardiovascular disease, and helped hundreds of other jurisdictions and eventually the U.S. Food and Drug Administration to implement such bans.[22,23]

Another approach to more effective research and intervention on CDOH is to employ participatory action research and community-based participatory research. These approaches engage those affected by a health problem in framing research questions, gathering and interpreting data, and presenting findings to policymakers and researchers.[24] By including community residents, workers, environmental activists, elected officials, and others in studying and addressing CDOH, researchers and public health professionals can ensure that the insights and experiences of these constituencies can inform both the findings and interpretation of this evidence. Baum et al.'s presentation of a community-informed process for conducting a corporate health impact assessment illustrates this strategy.[25]

A fifth methodological approach to the study of CDOH is to use data science, public health informatics, and what has been labeled "Big Data" to analyze and characterize how commercial actors influence health and also to synthesize the overwhelming accumulation of public, research, and commercial data into useable intelligence to guide public health practice. Lima and Galea's creation of the Corporate Permeation Index, a measure designed to compare the extent to which corporate influences have penetrated the policy arenas across industries and sectors, is an example of this approach.[26]

Finally, social discourse analysis, which combines political framing and social network analyses using publicly available media sources, has been used to study CDOH.[27] This recent approach offers an effective strategy for mapping industry practices across sectors.

In summary, academic programs can ensure that public health students can apply these six and other emerging approaches and methodology in practice to the study of CDOH and the development of policies and programs to reduce their harmful impact.

31.4 HOW TO TEACH

Infusing CDOH concepts, frameworks, and skills into the curricula of public health and other training programs will require developing a portfolio of teaching strategies from modest to more ambitious, as summarized in Table 31.2. The goal is to enable every faculty member and academic program to find something they can do to prepare their students. No program will be able to adopt every strategy listed in Table 31.2 to their degree program and students, but in our view, every program will be able to find something they can do to prepare their students to take on this fundamental influence on health. By matching the capacity and resources available to a specific school or academic program, faculty who want to strengthen their students' mastery of CDOH competencies can choose an appropriate mix of activities.

31.5 PEDAGOGICAL STRATEGIES

Whatever the course content and instructional format, any teaching/learning experience needs to engage learners in mastering, critically analyzing, and applying the knowledge presented in the classroom (whether in person or

Table 31.2 TEACHING STRATEGIES FOR CDOH

Teaching Approach	Advantages (+) and Disadvantages (−)	Examples
Lectures	+ Make it easier to reach learners outside academy and all students in a given discipline, rather than the few who choose a specialized elective. + Can be tailored to unique needs of learners' academic level and discipline. + By adding single lectures to several required courses, all students can get a systematic introduction of CDOH principles; incremental costs are low. − May lead to superficial coverage; lack of opportunities to learn with other disciplines; limited opportunities to practice application of new knowledge.	WHO and PAHO have offered lecture series and webinars on CDOH. LSHTM offers lectures and seminars on CDOH as part of core Master of Science modules.
Full courses	+ Enable students to develop and apply range of CDOH, exchange ideas with classmates from other disciplines, and practice skills in the classroom or in the community. + If required, courses ensure that all students in a program learn the material while electives offer interested students the opportunity to develop expertise. − May require additional resources and faculty expertise. Electives limit exposure to those who elect to take them.	CUNY offers Master of Public Health and Doctor of Philosophy interdisciplinary courses on corporations and health; University of Nevada, Reno, School of Public Health offers an undergraduate and graduate CDOH course; University of California, San Francisco offers a graduate course on CDOH; Erasmus University offers a graduate course on industrial epidemics; George Washington University Milken Institute School of Public Health offers a graduate course on CDOH.
Field placements	+ Offer students an opportunity to work with government agencies, civil society groups, businesses, and in other settings and to gain a practical knowledge and experience in addressing how CDOH influence health.	Field and work placements with unions, health departments, civil society groups, businesses, and global health agencies

(continued)

Table 31.2 CONTINUED

Teaching Approach	Advantages (+) and Disadvantages (–)	Examples
Research assignments	+ Allow students at various levels and in a variety of disciplines to develop research projects that provide knowledge and practice in its application of CDOH frameworks to solving public health problems.	Systemic reviews of literature on CDOH topics; corporate health impact assessments, case studies of successful and unsuccessful campaigns to modify CDOH
Dissertation projects	+ Provide an opportunity for in-depth examination of a problem (or solution) and for additional contributions to the literature.	A study of the health impact of precarious work in a sector and place
Degree programs	+ Degree programs could grant degrees in the field of CDOH. If created, these programs enable in-depth study of field. – May require more dedicated resources than the previous approaches.	None yet identified
Certificates	+ Certificates usually require three or four courses and can either be a component of a degree program or a stand-alone academic experience; can be interdisciplinary, ensuring that students get exposure to courses and faculty from more than one discipline.	None yet identified
Interdisciplinary workshops	Short courses, workshops, and symposia allow researchers and practitioners working in various setting to exchange ideas and develop skills.	Offered by a variety of academic institutions, WHO, and other organizations
Centers and institutes	Provide an institutional home for a team of researchers and practitioners to pursue ongoing research and intervention to address CDOH.	George Washington University Center on Commercial Determinants of Health LSHTM Commercial Determinants Research Group

CDOH, commercial determinants of health; CUNY, City University of New York; LSHTM, London School of Hygiene & Tropical Medicine; PAHO, Pan American Health Organization; WHO, World Health Organization.

virtually). Several pedagogical strategies may be appropriate for engaging learners in the study of CDOH, including the following:

Experiential learning: This approach immerses students in the actual situations they can expect to encounter in professional practice. By

critical analysis and reflection on these experiences, students cultivate new awareness and knowledge. Developed by Kolb, who defined
learning as "the process whereby knowledge is created through the
transformation of experience,"[28(p41)] experiential learning provides
students of CDOH with the opportunity to participate in and reflect
on efforts to take on these fundamental determinants of health. Its
emphasis on critical analysis and reflexivity distinguishes experiential learning from more traditional internships and service work.

Community-engaged pedagogy: This brings learners and faculty together
with community, labor, environmental, or other leaders and residents to deepen shared understanding of the causes and solutions
to a health problem under investigation. This approach is based on a
deep respect for the prior knowledge and experiences that community partners bring to the conversation.[29]

Team learning: Whether in classrooms or practice or research settings,
team learning offers students from various disciplines (e.g., history,
political science, business, law, medicine, and public health) or life
experiences an opportunity to exchange viewpoints, develop skills in
communicating across boundaries, and produce reports based on collective deliberations.[30] Each of these competencies also contributes
to addressing CDOH.

Case study teaching: This enables students to critically analyze specific
examples of commercial actors' influence on health and interventions to reduce harmful impact and to consider the relevance and ap-
plicability of this practice-based evidence. Several books and articles
provide material for comparative case study investigation of commercial influences,[31-33] and a number of document repositories are
available (e.g., the University of California, San Francisco's Industry
Document Library and the University of Bath's Stopping Tobacco
Organizations and Products).

31.6 CONCLUSION

For the past two centuries, public health professionals have worked with
reformers, government officials, clinicians, researchers, and social movements
to improve the living conditions, policies, and programs that shape health and
disease. Today, CDOH represent a fundamental cause of the world's most serious health, social, and environmental problems, from the COVID-19 pandemic, the climate emergency, and deaths of despair to the growing burden
of premature deaths and preventable illnesses from NCDs. Preparing public
health professionals who can apply the lessons from previous public health

successes to the 21st-century challenge of confronting harmful commercial influences on health has the potential to contribute to writing the next chapter of in the history of public health advances.

REFERENCES

1. Flynn MB. Global capitalism as a societal determinant of health: A conceptual framework. *Soc Sci Med*. 2021; 268: 113530.
2. Hall P. *Varieties of Capitalism, Emerging Trends in the Social and Behavioral Sciences: An Interdisciplinary, Searchable, and Linkable Resource*. Wiley; 2015.
3. West R, Marteau T. Commentary on Casswell (2013): The commercial determinants of health. *Addiction*. 2013; 108(4): 686–687.
4. Kickbusch I, Allen L, Franz C. The commercial determinants of health. *Lancet Glob Health*. 2016; 4(12): e895–e896.
5. Freudenberg N, Lee K, Buse K, et al. Defining priorities for action and research on the commercial determinants of health: A conceptual review. *Am J Public Health*. 2021; 111(12): 2202–2211.
6. Singh G, Cowden S. The intensification of neoliberalism and the commodification of human need: A social work perspective. *Crit Radical Social Work*. 2015; 3(3): 375–387.
7. Broad R, Cavanagh J. The corporate accountability movement: Lessons & opportunities. *Fletcher F World Aff*. 1999; 23: 151.
8. Biglan A. Corporate externalities: A challenge to the further success of prevention science. *Prev Sci*. 2011; 12(1): 1–11.
9. Steger MB. *Globalization: A Very Short Introduction*. Oxford University Press; 2017.
10. Fry M-L, Polonsky MJ. Examining the unintended consequences of marketing. *J Bus Res*. 2004; 57(11): 1303–1306.
11. Reich MR. Public–private partnerships for public health. *Nat Med*. 2000; 6(6): 617–620.
12. McNamara C. Trade liberalization and social determinants of health: A state of the literature review. *Soc Sci Med*. 2017; 176: 1–13.
13. Marmot M, Wilkinson R. *Social Determinants of Health*. Oxford University Press; 2005.
14. Maani N, Collin J, Friel S, et al. Bringing the commercial determinants of health out of the shadows: A review of how the commercial determinants are represented in conceptual frameworks. *Eur J Public Health*. 2020; 30(4): 660–664.
15. Schmidt H, Butter K, Rider C. Building digital tobacco industry document libraries at the University of California, San Francisco Library/Center for Knowledge Management. *D-Lib Magazine*. 2002; 8(9): 1–9.
16. Freudenberg N. ToxicDocs: A new resource for assessing the impact of corporate practices on health. *J Public Health Policy*. 2018; 39(1): 30–33.
17. Arnold RD, Wade JP. A definition of systems thinking: A systems approach. *Proc Comput Sci*. 2015; 44: 669–678.
18. Knai C, Petticrew M, Mays N, et al. Systems thinking as a framework for analyzing commercial determinants of health. *Milbank Q*. 2018; 96(3): 472–498.
19. Jayasinghe S. Social determinants of health inequalities: Towards a theoretical perspective using systems science. *Int J Equity Health*. 2015; 14(1): 1–8.

20. Lobb R, Colditz GA. Implementation science and its application to population health. *Annu Rev Public Health*. 2013; 34: 235–251.

21. Green LW, Allegrante JP. Practice-based evidence and the need for more diverse methods and sources in epidemiology, public health and health promotion. *Am J Health Promot*. 2020; 34(8): 946–948.

22. Brandt EJ, Myerson R, Perraillon MC, Polonsky TS. Hospital admissions for myocardial infarction and stroke before and after the trans-fatty acid restrictions in New York. *JAMA Cardiol*. 2017; 2(6): 627–634.

23. Ghebreyesus TA, Frieden TR. REPLACE: A roadmap to make the world trans fat free by 2023. *Lancet*. 2018; 391(10134): 1978–1980.

24. Ortiz K, Nash J, Shea L, et al. Partnerships, processes, and outcomes: A health equity–focused scoping meta-review of community-engaged scholarship. *Annu Rev Public Health*. 2020; 41: 177–199.

25. Baum FE, Sanders DM, Fisher M, et al. Assessing the health impact of transnational corporations: Its importance and a framework. *Global Health*. 2016; 12(1): 1–7.

26. Lima JM, Galea S. The Corporate Permeation Index—A tool to study the macrosocial determinants of non-communicable disease. *SSM Popul Health*. 2019; 7: 100361.

27. Hilton S, Buckton CH, Henrichsen T, Fergie G, Leifeld P. Policy congruence and advocacy strategies in the discourse networks of minimum unit pricing for alcohol and the soft drinks industry levy. *Addiction*. 2020; 115(12): 2303–2314.

28. Kolb DA. *Experience as the Source of Learning and Development*. Prentice Hall; 1984.

29. Rubin CL, Martinez LS, Chu J, et al. Community-engaged pedagogy: A strengths-based approach to involving diverse stakeholders in research partnerships. *Prog Community Health Partnerships*. 2012; 6(4): 481.

30. Reimschisel T, Herring AL, Huang J, Minor TJ. A systematic review of the published literature on team-based learning in health professions education. *Medical Teacher*. 2017; 39(12): 1227–1237.

31. Kenworthy N, MacKenzie R. *Case Studies on Corporations and Global Health Governance: Impacts, Influence and Accountability*. Rowman & Littlefield; 2016.

32. Quelch JA. *Consumers, Corporations, and Public Health: A Case-Based Approach to Sustainable Business*: Oxford University Press; 2016.

33. Freudenberg N, Picard Bradley S, Serrano M. Public health campaigns to change industry practices that damage health: an analysis of 12 case studies. *Health Educ Behav*. 2009; **36**(2): 230–249.

CHAPTER 32

Learning from Experience

Identifying Key Intervention Points Around Corporate Practices to Improve Health

MÉLISSA MIALON, JULIA ANAF, AND FRAN BAUM

32.1 INTRODUCTION

This chapter builds on the insights of previous chapters in this volume to examine how interventions designed to research, oppose, advocate against, regulate, and change the practices of corporations can be made. History demonstrates that corporate practices have long challenged health.[1] These practices include regulation of wages and working conditions, laws to reduce adverse environmental and health impacts of harmful products such as cigarettes and alcohol, and other harmful practices.[1] Researchers, journalists, activists, politicians, and public servants have worked over time to mitigate the harms of these products and practices to the end of protecting and improving population health.[1]

This chapter identifies key interventions that could help protect population health from the negative impacts of the commercial determinants of health (CDOH). It covers a mix of individual and collective options and presents the experiences of actors who have shown that it is possible to challenge corporate power and in doing so help protect population health. This chapter also focuses on the structural drivers of ill health and argues that, ultimately, the decision to address the CDOH must be taken collectively and will not result from individual actions alone. Four main sites of interventions to challenge the health harms caused by corporations are discussed: academic work,

Mélissa Mialon, Julia Anaf, and Fran Baum, *Learning from Experience* In: *The Commercial Determinants of Health.* Edited by: Nason Maani, Mark Petticrew, and Sandro Galea, Oxford University Press. © Oxford University Press 2023. DOI: 10.1093/oso/9780197578742.003.0032 investigative journalism, and civil society activism and regulation through public and institutional policies.

32.2 ACADEMIC WORK

One way of generating evidence on corporations and health is through research. There are researchers who, for example, study the harm caused by certain commodities, such as tobacco and ultra-processed foods.[2,3] Other research has posed the following questions[4-7]: What are corporations' market and political practices? How do they influence public policies? and What is their influence over the production of new knowledge? Such research on the practices of corporations has been facilitated through access to previously confidential documents from the tobacco industry, for example, with the public release of emails and minutes of meetings.[8] In the 1990s, attorneys in the United States sued five of the largest tobacco companies in the country.[9] The Tobacco Master Settlement Agreement forced companies to release their internal documents.[9] The documents are now known as the "Truth Tobacco Industry Documents" and are publicly accessible at the University of California.[8] Internal documents have helped the scientific community better understand the practices of the tobacco[10] and other harmful industries.[11,12] Where internal documents are scarce, publicly available information and interviews with key informants could help uncover relevant data.[7]

Nevertheless, researching CDOH has challenges that are unique to this field. Corporations often try to intimidate researchers. There are personal attacks, threats, and criticism of the researchers in question.[13,14] Spyware was installed on the phones of scientists advocating for the introduction of a soda tax in Mexico,[15] and an American academic, Marion Nestle, was followed by staff from Coca-Cola when she toured Australia giving public talks.[16] A further example is the researcher Lisa Bero, whose nutrition research has also been monitored by Coca-Cola.[17] Bero later wrote of the chilling effect such industry attention has on younger researchers.[18]

Research itself also might be questioned by corporations. Debate is a critical component of good science, but often corporations' questioning is unfounded and easily rebutted.[19] Although there is often no basis for industry claims, the damage to the scientific credibility of researchers, particularly when such criticism can be amplified by corporations, is real and not easy to challenge. It is therefore important that researchers are aware of and prepared to face such intimidation. Strong support needs to be given from senior researchers to encourage those early in their careers to see the benefits of taking up a career that involves critique of corporate products and practices. Senior researchers, often better placed to challenge industry critiques, could, for example, mentor and help protect early career researchers if there are unfair industry attacks on their research. A further means of support is by modeling the role of an academic who does high-quality work and ensures research findings are brought to the attention of civil society, industry, and government. It is also important that public policies and other mechanisms are put in place to protect those researching CDOH.[20] This will require research funding bodies to fund research on CDOH and universities to encourage such research and to protect the free speech of academics when they speak out about the damaging practices of corporations their research has uncovered.

In addition to intimidation, corporations also try to influence the topic of research and the careers of researchers and health profesionnals[21] by offering scholarships and influencing school and university curricula.[22,23] Teaching about CDOH is therefore important for translating that research into knowledge for the next generations of health and business professionals.

It is also of utmost importance that sources of scientific knowledge are free from financial conflicts of interest. History has taught us that once corporations start investing in research on their own products, they often create doubt about science.[24,25] When the tobacco industry discovered that cigarettes were carcinogenic, in its own laboratories, it invested in research to show that there were alternate explanations for the causes of cancers.[26] This led to delay in the acceptance by governments that smoking is harmful and of the need for tobacco control public policies, thus resulting in millions of deaths that could otherwise have been prevented.[27]

32.3 INVESTIGATIVE JOURNALISM

Investigative journalism also is a key intervention point for generating knowledge and action on corporate products and practices and their impacts on human health. In Brazil, *O Joio e o Trigo* is a blog created by two investigative journalists (now expanded to a dozen) to expose the harmful practices of the food industry in their country.[28] The blog receives support from civil society organizations, and the journalists are publishing books on the practices of other sectors, such as the tobacco industry and retailers.[29,30] In Australia, the activist group GetUp! launched a campaign to crowdsource funding for a journalist to investigate the predatory practices of companies benefitting from the privatized system of job agencies to help unemployed people find work.[31]

Well-respected newspapers also frequently report on corporations and their harmful products and practices. For example, in 2011, *The Guardian* published an article on how corporations target low- and middle-income countries with aggressive marketing practices; little research had been conducted on the subject at that time.[32] In 2016, the same newspaper reported on the ties between speakers at a United Nations (UN)/World Health Organization (WHO) panel on pesticides and cancer risks and the pesticide industry.[33] Recently, a journalist from *The New York Times* reported on the attacks faced by public health advocates, as described previously.[15,34] The release of the "Panama Papers," which exposed corporate tax havens, and associated reporting by the International Consortium of Investigative Journalists have resulted in some governments acting to retrieve some of the lost taxes.[35]

In addition to newspaper articles, there are also documentaries and movies on CDOH, which might help raising awareness about those issues in the mind of the public.[36]

32.4 CIVIL SOCIETY ACTIVISM

Civil society activism has been crucial for challenging corporate practices and CDOH in the past 50 years.[37] In the 1970s, for example, there was a boycott of Nestlé after the company was found to be responsible for the deaths of thousands of infants in Africa and Asia due to the use of aggressive marketing of infant formula in those regions.[38] The company was found to have contracted sales representatives, sometimes dressed as nurses, to freely distribute samples of its products in hospitals.[38] Parents were told about the supposed benefits of using infant formula, which thus discouraged many mothers from breast-feeding, with detrimental health impacts on their infants.[38] Due to poor living conditions, parents used unsafe water and often could not afford to pay for infant formula after all the free samples were used. Thus, in order to make their supply of formula last, they diluted it too much, and infants' nutritional needs were no longer met.[38] Civil society organizations, led by the International Baby Food Action Network and Corporate Accountability, launched a campaign to denounce these marketing practices and got the attention of the international community.[39] The work of those advocates eventually led to the adoption of the International Code for the Marketing of Breast-Milk Substitutes by WHO, with support from UNICEF, in 1981.[40] Infant formula companies are still regularly found to be breaching the Code, more than 40 years after its adoption, and civil society organizations still serve as a watchdog against such practices globally.[41]

Tobacco control is another example of success for civil society organizations in challenging corporations and their harmful products and practices, with the adoption of an international binding tool, the Framework Convention on Tobacco Control, in 2003 at the World Health Assembly.[42] This framework reflected many years of activism.[43,44]

Civil society collaborations also provide wide-ranging knowledge that can be the impetus for structural change through, for example, the development of sophisticated databases such as those on the extractives industry or industrial poisonings.[45,46] Trade unions are also part of civil society and have played active roles in challenging corporate practices, especially with regard to occupational health and safety—for example, in the case of the mining industry[47]—but also on broader issues including environmental impacts.[48] Within the health field, for many years the People's Health Movement, a global network of health activists, has identified corporate malpractice as a threat to health. Its founding People's Health Charter recognizes that corporations can act with such impunity because they are strongly supported by the global economic system.[49]

Civil society actors can also protest against corporations by opposing their expansion, as has been the case with proposals for new McDonald's fast-food outlets.[50] Another example is exposing the philanthropic activities of corporations, which in reality rest on contributions from the public while tax advantages accrue to the corporations.[51]

Importantly, civil society organizations often face challenges, including strategic litigation and discrediting of critics, when engaging in actions against corporations.[37] In Colombia, public health advocates are regularly intimidated in their work, a pattern repeated in Fiji and many other countries throughout the world.[34,37,52,53] A key challenge here is the power disparities between corporations and civil society actors, with the revenue of the largest corporations being greater than some national governments.[54] Here again, it is important to have mechanisms in place to protect civil society actors from the risks they face when engaging in their work on corporations and health. Networking and collaboration between different organizations are key,[55,56] as is international support from academics and international organizations, including the UN.

32.5 REGULATION THROUGH PUBLIC AND INSTITUTIONAL POLICIES

It is the duty of governments and international institutions to introduce mechanisms to protect population health from CDOH and also promote population health. This requires them to devise public and institutional policies to address all aspects of CDOH and minimize their detrimental impact on health. A proposed public policy agenda is discussed in the following chapters.

Public policy must ensure that existing regulations and mechanisms (e.g., the International Code of Marketing of Breast-Milk Substitutes or the Framework Convention on Tobacco Control, when they are translated in national law) are respected by corporations and that sanctions are applied in case of noncompliance. In addition, governments must also ensure an international tax compliance framework is in place and enforce the UN Binding Treaty on Business and Human Rights.[57]

Self-regulation, often promoted by the industry and even governments, is not sufficient, with industry often not complying with its own pledges.[58] For example, child labor is banned in many countries, but children still work on cocoa plantations for large global companies in Ivory Coast and other countries in Africa.[58]

Mechanisms to curtail corporations' influence on the development of public health policies should also be a key intervention point. Conflicts of interest policies were discussed previously in this book, and other mechanisms could be considered, such as the protection of whistleblowers, more transparency in the interactions between corporations and government officials and other actors working in the public sector, and codes of conduct for the independence and integrity of health professionals.[20] Many countries and institutions already have these mechanisms in place.[20] Here again, the implementation of such mechanisms, and the existence of sanctions when those are not respected, is crucial.

32.6 THE STRUCTURAL DRIVERS OF ILL HEALTH

In addition to the work of academics, investigative journalists, advocates from civil society, and government and international institutions in highlighting the harmful impacts of corporate activity, it is also important to question the structural drivers of ill health. Underpinning the political and economic power of corporations is an economic and political system that supports largely unregulated ways of operating.[59] These conditions have allowed companies to behave in ways that threaten human and ecological health, often with the support of national governments. Improved democratic processes are required to counteract the many ways in which powerful business interests can exert influence.

In the era of the COVID-19 pandemic, it is evident that public health systems perform best and that private systems are not as universal or effective.[60,61] Yet often public health systems are undermined by the power of the business lobby to convince governments to adopt market-based solutions instead of a human rights–based approach to health.[62] Corporate power has also been demonstrated in the refusal of pharmaceutical companies to remove intellectual property rights on COVID-19 vaccines even though much of their development has been publicly funded.[63] This points to broader structural issues of trade and economic agreements, which currently operate to protect businesses and not to consider human and ecological health.[64]

32.7 CONCLUSION

No single intervention can successfully address CDOH; rather, a myriad of options is required that together challenge harmful corporate products and practices throughout the world. It is important that corporate actions and their impacts on health are better understood so that we can act to mitigate those actions. Public debate on those issues is needed, particularly in the context of recovery from the COVID-19 pandemic. In many countries, there is an increased willingness of governments to intervene to support livelihoods, which has been shown to benefit both the health of the population and the economy. This has given a valuable space in which to consider capitalist and neoliberal systems and imagine a future that is not about growth at all costs but, rather, human flourishing.[65]

REFERENCES

1. Freudenberg N, Lee K, Buse K, et al. Defining priorities for research and action on the commercial determinants of health: A conceptual review. *Am J Public Health*. 2021; 111(12): 2202–2211.
2. Stuckler D, McKee M, Ebrahim S, Basu S. Manufacturing epidemics: The role of global producers in increased consumption of unhealthy commodities including processed foods, alcohol, and tobacco. *PLoS Med*. 2012; 9(6): 10. doi:10.1371/journal.pmed.1001235
3. Moodie R, Stuckler D, Monteiro C, et al. Profits and pandemics: Prevention of harmful effects of tobacco, alcohol, and ultra-processed food and drink industries. *Lancet*. 2013; 381(9867): 670–679. doi:10.1016/S0140-6736(12)62089-3
4. Ulucanlar S, Fooks GJ, Gilmore AB. The policy dystopia model: An interpretive analysis of tobacco industry political activity. *PLoS Med*. 2016; 13(9): e1002125. doi:10.1371/journal.pmed.1002125
5. Wiist WH. *The Bottom Line or Public Health: Tactics Corporations Use to Influence Health and Health Policy and What We Can Do to Counter Them*. Oxford University Press; 2010.
6. Freudenberg N. *Lethal but Legal: Corporations, Consumption, and Protecting Public Health*. Oxford University Press; 2014.
7. Mialon M, Swinburn B, Sacks G. A proposed approach to systematically identify and monitor the corporate political activity of the food industry with respect to public health using publicly available information. *Obes Rev*. 2015; 16(7): 519–530. doi:10.1111/obr.12289
8. University of California, San Francisco. Truth tobacco industry documents. 2017. https://www.industrydocumentslibrary.ucsf.edu/tobacco
9. U.S. Department of Justice, Office of the Attorney General of California. Master settlement agreement. 2017. http://oag.ca.gov/tobacco/msa
10. Bero L. Implications of the tobacco industry documents for public health and policy. *Annu Rev Public Health*. 2003; 24: 267–288. doi:10.1146/annurev.publhealth.24.100901.140813
11. Bond L. Access to confidential alcohol industry documents: From "Big Tobacco" to "Big Booze." *Australas Med J*. 2009; 1(3): 1–26. doi:10.4066/AMJ.2009.43
12. Hawkins B, McCambridge J. Can internal tobacco industry documents be useful for studying the UK alcohol industry? *BMC Public Health*. 2018; 18(1): 808. doi:10.1186/s12889-018-5722-0

13. Mialon M, Swinburn B, Allender S, Sacks G. "Maximising shareholder value": A detailed insight into the corporate political activity of the Australian food industry. *Aust N Z J Public Health*. 2017; 41(2): 165–171. doi:10.1111/1753-6405.12639

14. Mialon M, Corvalan C, Cediel G, Scagliusi FB, Reyes M. Food industry political practices in Chile: "The economy has always been the main concern." *Glob Health*. 2020; 16(1): Article No. 107. doi:10.1186/s12992-020-00638-4

15. Perlroth N. Spyware's odd targets: Backers of Mexico's soda tax. *The New York Times*. February 11, 2017. https://www.nytimes.com/2017/02/11/technology/hack-mexico-soda-tax-advocates.html

16. Wilson W. Hillary Clinton campaign officials helped Coca-Cola fight soda tax. Keep Fitness Legal. October 12, 2016. Accessed April 14, 2021. https://keepfitnesslegal.crossfit.com/2016/10/12/hillary-clinton-campaign-officials-helped-coca-cola-fight-soda-tax

17. Strom M. Coca-Cola's secret plan to monitor Sydney University academic Lisa Bero. *The Sydney Morning Herald*. October 21, 2016. Accessed April 28, 2021. https://www.smh.com.au/technology/cocacolas-secret-plan-to-monitor-sydney-university-academic-lisa-bero-20161020-gs6m4a.html

18. Cochrane Australia. Lisa Bero says public will increasingly demand less wining and dining, more independence from health professionals. n.d. Accessed April 28, 2021. https://australia.cochrane.org/news/lisa-bero-says-public-will-increasingly-demand-less-wining-and-dining-more-independence-health

19. Monteiro CA, Cannon G, Moubarac J-C, Levy RB, Louzada MLC, Jaime PC. Ultra-processing. An odd "appraisal." *Public Health Nutr*. 2018; 21(3): 497–501. doi:10.1017/S1368980017003287

20. Mialon M, Vandevijvere S, Carriedo-Lutzenkirchen A, et al. Mechanisms for addressing and managing the influence of corporations on public health policy, research and practice: A scoping review. *BMJ Open*. 2020; 10(7): e034082. doi:10.1136/bmjopen-2019-034082

21. Mitchell G, McCambridge J. The "snowball effect": Short- and long-term consequences of early career alcohol industry research funding. *Addict Res Theory*. 2021; 30(2): 119–125. https://eprints.whiterose.ac.uk/175591

22. Powell D. *Schools, Corporations, and the War on Childhood Obesity* (Critical Studies in Health and Education). Routledge; 2019.

23. Holloway K. Uneasy subjects: Medical students' conflicts over the pharmaceutical industry. *Soc Sci Med*. 2014; 114: 113–120. doi:10.1016/j.socscimed.2014.05.052

24. Proctor RN. *Golden Holocaust: Origins of the Cigarette Catastrophe and the Case for Abolition*. University of California Press; 2012. doi:10.1136/medhum-2012-010202

25. Oreskes N, Conway E. Merchants of doubt: How a handful of scientists obscured the truth on issues from tobacco smoke to global warming. *Choice Rev Online*. 2011; 48(11): 48-6243–48-6243. doi:10.5860/choice.48-6243

26. Brandt AM. Inventing conflicts of interest: A history of tobacco industry tactics. *Am J Public Health*. 2012; 102(1): 63–71. doi:10.2105/AJPH.2011.300292

27. Peto R, Lopez AD, Boreham J, Thun M. *Mortality from Smoking in Developed Countries 1950–2000*. 2nd ed. Oxford University Press; 2006.

28. Peres J. Big Food targets Brazilian researcher. *O Joio e o Trigo*. 2017. http://ojoioeotrigo.hospedagemdesites.ws/2017/12/ultra-attack-brazilian-researcher-targets-transnational-food/

29. Peres J, Moriti N. Roucos e *Sufocados*. Editora Elefante; 2008. https://elefanteeditora.com.br/produto/roucos-e-sufocados

30. Matioli V, Peres J. Donos do *Mercado*. Editora Elefante; 2020. https://elefanteedit ora.com.br/produto/donos-do-mercado

31. Get Up! Help Michael West expose predatory job agencies! n.d. Accessed April 28, 2021. https://www.getup.org.au/campaigns/unemployment-services/mich eal-west-report-employment-services/help-michael-west-expose-predatory-job-agencies?secure_token=ff0c6817e656018b74b0f95d06c7f801b16d8f93eae3a c03c943820d54d1d7af&t=GLkGT0J2&utm_campaign=Will_you_support_in-dependent_journalism___NAME_friends__&utm_content=30671&utm_med ium=email&utm_source=blast

32. Lawrence F. Alarm as corporate giants target developing countries. *The Guardian*. November 23, 2011. http://www.theguardian.com/global-development/2011/ nov/23/corporate-giants-target-developing-countries

33. Nelsen A. UN/WHO panel in conflict of interest row over glyphosate cancer risk. *The Guardian*. May 17, 2016. https://www.theguardian.com/environment/2016/ may/17/unwho-panel-in-conflict-of-interest-row-over-glyphosates-cancer-risk

34. Jacobs A, Richtel M. She took on Colombia's soda industry. Then she was silenced. *The New York Times*. November 13, 2017. https://www.nytimes.com/2017/11/ 13/health/colombia-soda-tax-obesity.html

35. The International Consortium of Investigative Journalists. The Panama papers: Exposing the rogue offshore finance industry. 2021. Accessed April 28, 2021. https://www.icij.org/investigations/panama-papers

36. Horel S. Les alimenteurs. 2013. http://www.allocine.fr/film/fichefilm_gen_cf ilm=213593.html

37. Anaf J, Baum F, Fisher M, Friel S. Civil society action against transnational corporations: Implications for health promotion. *Health Promot Int*. 2020; 35(4): 877–887. doi:10.1093/heapro/daz088

38. Muller M. The baby killer: A War on Want investigation into the promotion and sale of powdered baby milks in the Third World. War on Want. 1974. http://arch ive.babymilkaction.org/pdfs/babykiller.pdf

39. Cumming LS. International Baby Food Action Network (IBFAN). In: Anheier HK, Toepler S, eds. *International Encyclopedia of Civil Society*. Springer; 2010: 880–881. doi:10.1007/978-0-387-93996-4_813

40. World Health Organization. International Code of Marketing of Breast-Milk Substitutes. 1981. https://apps.who.int/iris/rest/bitstreams/48415/retrieve

41. International Baby Food Action Network, International Code Documentation Centre. *Breaking the rules, stretching the rules 2017: Evidence of violations of the International Code of Marketing of Breast-Milk Substitutes and subsequent resolutions*. International Baby Food Action Network; 2017.

42. Mamudu HM, Glantz SA. Civil society and the negotiation of the Framework Convention on Tobacco Control. *Glob Public Health*. 2009; 4(2): 150–168. doi:10.1080/17441690802095355

43. Chapman S. Public Health Advocacy and Tobacco Control: Making Smoking History. Wiley-Blackwell; 2008. https://www.wiley.com/en-al/Public+Health+ Advocacy+and+Tobacco+Control%3A+Making+Smoking+History-p-978047 0691632

44. Collin J. Taking steps toward coherent global governance of alcohol: The challenge and opportunity of managing conflict of interest. *J Stud Alcohol Drugs*. 2021; 82(3): 387–394. doi:10.15288/jsad.2021.82.387

45. ToxicDocs. Project ToxicDocs. n.d. Accessed April 28, 2021. https://www.toxicd ocs.org

46. Environmental Justice Organisations, Liabilities and Trade. Mapping environmental justice. n.d. Accessed April 28, 2021. http://www.ejolt.org
47. Anaf J, Baum F, Fisher M, London L. The health impacts of extractive industry transnational corporations: A study of Rio Tinto in Australia and Southern Africa. *Glob Health*. 2019; 15(1): 13. doi:10.1186/s12992-019-0453-2
48. Pearce S. Tackling climate change a new role for trade unions in the workplace. ACAS. 2012. Accessed July 26, 2021. https://www.bl.uk/collection-items/tackling-climate-change-a-new-role-for-trade-unions-in-the-workplace
49. People's Health Movement. The People's Charter for Health. n.d. Accessed April 28, 2021. https://phmovement.org/the-peoples-charter-for-health
50. Anaf J, Baum FE, Fisher M, Harris E, Friel S. Assessing the health impact of transnational corporations: A case study on McDonald's Australia. *Glob Health*. 2017; 13(1): 7. doi:10.1186/s12992-016-0230-4
51. Simon M. Clowning around with charity: How McDonald's exploits philanthropy and targets children. Eat Drink Politics. 2013. http://www.eatdrinkpolitics.com/2013/10/29/clowning-around-with-charity-how-mcdonalds-exploits-philanthropy-and-targets-children
52. Mialon M, Gaitan Charry DA, Cediel G, Crosbie E, Baeza Scagliusi F, Pérez Tamayo EM. "The architecture of the state was transformed in favour of the interests of companies": Corporate political activity of the food industry in Colombia. *Glob Health*. 2020; 16(1): 97. doi:10.1186/s12992-020-00631-x
53. Mialon M, Swinburn B, Wate J, Tukana I, Sacks G. Analysis of the corporate political activity of major food industry actors in Fiji. *Glob Health*. 2016; 12(1): Article No. 18. doi:10.1186/s12992-016-0158-8
54. Global Justice Now. 69 of the richest 100 entities on the planet are corporations, not governments, figures show. October 17, 2018. Accessed April 28, 2021. https://www.globaljustice.org.uk/news/69-richest-100-entities-planet-are-corporations-not-governments-figures-show
55. Mialon M, Fooks G, Cullerton K, et al. Corporations and Health: the need to combine forces to improve population health. *Int J Health Policy Manag*. 2022.
56. Nakkash R, Mialon M, Makhoul J, et al. A call to advance and translate research into policy on governance, ethics, and conflicts of interest in public health: The GECI-PH network. *Glob Health*. 2021; 17(1): 1–4. doi:10.1186/s12992-021-00660-0
57. BindingTreaty.org. Global InterParliamentary Network in support of a binding treaty. UN Binding Treaty on Transnational Corporations and Human Rights. n.d. Accessed April 28, 2021. https://bindingtreaty.org
58. Hershey, Nestle and Mars broke their pledges to end child labor in chocolate production. *The Washington Post*. 2019. Accessed April 15, 2021. https://www.washingtonpost.com/graphics/2019/business/hershey-nestle-mars-chocolate-child-labor-west-africa/
59. Mialon M. An overview of the commercial determinants of health. *Glob Health*. 2020; 16: Article No. 74. doi:10.1186/s12992-020-00607-x
60. United Nations Department of Economic and Social Affairs. UN/DESA Policy Brief 79: The role of public service and public servants during the COVID-19 pandemic. June 11, 2020. Accessed April 29, 2021. https://www.un.org/development/desa/dpad/publication/un-desa-policy-brief-79-the-role-of-public-service-and-public-servants-during-the-covid-19-pandemic
61. Baum F, Freeman T, Musolino C, et al. Explaining COVID-19 performance: What factors might predict national responses? *BMJ*. 2021; 372: n91. doi:10.1136/bmj.n91

62. Bakh U, Sahacic A. Human rights based approach to tobacco control as an effective tool for building strategic alliances and political will: Experience from Bosnia and Herzegovina. *Tob Induc Dis*. 2018; 16(1). doi:10.18332/tid/84041

63. It's time to consider a patent reprieve for COVID vaccines. Nature. 2021; 592(7852): 7. doi:10.1038/d41586-021-00863-w

64. Gleeson D, Friel S. Emerging threats to public health from regional trade agreements. *Lancet*. 2013; 381(9876): 1507–1509. doi:10.1016/S0140-6736(13)60312-8

65. Jackson T. Post Growth: Life *After* Capitalism. Polity; 2021.

CHAPTER 33

A Policy Agenda for the Commercial Determinants of Health

SALLY CASSWELL

33.1 A POLICY AGENDA

A nexus of powerful actors benefits from the products and business practices described in this book as part of the commercial determinants of health
(CDOH). This nexus is both broad and dense, with linkages between investment companies, extractive industries, producers of hazardous products and
the organizations they fund such as Phillip Morris' Foundation for a Smoke-
Free World, numerous think tanks, retailers and marketers including digital
platforms, and organizers of branded events such as Coca-Cola's Olympics and
Heineken's Formula 1. These linkages also encompass policymakers whose
accountabilities include protection of the health and well-being of their populations but who may also have competing interests—personal, financial (see
Chapter 23), and ideological (see Chapter 30). These commercial interests
penetrate intergovernmental organizations and multisectoral public–private
partnerships (PPPs). Together, they represent a formidable array of actors
with overlapping interests and considerable resources, and they provide a
significant challenge for public health actors who propose an evidence-based
policy agenda in the interests of population health.

Redressing the discursive power of commercial interests is identified as a
priority for a public health policy agenda in this chapter. The political and institutional architectures intrinsically enmeshed at global and national levels
create a system that supports and maintains the negative consequences of
CDOH; a public health policy agenda must address all parts of the system.
Some elements in the political economy suggest positive change is possible

Sally Casswell, A Policy Agenda for the Commercial Determinants of Health In: The Commercial Determinants of Health.
Edited by: Nason Maani, Mark Petticrew, and Sandro Galea, Oxford University Press. © Oxford University Press 2023.
DOI: 10.1093/oso/9780197578742.003.0033

but considerable uncertainty exists, not least given the unknown implications of response to the COVID-19 pandemic.

33.2 ADDRESSING DISCURSIVE POWER

Discursive power—the ability of contributors to communication spaces to introduce, amplify, and maintain framings and shape public discourses and controversies—has long been a key way in which commercial interests have acquired a privileged, albeit contested, position in the overall political arena. Global governance is the material expression of an ideology[1] that privileges economics over health and legitimizes commercial entities as "partners" in a "whole of society" framing. Coherent and consistent messaging takes place across different CDOH sectors, with themes of individual freedom and responsibility. The framings used by commercial sector actors are "weapons of advocacy" to promote policies aligned with their interests.[2] Reframing the narrative within which the policy agenda is created may be one of the strongest approaches available to the public health community.

33.3 CONFLICTS OF INTEREST

Attributing responsibility for ill health of people and the planet to the nexus of commercial interests and undermining their acceptability as partners in setting the policy agenda require a process of denormalization of the industry, such as occurred in relation to the tobacco industry in the decades leading up to the Framework Convention on Tobacco Control (FCTC). Common tropes in tobacco control were that tobacco "when used as the manufacturer directed" resulted in death and there is "no safe level" of tobacco use. Although technically open to challenge, these statements powerfully defined tobacco as deadly. At the same time, the tobacco industry was shown to be prioritizing profits over people's health by marketing a product they knew to be lethal.[3] A consensus developed on the tobacco industry's conflict of interest.

In contrast, the alcohol industry, learning from tobacco's experience, actively promoted the narrative that alcohol in moderation is good for you and worked hard to establish a role as part of the solution to alcohol harm.[4] The industry's claim that it does not promote heavy drinking can, however, be challenged by promulgating evidence of its reliance on extremely heavy drinking occasions for large shares of its profits.[5] Similarly, the industry's claim to authentic partnership is challenged by the considerable evidence of its subversion of effective policy along with tobacco and unhealthy food industries.[6]

Extractive industries, particularly the fossil fuels industry, have used a rhetoric of climate "risk" rather than reality, an emphasis on consumers' demand for energy, and unreliability of renewable energy sources to normalize fossil fuel lock-in and individualize responsibility.[7] Like the tobacco industry, documented awareness of the reality of climate change due to fossil fuels while the industry used its resources to promote misinformation has been used to denormalize the fossil fuel industry. The extent of the industry's donations to policymakers, harm to those employed in the industry, and extreme events such as bush fires and flooding have shifted the narrative. Furthermore, examples of best practice in moving to renewable energy are now available.[8]

The narrative on unhealthy food has included a food industry focus on the role of physical activity as the primary modulator of obesity[9] along with the commonsense notion that "we all have to eat." Differentiating healthy food and eco-friendly supply chains from high-profit, ultra-processed unhealthy food products and highlighting the market power and business practices that promote overconsumption are necessary to change this narrative.

Oversupply and extensive marketing, especially to disadvantaged groups, are business practices indicative of the need for commercial interests to put "profits before people." Making visible the business practices of industry is essential to challenge the current acceptance of engagement with commercial interests at both national and global levels and to undermine the logic of the PPP when hazardous products are involved.

33.4 ADDRESSING INEQUITIES IN NEGATIVE EXTERNALITIES— INCREASING FAIRNESS

An important lens is the unequal distribution of costs and benefits generated from market transactions of CDOH actors. The global soft drink industry disproportionately affects groups of lower socioeconomic status, as does pollution from fossil fuel industries located in poorer neighborhoods. Similarly, alcohol harm is disproportionately experienced by these and other vulnerable groups such as colonized Indigenous Peoples. On the other hand, it is the elites who make up the shareholders and corporate executives who largely benefit from the wealth generated from these industries.[10]

Building a policy agenda on a narrative that explains the way regulating the practices of commercial interests increases fairness may be influential, depending on prevalent normative values. For example, in the case of disproportionate harm to colonized Indigenous People in New Zealand, a claim against the government that it had failed to protect Māori from alcohol harm[11] contributed to elevating reform of alcohol legislation on the policy agenda. Similarly, a legal challenge based on the constitutional protection of human rights successfully increased smoke-free environments and restrained marketing of tobacco in India.[12]

33.5 EXPANDING THE NARRATIVE ON MARKETING TO INCLUDE THE DIGITAL ECOSYSTEM AND MOVE BEYOND PROTECTION OF CHILDREN

Marketing is essential for producers of hazardous products in particular, and much policy focus has been to avoid effective regulation. The past two decades have seen a significant shift of marketing resources to digital platforms that allow for targeting of consumers and integration of marketing and purchase to an unprecedented extent. Much marketing is now "dark" in that it is not accessed by others than those targeted, ephemeral in that no record is kept, and dynamic because the algorithms targeting the marketing are continually revised to sell more products.[13] These characteristics mean it is not well understood and not easily subject to regulation. The public health narrative of protection of children is now even more misguided given the increased ability to identify and target marketing messages to vulnerable adults. The focus on children was aligned with a neoliberal ideology in which personal responsibility was privileged, and agreement on the need for protection could be reached only with regard to children. In the absence of any feasible way to control this digital ecosystem, complete bans on marketing of such unhealthy products, as are in place for tobacco with positive results,[14] are needed to achieve freedom from misinformation and manipulation by consumer marketing.[15]

33.6 REBALANCING GLOBAL ARCHITECTURE

Processes of globalization, supported by neoliberal ideology, have allowed the development of corporations into large and powerful entities designed primarily for the accumulation of wealth via profits. Transnational corporations (TNCs) command financial and human resources of a magnitude previously unknown, with market and political implications.

There is virtually no global regulation of TNCs to restrain their influence in global governance. An attempt by low- and middle-income countries (LMICs) to initiate a legally binding agreement to regulate TNCs failed in the 1970s, and three decades later, in a context with much greater engagement with TNCs, the UN's global compact promoted corporate social responsibility and voluntarism.[16] Corporate social responsibility activities and particularly PPPs have become influential in global governance and were included in the only Sustainable Development Goal that addressed mechanisms to achieve the goals.[17]

Trade and investment agreements (TIAs) are extremely influential. They promote narratives of the primacy of economic interests and are particularly powerful elements of global governance given processes of compulsory resolution of disputes and the application of sanctions. Such TIAs constrain government's willingness to enact regulation that may be challenged and result in expensive litigation. This is particularly true for LMICs, which have limited resources to either examine the implications of TIAs before they sign or challenge corporations' interpretation of them. These TIAs have also included articles that protect global digital platforms from national legislation.[18] In 2021, the World Trade Organization (WTO) reported there were 348 regional trade agreements in force.

In contrast, there is only one legally binding health treaty in place that acknowledges the commercial determinants of health—the FCTC. Even as the FCTC was being negotiated, the value of a similar approach for another hazardous product, alcohol, was noted. Since then, the value of the FCTC has been demonstrated in countries adopting stronger tobacco control measures faster, as has its normative influence in trade negotiations.[19] New marketing developments, including new products, mean such treaties need revision to meet changing circumstances, but this does not negate their value.

There have been numerous calls for a framework convention on alcohol[20] and on food systems to support better health, environmental sustainability, and greater equity.[21] Most recently, the response to the COVID pandemic has included the call for a framework convention on pandemic control.[22] An expansion of a network of health treaties equivalent to the FCTC is a key element of the policy agenda to respond to CDOH by rebalancing the global architecture. Achieving this major impact on the policy agenda will require a concerted effective alliance between LMICs and civil society.

LMICs are emerging markets for producers of hazardous products where there is ample opportunity to recruit new users. In intergovernmental institutions, high-income countries (HICs), where many of the TNCs producing and marketing these products are headquartered and owned, have consistently rejected policy suggestions, often made by LMICs, that would constrain TNCs.[23] A failure to engage in democratic debate means the opportunity to advance knowledge of the harms and possible responses is lost. Support from civil society for the voices of governments from LMICs could redress this epistemic–democratic deficit of global governance.[24] This makes the need to provide resource for civil society to operate at the global level a high priority as part of a CDOH policy agenda, and there are currently few examples of such funding from philanthropists or development agencies. Resource is also needed to enhance the capacity of LMICs to engage in global governance as well as improve national-level activities (see Chapter 28).

The World Health Organization (WHO) has been the major policyholder in relation to many of the risk factors and diseases that are a consequence of CDOH, although other UN agencies and rapporteurs, and normative documents such as the Sustainable Development Goals, are also relevant. Intergovernmental agencies are member state–led, but case studies of multilateral negotiations have revealed the active role of the bureaucrats who staff international organizations, showing that they are able to exercise influence on the policy agenda "by forging strategic alliances, sponsoring research, mobilizing technical expertise, raising public awareness and playing a leadership role in negotiations."[25]

In some cases, the WHO secretariat has proved more resistant to change than member states were subsequently shown to be, such as the substantial resistance to the initial proposal from consultants that a Framework Convention on Tobacco Control be developed.[12] However, key players in WHO, including the Director General, subsequently took on roles of policy entrepreneurs, crucial for the achievement of the FCTC. The WHO secretariat, in a context of UN support for PPPs and normalized alcohol use in many HICs, have so far failed to provide strategic support to LMICs that have attempted to place a Framework Convention on Alcohol Control on the policy agenda,[23] and the necessary policy entrepreneur(s) in the UN system has not yet emerged. Opportunities within global governance may go beyond WHO; for example, a UN treaty, the International Covenant on Economic, Social and Cultural Rights (ICESCR), provides the most comprehensive coverage of the right to health under international human rights law. Many UN agencies have the possibility to affect health, and greater institutional linkages and focus on shared action for health are needed,[26] but this is hampered by only rudimentary interfaces between agencies such as WHO and WTO.[27] Stronger normative pressure from civil society, LMICs, and supportive HICs is urgently needed.

A priority for a policy agenda to rebalance global architecture is accountability and reporting mechanisms to make visible industry practices. The current reliance on informal monitoring and dissemination by nongovernmental organizations (NGOs) is insufficient. The International Code of Marketing of Breast-Milk Substitutes provides a model in which governments were tasked with reporting regularly to the World Health Assembly any violations of the code, and since 2014 an international collaboration builds capacity to support monitoring implementation of the code. Similarly, monitoring compliance with states obligations under ICESCR is carried out via reports and the submission of relevant documentation from UN specialized agencies, other UN bodies, and NGOs to permit independent verification of information received from states.[28]

33.7 NATIONAL CDOH POLICY AGENDAS

Policy agendas at the national level are constrained in many jurisdictions by the electoral cycle, politicians' desire to avoid controversial policies, and the chilling effect of TIAs. The hegemony of economic interests means the health sector often operates from a less powerful position than trade and industry sectors, and the narrative commonly promulgated—that of individual responsibility—often gives responsibility to Ministry of Health to educate and raise awareness about problems rather than address their upstream causes.[29] To the extent that the prevailing narrative can be influenced to include the role of availability, affordability, and marketing of hazardous products as causes of harm, there is a greater likelihood of a multisectoral response and achieving policy coherence across the different government sectors. However, a common multisectoral response is to produce a national policy statement, which may be weakened by influence from commercial interests[30] and, even without this, may reflect a "lowest common denominator" of what all government sectors can agree to.

Therefore, it might be argued the primary focus for advocacy should be linking harm from CDOH to the need for legislation. Two recent successful examples of legislation were the passing of minimum unit pricing for alcohol in Scotland[31] and the sugar-sweetened beverage tax in Mexico.[32] Analysis has identified common elements, including the consistent promulgation by key players of the characteristics of the problem: an obesity epidemic in Mexico and levels of alcohol harm higher in Scotland than in neighboring England plus, in the latter case, the price of alcohol being less than the price of water. Using these framings to get these policies onto the agenda was achieved by collaborative action, including media advocacy by coalitions of academia and NGOs and also, in Mexico, consumer protection societies. Both successes took advantage of a supportive political context: in Mexico, a new government with a need for new revenue streams, the successful alliance built with the finance ministry, and in Scotland, a supportive government that was unable to set direct taxes. Technical policy development to ensure the policy was seen to be feasible and effective was supported by academia in both countries and, in Mexico's case, the Pan American Health Organization and philanthropic funding.

In other environments, the influence of commercial interests has prevailed, in part reflecting the long-term and dense relationships between industry actors and politicians.[33] Anti-corruption and transparency regulation may be a necessary precursor of effective CDOH policy.[34]

In addition to public health pricing policies, government industrial policy can redress the impact of lower prices due to the productive efficiency of health-harming corporations by supporting organizations that produce healthier and more sustainable alternatives.[10] The expansion of large retail outlets that reduce prices is also relevant to a CDOH policy agenda; the proliferation of Walmart Supercenters has been associated with a 10.5% increase in obesity in the United States since the late 1980s.[35] Government policy can support investment in infrastructure that supports local food supply chains for perishable products, supporting farmers to engage in direct sales in produce markets and alternative food business models such as food cooperatives.[10]

How profits and externalized costs are distributed among corporations, society at large, and the environment can inform and support a public health policy agenda. In jurisdictions in which taxpayers pay for services, such as health, justice, corrections, police, and local government, contrasts between the profits of the TNCs and efforts to minimize their corporate taxes, on the one hand, and the external costs to society, on the other hand, are a relevant narrative for policymakers. The contributions of harmful product manufacturers to the economy through employment, corporate social responsibility (CSR) contributions, and taxes are arguments used against regulation of hazardous products. Accurate data on these are not readily available in many settings but are very relevant to the CDOH policy agenda.

33.8 THE VALUE OF CROSS-ANALYSIS OF CDOH VERSUS SPECIFIC ISSUE ADVOCACY?

Communicating the nature of conflicts of interest may be enhanced by examining business practices across a range of industries, as this book sets out. A joined-up response to CSR might include a consistent narrative that values CSR activities, such as minimizing impact on the environment and providing good working conditions for employees, but maintains strong critique of the branding (either product or corporate) of "good works" and demands robust and independent evaluation. Similarly, a collaborative focus could challenge PPPs between national and global agencies and the producers and marketers of hazardous products. The issue of reformulation of products is more prominent in relation to unhealthy food, but the growth in marketing of low-alcohol products and the tobacco industry's role in the vaping industry represent common elements. The importance of food systems for climate change, freshwater use, land use, biodiversity loss, and chemical pollution is an emerging part of the narrative on unhealthy food, and depletion of water sources is an issue for soft drink and alcohol production. However, because alcohol products are psychoactive, carcinogenic, and dependence producing, they may align more closely in some narratives with tobacco than with unhealthy food.

33.9 LINKAGES AND COALITION-BUILDING

At national and global levels, civil society can make a contribution to setting the policy agenda. Although it is apparent that there are conspicuous asymmetries in power, in cases of highly visible and contested short-term political struggles, civil society may be the decisive voice. In 2018, the Global Fund's partnership with Heineken to use its extensive retail networks to deliver vaccines and medicines was suspended following a collaborative social media campaign on the part of several NGOs illustrating the value of both coalitions and response agility.[36] However, across the CDOH more broadly, there are few examples of joined-up advocacy compared with the interrelationships between commercial actors. Engaging a broader range of civil society interests in horizontal linkages, including those addressing corporate power more generally, and working collaboratively with investigative journalists would strengthen the CDOH policy agenda.

33.10 THE WAY FORWARD—GROUNDS FOR OPTIMISM?

The ideology of neoliberalism is waning in many areas of the world, reflecting concern regarding the market-led impacts on climate change, inequality, and the increasing power of emerging economies, some of which eschew neoliberalism.[37] Recent events in global governance suggesting reduced hegemony include the insistence by countries with emerging economies to exclude some of the protections for TNCs in the 2020 multilateral agreement covering half of the world's population—the Regional Comprehensive Economic Partnership. In a different context, a UK Supreme Court's interpretation of European Union (EU) law in 2017 stated that courts should give national governments considerable discretion in their valuation of health relative to free trade.[38] Industrial policy is also being used to challenge some of the TNCs, such as the EU's anti-trust investigation of Coca-Cola, and the use of data by the digital platforms.[39] Although these are not responses to health concerns, the challenge to market power may be relevant. However, at this stage, there is little sign of a loss of hegemony in the ideological support for PPPs, with the WHO Foundation currently in receipt of funding from Nestlé[40] and open to funding from the alcohol industry.[41]

Central to the development of a policy agenda for CDOH is a question: How much do corporate capitalism and surveillance capitalism[42] have to change in order to achieve real improvement in health and equity? Emerging movements such as the Green New Deal[43] openly endorse critiques related to the production of hazardous products, and the global attention to climate change and inequality provides an opportunity for change. However, such trends do not guarantee any challenge to the oversupply and marketing of unhealthy commodities; a window of opportunity may exist, but the public health field will need to engage creatively with the opportunity to make real change.[44] It is not clear what the implications of the response to the COVID-19 pandemic will be in shaping intergovernmental action or unilateralism and whether the rhetoric of "build back better" will have real implications for efforts to reshape global architecture to value health and well-being. However, the emergence in the past two decades of a global governance that is more intrusive and with more demanding normative principles[27] may provide grounds for some optimism.

REFERENCES

1. Payne A, Phillips N, eds. *Handbook of the International Political Economy of Governance.* Elgar; 2014.
2. Ralston R, Hill SE, da Silva Gomes F, Collin J. Towards preventing and managing conflict of interest in nutrition policy? An analysis of submissions to a consultation on a draft WHO tool. *Int J Health Policy Manag.* 2021; 10(5): 255–265.
3. Palazzo G, Richter U. CSR business as usual? The case of the tobacco industry. *J Bus Ethics.* 2005; 61(4): 387–401.
4. Casswell S. Vested interests in addiction research and policy. Why do we not see the corporate interests of the alcohol industry as clearly as we see those of the tobacco industry? *Addiction.* 2013; 108(4): 680–685.
5. Casswell S, Callinan S, Chaiyasong S, et al. How the alcohol industry relies on harmful use of alcohol and works to protect its profits. *Drug Alcohol Rev.* 2016; 35(6): 661–664.
6. World Health Organization. Preparation for the third High-level Meeting of the General Assembly on the Prevention and Control of Non-communicable Diseases, to be held in 2018 (Report by the Director-General). Executive Board EB142/15, 142nd session, Provisional agenda item 3.8. 2017. Updated December 22, 2017. Accessed March 12, 2019. http://apps.who.int/gb/ebwha/pdf_files/EB142/B142 _15-en.pdf
7. Supran G, Oreskes N. Rhetoric and frame analysis of ExxonMobil's climate change communications. *One Earth.* 2021; 4(5): 696–719.
8. McGreevy M, Baum F. Against the odds, South Australia is a renewable energy powerhouse. How on Earth did they do it? The Conversation. February 24, 2021. Updated February 25, 2021. Accessed November 22, 2021. https://theconversat ion.com/against-the-odds-south-australia-is-a-renewable-energy-powerhouse-how-on-earth-did-they-do-it-153789
9. Klein JD, Dietz W. Childhood obesity: The new tobacco. *Health Aff.* 2010; 29(3): 388–392.
10. Wood B, Williams O, Baker P, Nagarajan V, Sacks G. The influence of corporate market power on health: Exploring the structure–conduct–performance model from a public health perspective. *Global Health.* 2021; 17(1): 41.
11. Ratu D. *A Claim to the Waitangi Tribunal Under the Treaty of Waitangi Act 1975 in Relation to WAI 2575—The Health Inquiry.* The Waitangi Tribunal; 2017.
12. Crow ME. Smokescreens and state responsibility: Using human rights strategies to promote global tobacco control. *Yale J Int Law.* 2004; 29: 209–250.
13. Carah N, Brodmerkel S. Alcohol marketing in the era of digital media platforms. *J Stud Alcohol Drug.* 2021; 82: 18–27.
14. Buchanan L, Kelly B, Yeatman H, Kariippanon K. The effects of digital marketing of unhealthy commodities on young people: A systematic review. *Nutrients.* 2018; 10(2): Article No. 148.
15. Petticrew M, Maani N, Pettigrew L, Rutter H, Van Schalkwyk MC. Dark nudges and sludge in Big Alcohol: Behavioral economics, cognitive biases, and alcohol industry corporate social responsibility. *Milbank Q.* 2020; 98(4): 1290–1328.

16. Lim A. Global fields, institutional emergence, and the regulation of transnational corporations. *Soc Forces*. 2020; 99(3): 1060–1085.

17. Collin J, Casswell S. Alcohol and the Sustainable Development Goals. *Lancet*. 2016; 387: 2582–2583.

18. Kelsey J. How might digital trade agreements constrain regulatory autonomy: The case of regulating alcohol marketing in the digital age. *N Z Univ Law Rev*. 2020; 29: 153–179.

19. O'Brien P. Missing in action: The global strategy to reduce the harmful use of alcohol and the WTO. *Eur J Risk Regul*. 2020: 1–22. doi:10.1017/err.2020.1067

20. Casswell S. Current developments in the global governance arena: Where is alcohol headed? *J Glob Health*. 2019; 9(2): 020305. doi:10.7189/jogh.7109.020305

21. Swinburn BA, Kraak VI, Allender S, et al. The global syndemic of obesity, undernutrition, and climate change: The Lancet Commission report. *Lancet*. 2019; 393(10173): 791–846.

22. The Independent Panel for Pandemic Preparedness & Response. COVID-19: Make it the last pandemic. May 2021. https://theindependentpanel.org/wp-content/uploads/2021/05/COVID-19-Make-it-the-Last-Pandemic_final.pdf

23. Casswell S, Rehm J. Reduction in global alcohol-attributable harm unlikely after setback at WHO Executive Board. *Lancet*. 2020; 395: 1020–1021.

24. Stevenson H. The wisdom of the many in global governance: An epistemic–democratic defense of diversity and inclusion. *Int Stud Q*. 2016; 60(3): 400–412.

25. Michie J. *The handbook of globalisation*. 3rd ed. Elgar; 2019.

26. Gopinathan U, Watts N, Lefebvre A, Cheung A, Hoffman SJ, Røttingen J-A. Global governance and the broader determinants of health: A comparative case study of UNDP's and WTO's engagement with global health. *Glob Public Health*. 2019; 14(2): 175–189.

27. Zürn M. *A Theory of Global Governance: Authority, Legitimacy, and Contestation*. Oxford University Press; 2018.

28. Heymann J, McNeill K, Raub A. Rights monitoring and assessment using quantitative indicators of law and policy: International Covenant on Economic, Social and Cultural Rights. *Hum Rights Q*. 2015; 37(4): 1071–1100.

29. Patay D. Navigating conflicting mandates and interests in the governance of the commercial determinants of health: The case of tobacco in Fiji and Vanuatu [Doctoral thesis]. Australian National University; 2021.

30. Juma PA, Mapa-Tassou C, Mohamed SF, et al. Multi-sectoral action in non-communicable disease prevention policy development in five African countries. *BMC Public Health*. 2018; 18(1): 953.

31. Katikireddi SV, Hilton S, Bonell C, Bond L. Understanding the development of minimum unit pricing of alcohol in Scotland: A qualitative study of the policy process. *PLoS One*. 2014; 9(3): e91185.

32. James E, Lajous M, Reich MR. The politics of taxes for health: An analysis of the passage of the sugar-sweetened beverage tax in Mexico. *Health Syst Reform*. 2020; 6(1): e1669122.

33. Casswell S. Development of alcohol control policy in Vietnam: Transnational Corporate Interests at the Policy Table, Global Public Health Largely Absent. *Int J Health Policy Manag*. 2022; published online June 1. doi:10.34172/ijhpm.2022.6625

34. Tangcharoensathien V, Srisookwatana O, Pinprateep P, Posayanonda T, Patcharanarumol W. Multisectoral actions for health: Challenges and

opportunities in complex policy environments. *Int J Health Policy Manag.* 2017; 6(7): 359–363.

35. Courtemanche C, Carden A. Supersizing supercenters? The impact of Walmart Supercenters on body mass index and obesity. *J Urban Econ.* 2011; 69(2): 165–181.

36. Bonafont LC. Interest groups and agenda setting. In: Zahariadis N, ed. *Handbook of Public Policy Agenda Setting.* Elgar; 2016: 200–216.

37. Phillips N, Payne A. Introduction: The international political economy of governance. In: Payne A, Phillips N, eds. *Handbook of the International Political Economy of Governance.* Elgar; 2014: 1–11.

38. Meier P, Brennan A, Angus C, Holmes J. Minimum unit pricing for alcohol clears final legal hurdle in Scotland. *BMJ.* 2017; 359: j5372.

39. Bundeskartellamt. Bundeskartellamt prohibits Facebook from combining user data from different sources. 2019. Updated February 7, 2020. Accessed August 10, 2020. https://www.bundeskartellamt.de/SharedDocs/Meldung/EN/Pressem itteilungen/2019/07_02_2019_Facebook.html

40. Maani N, Van Schalkwyk MC, Petticrew M, Ralston R, Collin J. The new WHO Foundation—Global health deserves better. *BMJ Glob Health.* 2021; 6(2): e004950.

41. June Yue Yan L, Casswell S. The WHO Foundation should not accept donations from the alcohol industry. *BMJ Global Health* 2022; 7.5: e008707.

42. Zuboff S. *The Age of Surveillance Capitalism: The Fight for the Future at the New Frontier of Power.* Profile Books; 2019.

43. Congress.gov. H.Res.109—Recognizing the duty of the federal government to create a Green New Deal. 116th Congress (2019–2020). 2019. Accessed November 22, 2021. https://www.congress.gov/bill/116th-congress/house-res olution/109/text

44. Lencucha R, Thow AM. Intersectoral policy on industries that produce unhealthy commodities: Governing in a new era of the global economy? *BMJ Glob Health.* 2020; 5(8): e002246.

CHAPTER 34

Commercial Determinants of Health

A Research and Translational Agenda

NASON MAANI, MARK PETTICREW, AND SANDRO GALEA

34.1 INTRODUCTION

The chapters of this book provide a grounding for the reader interested in the commercial determinants of health (CDOH). This includes definitions and arguments as to why these forces constitute a foundational component of the social determinants of health, a rationale for the systematic study of the potential harms associated with these determinants, and how such study might be pursued. Through a range of disciplinary lenses, the chapters have described the various ways in which commercial actors shape the upstream drivers of health, such as through shaping policy, evidence, norms, and public discourse. Having developed this broader interdisciplinary lens for the reader, the book also provides examples of how this lens can be applied to a variety of industries that serve as case studies. In some cases, these are areas in which the evidence base is relatively well developed. In others, such as gambling or fossil fuels, the case studies serve as examples of how useful the triangulation of evidence and theory from other arenas might be in the study of these less well-researched industries. They offer glimpses into the extent to which there are commonalities between such industry sectors that merit further research, and lessons that can inform advocacy and regulatory approaches, such as in areas of trade, law, governance, conflicts of interest, the evaluation of industry-funded interventions and evidence, and the aims and effects of various forms of corporate social responsibility.

Nason Maani, Mark Petticrew, and Sandro Galea, *Commercial Determinants of Health* In: *The Commercial Determinants of Health*. Edited by: Nason Maani, Mark Petticrew, and Sandro Galea, Oxford University Press. © Oxford University Press 2023. DOI: 10.1093/oso/9780197578742.003.0034

Having given examples of the similarities and differences of a range of different commercial sectors, the next part of the book widened its perspective to consider the cumulative, distal effects of such commercial activities, beyond individual sectors, on health and equity. This included cumulative effects on policy, the evidence base, and public discourse. Taken together, it is hoped this will provide the reader a firm grasp of the conceptual and empiric state of the field and what the implications might be for policy.

It is important to acknowledge that this is a field in development and, as with the social determinants of health more broadly, contains multitudes of meanings depending on the orientation of the observer and a range of potential research and translational directions. In this chapter, from our perspective as editors who have had the privilege of reading and learning from the breadth and depth of knowledge made available by this diverse and highly dedicated author group, we reflect on the potential research and translational directions that seem of particular interest as this field develops. It is hoped that these might help the reader consider the possible journeys available in this field in addressing knowledge gaps and, through doing so, conduct work that is as beneficial as possible to the wider world. We offer three main reflections in this vein.

34.2 SEEING BOTH THE FOREST AND THE TREES

First, as the field develops, it seems critical that scholarship on CDOH both includes research on defining and describing the cumulative effects of commercial activity on health (i.e., the forest) and also advances empiric and conceptual understanding regarding individual companies, practices, and industries (i.e., the trees).

Through this book, various chapters have shown the value of wider definitions of CDOH (e.g., see Chapters 2 and 21) while also showing just how much remains to be understood about industries that have been a focus for some time, such as the tobacco industry (see Chapter 11). The reasons for gaps in understanding include a lack of available data, direct obstruction, the threat of legal action, and a lack of interest among research funders. This is particularly the case in many low- and middle-income countries (see Chapter 28), even though the adverse health and governance impacts of large-scale commercial actors in such settings are both less well-described and potentially more harmful.

Seeing the forest and the trees in commercial determinants of health research is also of critical importance when considering how potential definitions and research objectives might map onto translational opportunities. For example, the book reveals clear commonalities in how different harmful product industries resist policy "best buys" through a variety of means, even though for some harmful product industries (e.g., alcohol, gambling, or fossil fuels, discussed in this book), empirical evidence remains relatively limited and, perhaps more important, has not been widely recognized among the public and policymakers in the same way the activities of the tobacco industry have. Research and advocacy in these areas, particularly when it translates the cross-industry evidence that does exist into shifts in public understanding, may well yield the greatest return, in the shortest time, to population health.

It has been argued, both in chapters in this book and elsewhere, that part of the "forest" we often fail to see are the health benefits provided by the private sector. Indeed, it is the case that directly through the provision of goods and services, and indirectly through providing employment and income, the private sector performs important social functions that are accompanied by health benefits. Crucially, however, we must acknowledge that these benefits are a consequence of profit-seeking, often constrained in health-protecting ways through regulation. That is not to cast a moral judgment on profit-seeking itself but, rather, to acknowledge what is the reality of commercial activity. In the pursuit of profits, companies affect population health in positive or negative ways, commensurate to their scale and influence, and the nature of the products and services they produce, market, and sell. At core, where companies impact positively on health, they do so because it is profitable. Where companies affect health adversely, again, they do so because it is profitable. It seems therefore reasonable to both acknowledge that commercial activity can have positive effects that are already incentivized through profit and also recognize that empirical research and scholarship on areas in which profit and health are misaligned may lead to the greatest net benefit to health in the short term.

Similarly, it has been argued that many economic operators are informal, or small to medium-sized businesses, whereas the focus of much CDOH research to date has been on multinational companies. There is clearly a need for greater granularity in our understanding on this topic. At the same time, in areas in which activity has been heavily consolidated, there may be greater value to science and society in focusing on the effects of the largest, most powerful entities rather than hundreds of small entities representing a small fraction of overall health impact.

34.3 THE VALUE OF BREAKING DOWN SILOS

In acknowledgment of the challenges encountered in pursing CDOH research, there is a need to learn from what has already been done in fields outside public health. In this book, we included a range of perspectives from legal scholars, political scientists, trade researchers, social scientists, food scientists, epidemiologists, and advocates. This has, we hope, widened the lens of what CDOH scholarship could be and, therefore, the breadth and type of evidence and scholarship that might be considered in future research. There is, however, scope to go much further with regard to cross-disciplinary work.

A field such as CDOH, which considers the social, political, economic, and health impacts of companies and industries that can be transnational in nature, must by necessity be characterized by "edge-dwelling" between disciplines and topic areas, if only to help build a true picture of these effects. This has several potential benefits. First, it avoids repeating work unnecessarily so that we might maximize the impact of the relatively small amounts of funding available by applying them to important gaps in our understanding. Second, it allows for the building of a greater coalition of researchers and advocates collectively interested in this topic area, widening the lens of possible research approaches, evidence reviews, and translational opportunities. Third, it helps the next generation of CDOH researchers. If we focus on building cross-disciplinary bridges as part of this research area, future doctoral students and scholars will find them easier to traverse, more intuitive, and, therefore, will go further than we can ourselves.

Although this book may contribute toward such efforts, other critical elements are required—such as the building of a global community of practice, the developing of larger scientific organizations and conferences, and the launching of one or more journals with a focus on this area—that might truly help bring a diversity of disciplines and topic areas together to the benefit of the field and wider society.

34.4 CONDUCTING CDOH RESEARCH OF CONSEQUENCE

A theme that underpins the book and the future of CDOH is the importance of identifying areas of CDOH research that can be of the greatest consequence to wider society. Considering, on the one hand, the vastness of corporate power in the modern era and its pervasive yet largely invisible influence on our norms, structures, and health at a global level and, on the other hand, the relatively limited resources available to CDOH researchers, it seems critical that our research be conducted with a view to societal impact.

This might seem obvious, but in reality, the coalescing of any new field of research represents both an opportunity, in terms of the cross-disciplinary fertilization mentioned above, and a challenge, because it risks becoming an academic silo of its own, with its own language, norms, and methods. At times, subdivisions within the field may also remain and hinder collective progress, as have been observed in One Health[1] and global health.[2] As noted in the context of epidemiological research, as time passes, standards of good research may drift toward being overly focused on identifying and cataloguing the causes of particular health problems rather than seeking to provide the solutions to said problems.[3]

In considering the breadth and scope of commercial influence on our world as outlined in this book, it seems clear that CDOH serves the greatest social good by being a diverse, consequentialist, self-critical, and outward-looking field, in which academic progress is informed by, communicated to, and forms part of wider societal progresses.

34.5 CONCLUSION

Science has always helped society bear witness to the forces that shape the world around us. As we look to build back better following a global pandemic and its consequences, it is perhaps more prudent than ever to bear witness to the commercial forces that shaped the world around us and, by extension, our health.[4–6] Research on CDOH has therefore never been more relevant, nor more likely to be heavily contested by a range of competing interests.[4] The chapters of this book demonstrate the value of this approach in shaping our understanding, the challenges inherent in it, and how we might overcome them through capacity-building, education, research, policy, and advocacy.

REFERENCES

1. Manlove KR, Walker JG, Craft ME, et al. "One Health" or three? Publication silos among the One Health disciplines. *PLOS Biol*. 2016; 14(4): e1002448.
2. Abdalla SM, Solomon H, Trinquart L, Galea S. What is considered as global health scholarship? A meta-knowledge analysis of global health journals and definitions. *BMJ Global Health*. 2020; 5(10): e002884.
3. Galea S. An argument for a consequentialist epidemiology. *Am J Epidemiol*. 2013; 178(8): 1185–1191.
4. van Schalkwyk MCI, Maani N, McKee M. Public health emergency or opportunity to profit? The two faces of the COVID-19 pandemic. *Lancet Diabetes Endocrinol*. 2021; 9(2): 61–63.
5. Maani N, Van Schalkwyk MC, Petticrew M, Galea S. The commercial determinants of three contemporary national crises: How corporate practices intersect with the COVID-19 pandemic, economic downturn, and racial inequity. *Milbank Q*. 2021; 99(2): 503–518.
6. Van Schalkwyk MC, Maani N, Cohen J, McKee M, Petticrew M. Our postpandemic world: What will it take to build a better future for people and planet? *Milbank Q*. 2021; 99(2): 467–502.

CONFLICTS OF INTEREST STATEMENTS

Chapter	Conflicts of Interest
1	NM and MP are members of the UK SPECTRUM research consortium, funded by the UK Prevention Research Partnership. NM has received consulting fees from the World Health Organization. SG receives royalties from academic publishers for several books and serves on the board of Sharecare.
2	No relevant conflicts of interest were declared.
3	FB is Co-chair of the Global Steering Council of the People's Health Movement. No other relevant conflicts of interest were declared.
4	No relevant conflicts of interest were declared.
5	No relevant conflicts of interest were declared.
6	NM and MP are members of the UK SPECTRUM research consortium, funded by the UK Prevention Research Partnership. NM has received consulting fees from the World Health Organization. No other relevant conflicts of interest were declared.
7	No relevant conflicts of interest were declared.
8	No relevant conflicts of interest were declared.
9	No relevant conflicts of interest were declared.
10	TS has received research funding, travel expenses, and occasional minor personal fees for work commissioned by government alcohol monopolies in Canada, Finland, and Sweden. In each case, the funded research involved estimating the potential impacts of alternative measures to improve public health and safety outcomes from alcohol consumption. No other relevant conflicts of interest were declared.
11	No relevant conflicts of interest were declared.
12	NM and MP are members of the UK SPECTRUM research consortium, funded by the UK Prevention Research Partnership. NM has received consulting fees from the World Health Organization. No other relevant conflicts of interest were declared.

Chapter	Conflicts of Interest
13	No relevant conflicts of interest were declared.
14	No relevant conflicts of interest were declared.
15	No relevant conflicts of interest were declared.
16	No relevant conflicts of interest were declared.
17	No relevant conflicts of interest were declared.
18	No relevant conflicts of interest were declared.
19	No relevant conflicts of interest were declared.
20	NK has an immediate family member who works for, and receives stock compensation from, Microsoft. They have no direct work with any of the technologies discussed in this chapter. No other relevant conflicts of interest were declared.
21	JL-N has received funding from the Victorian Health Promotion Foundation and The George Institute for Global Health. She is a member of the People's Health Movement and the Healthy Food Systems Australia advocacy group. The views expressed in this chapter are hers alone and not necessarily those of the above organizations. No other relevant conflicts of interest were declared.
22	JML is an employee of the World Health Organization (WHO); however, this chapter relates to work conducted in the course of her doctoral studies, prior to her engagement with WHO. The views expressed in the chapter are her own and do not reflect those of WHO.
23	No relevant conflicts of interest were declared.
24	No relevant conflicts of interest were declared.
25	No relevant conflicts of interest were declared.
26	WHW declares royalties from a related textbook and also personal financial donations to not-for-profit corporate and democracy research and reform advocacy organizations.
27	No relevant conflicts of interest were declared.
28	No relevant conflicts of interest were declared.
29	PJA has never accepted funding directly from gambling, alcohol, or other unhealthy commodity industries. He participated in research projects in the 1990s funded by two hypothecated funding sources—money levied from alcohol consumption and administered by New Zealand's Alcohol Advisory Council, an Autonomous Crown Entity (established by an Act of Parliament in 1976 and disbanded in 2012), and money levied from gambling consumption and administered by the NZ Ministry of Health. Since 2004, he has not accepted funding from hypothecated sources.
30	No relevant conflicts of interest were declared.
31	No relevant conflicts of interest were declared.

Chapter	Conflicts of Interest
32	No relevant conflicts of interest were declared.
33	No relevant conflicts of interest were declared.
34	NM and MP are members of the UK SPECTRUM research consortium, funded by the UK Prevention Research Partnership. NM has received consulting fees from the World Health Organization. SG receives royalties from academic publishers for several books and serves on the board of Sharecare.

INDEX

For the benefit of digital users, indexed terms that span two pages (e.g., 52–53) may, on occasion, appear on only one of those pages.

Tables, figures, and boxes are indicated by *t*, *f*, and *b* following the page number

branding, 35, 103, 144, 179, 348
Brandt, A, 63
Brazil National Cancer Institute 3Ps,
    237, 238t
breast cancer charities,
    "pinkwashing," 52
British American Tobacco, 287–88
    "Better Regulation" campaign, 73
    cost–benefit analysis, 165
    secondhand smoke research,
        internal, 72
    upstream policy influence, 103
    Uzbekistan, 223
British colonies, North American, 264
British Petroleum, 111, 117
    Helios Power, 116
Brussels Declaration, 233
Bruun, Kettil, *Alcohol Control Policies in
    Public Health Perspective*, 91–92
bubonic plague, spread via trade, 59–60
Burke L, 154–55
Burwell v. Hobby Lobby, 180
business costs overestimation, 167–68

Canada
    alcohol minimum prices, 94–95
    alcohol sales, privatization, 93
    high-fructose corn syrup, trade
        deal, 80–81
    Low Risk Drinking Guidelines, 91
    video lottery terminals, 123–24
cancer
    from alcohol, 50, 51, 61–62,
        90, 144–45
    industry denial, 50, 51
    asbestos, 71, 72–73
    responsibility, industry
        displacement, 53
    from tobacco, 61–63
capitalism. *See also specific topics*
    definition, 322t
    financialized, 23
        reduced taxation, 23
    intellectual monopoly, 227–28
    philanthrocapitalism, 227
    predatory, 178
    state-centric, 23
    surveillance, 126, 349–50
Carbon Democracy (Mitchell), 111–12
case study teaching, 327

causality, 246, 248, 258, 269
causal relationships, public health, 124
    denialism, 51
    gambling industry, 122–24
cause marketing, 157t
causes of the causes, 321
Center for Economic and Policy
        Research, *Agency Spotlight*, 270
change, resistance to, and (re)producing
        void of knowledge, 127–28, 128f
charitable and in-kind giving, 157t
charities. *See also specific topics and types*
    industry-funded, 52
China, 23
    advertising and economic
        prosperity, 58
    Coca-Cola promotion, 58, 61
    Nestlé milk market control, 284–85
chronic disease, risk factors. *See also*
        noncommunicable disease
    equity of access, 18
    health behaviors and choices, 18
*Citizens United v. Federal Election
        Commission*, 179–80, 182, 266
civil society
    activism, 333–34
    power, 23–24
climate activism, anti-
        consumption, 65–66
climate change, corporate role, 178
    responsibility, industry
        displacement, 53
coal industry. *See also* fossil fuels industry
    doubt, manufacturing, 114
    rhetorical strategies, 114–15
coalition-building, 348–49
Coca-Cola. *See also* sugar-sweetened
        beverage industry
    anti-trust investigation, EU, 349
    China, promotion, 58, 61
    corporate social responsibility, 157t
    denialism, 70–71
    Global Energy Balance Network, 70–
        71, 134
    goods and services, 216
    international market expansion,
        61, 62–63
    trade domination, 78
    World War II, for American
        soldiers, 61